An Introduction to
Biomaterials
Science and Engineering

Other World Scientific Titles by the Author

An Introduction to Electrospinning and Nanofibers
ISBN: 978-981-256-415-3
ISBN: 978-981-256-454-2 (pbk)

An Introduction to Biocomposites
ISBN: 978-1-86094-425-3
ISBN: 978-1-86094-426-0 (pbk)

Polymer Membranes in Biotechnology: Preparation, Functionalization and Application
ISBN: 978-1-84816-379-9
ISBN: 978-1-84816-380-5 (pbk)

The Changing Face of Innovation: Is it Shifting to Asia?
ISBN: 978-981-4291-58-3 (pbk)

Additive Manufacturing: Foundation Knowledge for the Beginners
ISBN: 978-981-122-481-2
ISBN: 978-981-122-624-3 (pbk)

An Introduction to
Biomaterials
Science and Engineering

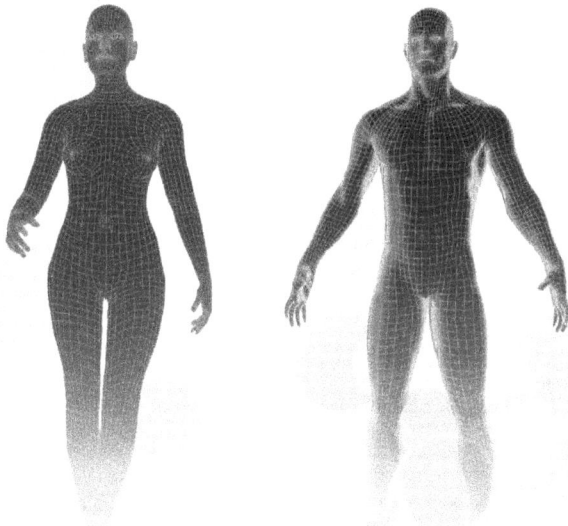

A Sandeep Kranthi Kiran
Seeram Ramakrishna

National University of Singapore, Singapore

World Scientific

NEW JERSEY · LONDON · SINGAPORE · BEIJING · SHANGHAI · HONG KONG · TAIPEI · CHENNAI · TOKYO

Published by

World Scientific Publishing Co. Pte. Ltd.

5 Toh Tuck Link, Singapore 596224

USA office: 27 Warren Street, Suite 401-402, Hackensack, NJ 07601

UK office: 57 Shelton Street, Covent Garden, London WC2H 9HE

Library of Congress Cataloging-in-Publication Data
Names: Kiran, A. Sandeep Kranthi, author. | Ramakrishna, Seeram, author.
Title: An introduction to biomaterials science and engineering /
    A. Sandeep Kranthi Kiran, Seeram Ramakrishna.
Description: Hackensack, NJ : World Scientific, [2021] |
    Includes bibliographical references and index.
Identifiers: LCCN 2020041070 | ISBN 9789811228179 (hardcover) |
    ISBN 9789811228186 (ebook) | ISBN 9789811228193 (ebook other)
Subjects: MESH: Biocompatible Materials | Biomedical Engineering |
    Equipment and Supplies
Classification: LCC R857.B54 | NLM QT 37 | DDC 610.28--dc23
LC record available at https://lccn.loc.gov/2020041070

British Library Cataloguing-in-Publication Data
A catalogue record for this book is available from the British Library.

For any available supplementary material, please visit
https://www.worldscientific.com/worldscibooks/10.1142/12038#t=suppl

Desk Editor: Shaun Tan Yi Jie

Typeset by Stallion Press
Email: enquiries@stallionpress.com

Preface

This is undoubtedly an exciting time to be studying *An Introduction to Biomaterials Science and Engineering*. Biomaterials is a dynamic field that has a massive influence on modern-day medicine. The chapters of this book reflect the emergence of this field, and help the students to understand, enhance, and broaden their expertise in this rapidly developing area. We bring myriad facets together and provide a collective understanding of the field of biomaterials to the younger generation. Topics presented in this book cover a wide range of themes, outlined in 13 chapters, starting from the basis of all living things to 3D bioprinting of tissues and organs. Overall, we expect this book will be an excellent reference to experts, researchers, Ph.D. and M.Sc. scholars, and, more importantly, to the graduate and postgraduate students who are entering or want to enter the field of biomaterials.

Life has been dissected to the smallest molecules and is synonymous with cells. Therefore, the first chapter covers the fundamental concepts of cell structures and their functions. This chapter module also introduces the structure and functions of the human body. The next chapter offers comprehensive glossary in tabular and text form relating to typical human disorders, infectious and non-infectious diseases. The list of various kinds of materials and medical devices employed to treat those diseases and disorders are also discussed in detail. In chapter 3, we introduce the basics of stem cells, which have the capability to become almost any type of cell in the body. Additionally, understanding of the primary tissues, such as epithelium, connective tissue, muscle, and nervous tissues, is also aided by notes on the extracellular matrix and growth factors.

Biomaterials such as implants and scaffolds work in conjunction with living matter and serve to replace or repair parts of the functional system.

This raises several specific obligations for their specific properties. Therefore, chapters 4 to 7 discuss the complex field of biomaterials engineering and explore new materials related to polymers, ceramics, biometals, and much more.

Biomaterials are integral parts of medical devices. The term "medical devices" includes a considerable range of equipment, from simple tongue depressors and blood glucose meters to the hemodialysis machine. However, medical device risks associated with severity, contact length, and impact on the infected body system are regulated by constituttional laws laid down by government authorities. Chapter 8 discusses these various medical regulations associated with the U.S.A., Europe, China, Singapore, and India. This chapter also facilitates the students to understand the importance of medical device sterilization. Surface modification of materials is a broad subject with many different considerations. Thus, in chapter 9, we describe the development of principal surface engineering techniques concerning surface topographical, structural, mechanical, and cellular adhesion and proliferation perspectives. All the surface engineering techniques performed on polymeric, ceramic, and metallic biomaterials are presented as separate sections.

Over the last two decades, the field of tissue engineering has improved considerably, offering regeneration capacity to almost all the human body's tissues and organs. Accordingly, in chapter 10, we introduce tissue engineering and regenerative medicine, emphasizing the progress made in scaffold materials, tissue-specific strategies, fabrication approaches, and development of tissue-engineered medical products. Due focus is also given to explain the wound healing process, cell-material interactions, as well as cell-extracellular matrix interaction with human tissues. Moving forward, advances in nanotechnology have led to the development of engineered drug delivery constructions, which have heralded a new age in the healthcare industry. In view of this, in chapter 11, different aspects to design novel drug delivery systems and breakthrough advances in therapeutics and diagnostics are presented. Chapter 12 provides the basics of the core concepts, methods, and instrumentation of biosensors. In the final chapter, we discuss the fundamentals, principles, and applications of sophisticated 3D bioprinting technologies. Bioprinting has promoted tissue engineering as a practical treatment alternative for patients suffering from tissue and organ failure by biomanufacturing tissue constructs, tissues, and organs using living cells.

Due care has been taken in writing this first edition of the book. However, inadvertently there will be some errors, or some topics left unattended or overlooked. We, as authors, would appreciate any such notices, contributions, and/or criticisms. They will be dealt with accordingly in the second edition of this book.

Finally, the authors would like to thank Lloyd's Register Foundation, U.K. (Project Number R265000553597 Nanotechnology in Sub-Sea Power Transmission), for supporting this project.

Sandeep Kranthi Kiran A
Seeram Ramakrishna

About the Authors

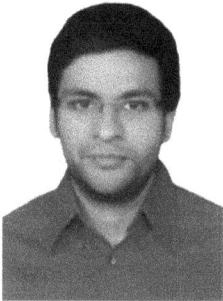

Dr. A Sandeep Kranthi Kiran is a Post-Doctoral Fellow at the Department of Mechanical Engineering, National University of Singapore (NUS). He received his PhD degree from Indian Institute of Technology (IIT) Madras, India and NUS, Singapore under the prestigious "*IIT Madras-NUS Joint Ph.D. Doctoral Programme*". For the year 2019–2020 he received the *Institute Research Award* from IIT Madras on recognition of quantity and quality of research work done in his doctoral studies. His research interests include the fabrication of electrospun nanostructure materials, 3D printing, metallic nanostructured biomaterials, and antimicrobial ceramic coatings. He is currently working on the development of anti-viral coatings for 3D printed facemasks.

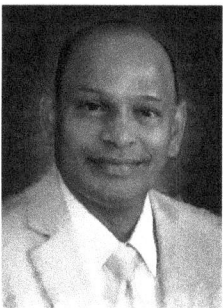

Professor Seeram Ramakrishna, *FREng* is the Director of Center for Nanofibers and Nanotechnology at National University of Singapore (https://www.nature.com/articles/nj0232. pdf?draft=marketing). He is regarded as the guru of electrospinning and nanofibers (http://nart2020. com/conferenceinfo/). Microsoft Academic ranked him among the top 36 salient authors out of three million materials researchers worldwide (https:// academic.microsoft.com/authors/192562407). He is named among the World's Most Influential Minds (Thomson Reuters), and the Top 1% Highly Cited Researchers in materials science and cross-field categories

(Clarivate Analytics). He received his PhD from University of Cambridge, UK and TGMP from Harvard University, USA. He is appointed as the Honorary Everest Chair of MBUST, Nepal. He is an elected Fellow of UK Royal Academy of Engineering (*FREng*); Singapore Academy of Engineering; Indian National Academy of Engineering; ASEAN Academy of Engineering & Technology; International Union of Societies of Biomaterials Science and Engineering (*FBSE*); Institution of Engineers Singapore; ISTE, India; Institution of Mechanical Engineers and Institute of Materials, Minerals & Mining, UK; American Association of the Advancement of Science; ASM International; American Society for Mechanical Engineers; American Institute for Medical & Biological Engineering; and International Association of Advanced Materials (FIAAM). He chairs the Circular Economy taskforce at NUS, and is a member of Enterprise Singapore's and International Standards Organization's Committees on ISO/TC323 Circular Economy and Circularity. He is the Editor-in-Chief of Springer NATURE journal *Materials Circular Economy*. He is an editorial board member of Springer NATURE journal *Advanced Fiber Materials*; Elsevier Journal *Current Opinion in Biomedical Engineering*; and NATURE *Scientific Reports*. He is an opinion contributor to the Springer Nature Sustainability Community (https://sustainabilitycommunity.springernature.com/users/98825-seeram-ramakrishna/posts/looking-through-covid-19-lens-for-a-sustainable-new-modern-society).

Contents

Chapter 1
Functions of human body systems

1.1 Cells

The cell is one of the most complex systems humankind has ever encountered. Life is synonymous with the cell because it undergoes *mitosis*, a process by which another cell is formed. A cell and its nucleus (Figure 1.1) are the smallest functional units in a living organism that work in conjunction. The different cell organelles, along with their principal functions, are tabulated in Table 1.1. All surviving organisms are made up of one (unicellular) or more cells (multicellular), which are fused together in groups (tissues); then tissues form organs, organs make up organ systems, and organ systems act as a group to establish a fully shaped entity and keep it alive and functioning. A functional tissue/organ contains trillions of coordinated cells that are mobilized in tandem to perform required physiological tasks. Carrying immense, organism-specific genetic knowledge compacted in their nuclei, cells coordinate with adjacent cells to provide the tissue with specific functions.

Over 200 different cell types are present in the human body (Table 1.2) with a variety of sizes and shapes, but all have certain common features. A few cell types are shown in Figure 1.2. Each cell comprises DNA as the hereditary material, a nucleus, and a cytoplasm. Cells also possess many other components, such as organelles and ribosomes, that execute different functions.

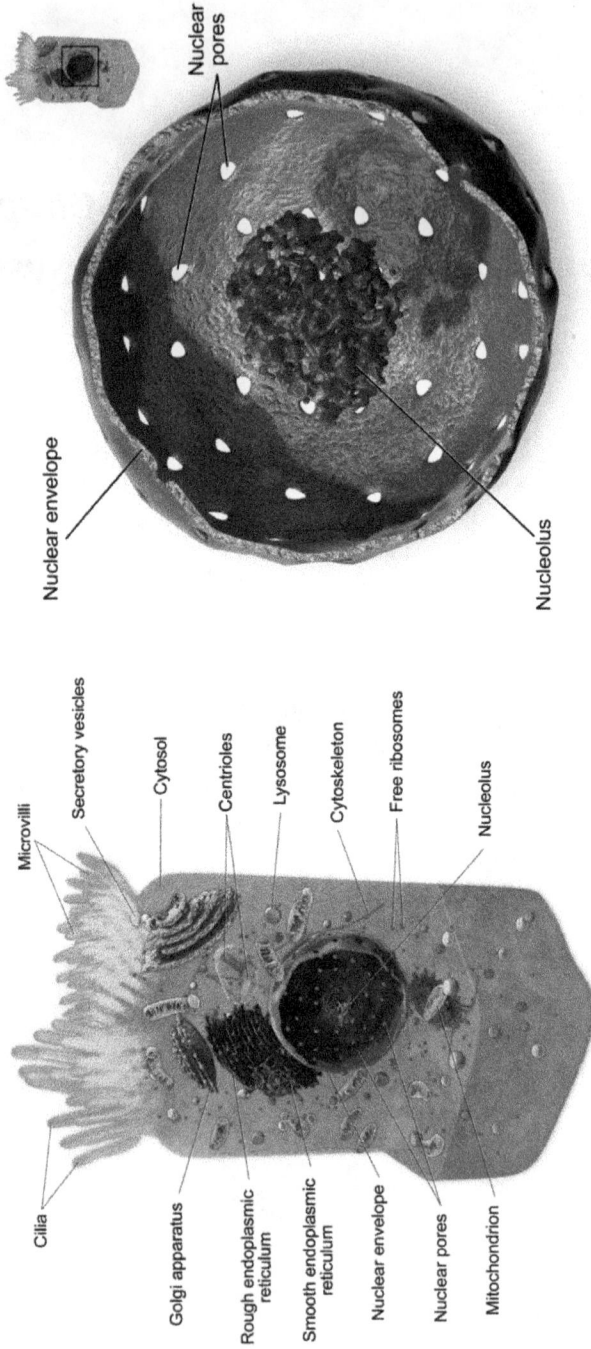

Figure 1.1:   Anatomy of the cell and its nucleus (Blaus, 2014).

Table 1.1: Cell organelles and their functions.

Cell organelle	Functions
Nucleolus	Considered as the brain of the nucleus; engaged in regulating cellular activities and cellular reproduction
Nuclear membrane	The envelope that surrounds and protects the nucleus
Endoplasmic reticulum	Involved in calcium storage, modification, synthesis, transportation of proteins and lipid metabolism
Golgi apparatus	Involved in the transportation of materials within the cell
Ribosomes	Make proteins; proteins are essential for mending damage and regulating chemical processes
Mitochondria	Responsible for generating chemical energy needed to power the cell's biological and chemical reactions
Lysosomes	Considered as the *"digestive system"* of the cell because they are responsible for the inter- and extracellular breakdown of substances using enzymes
Cilia	Responsible for moving a cell or group of cells; also assists in transporting fluid or materials
Cytoskeleton	Helps the cell to maintain its internal shape and organization

Table 1.2: Human cell types and their functions.

Cell type	Cell subtype	Main function
Stem cells	Embryonic stem cells Adult stem cells	Stem cells are the body's raw materials. Depending on the organism and tissue type, stem cells have the capability to differentiate into various distinct cell types and provide new cells for the body as it grows.
Red blood cells	Erythrocytes	Red blood cells transport fresh oxygen from the lungs to all sections of the body and carry away carbon dioxide from other tissues to discharge in the lungs.
White blood cells	Granulocytes Agranulocytes	These are the cells of the immune system, which shield the body from contagious, infectious, and virulent diseases and foreign bodies.
Nerve cells	Neurons Glial cells	Nerve cells are responsible for transmitting electrical messages and signals throughout the body and helping it to respond appropriately.

(Continued)

Table 1.2:   *(Continued)*

Cell type	Cell subtype	Main function
Muscle cells	Skeletal Cardiac Smooth	Muscle cells make up the tissues of the muscles, which facilitate the movement of the body.
Cartilage cells	Chondrocytes	Cartilage is a resilient and smooth elastic tissue that is vital to the body's structure. Chondrocytes are highly specialized cells that generate large amounts of extracellular matrix consisting of collagen fibres, proteoglycan, and elastin fibers. Cartilage provides support and allows flexibility of movement.
Bone cells	Osteoblasts Osteoclasts Osteocytes Bone lining cells	Bone cells help in bone development, retaining and maintaining of the mineral concentration of matrix, and bone resorption.
Skin cells	Keratinocytes Melanocytes Merkel cells Langerhans cells	Skin cells protect the body by blocking toxins and pathogens. They act against UV radiation and minimize heat, solute, and water loss. They also help in the determination of skin color.
Endothelial cells		These cells form the lining of blood vessels and are the main regulator of vascular homeostasis. They release substances that control vascular relaxation and contraction, and control the localization of the inflammatory response as well.
Epithelial cells		Epithelial cells form the lining of cavities in the body. They are specialized for secretion, selective absorption of nutrients, protection, transcellular transport, and sensing.
Fat cells	White adipocytes Brown adipocytes	Fat cells provide insulation and serve as an energy store. They also aid in transforming energy from food into heat.
Sex cells	Sperm cells Ovum cells	Sex cells are central to the reproduction process.

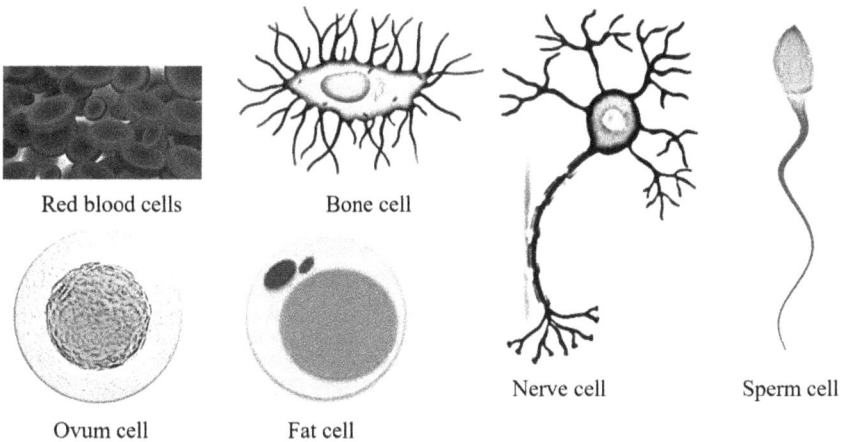

Red blood cells   Bone cell

Nerve cell   Sperm cell

Ovum cell   Fat cell

Figure 1.2: Examples of human cells.

Key points

Cells
- The cell is the fundamental building block and smallest common denominator of all organisms.
- The nucleus controls cell growth and reproduction.
- Eukaryotic and prokaryotic cells are the two main types of cells.

1.2 Human body

The immense complexity, as well as flexibility of a functioning human body and emergent mind, are an inspiration to the futuristic computers, artificial intelligence, and intelligent materials. The human body is the physical component consisting of living cells as well as extracellular materials and arranged into tissues, organs, and systems. It is an amazing biological product that is endorsed and supported by well-structured and mutually dependent systems and their distinctive organs. All components contribute in various ways to a human being's biological, physical, mental, and emotional wellbeing. The body has structural layers that build upon one another where cells form tissues, tissues form organs, and organs make up itself. To keep itself active, living, and running, it executes millions of complicated functions every minute. Thousands of biochemical and physical interactions between various factors and components occur at the same time. These reactions and interactions keep the body '*alive*' and is known as metabolism.

1.2.1 *Elements of the human body*

On Earth, there are 94 naturally occurring elements. Of these 94, only 11 are identified in living beings in greater quantities than trace amounts. Most of the human body consists of water, where cells comprise about 65–90 wt.% of it. There is about 75–80% of water in a baby. As a person grows older, this percentage falls to about 60–65% for men and 50–60% for women. Figure 1.3 and Table 1.3 demonstrate the 11 typical elements found in the human body and their proportion of total body weight.

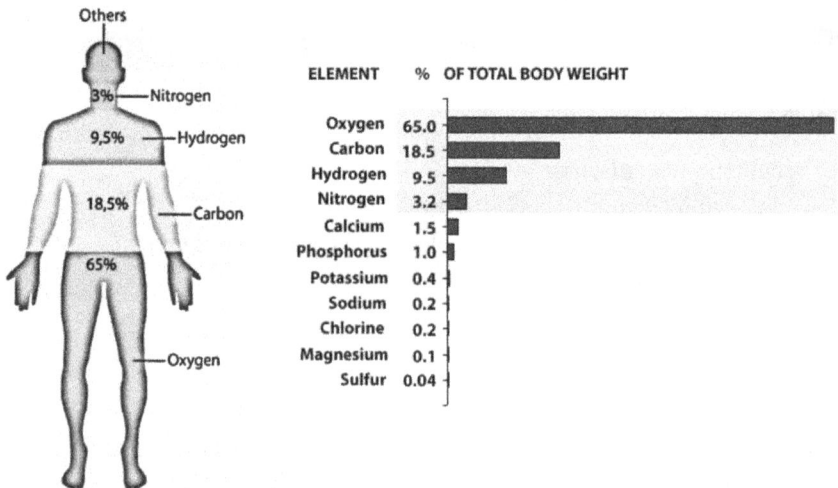

Figure 1.3: The common elements observed in the human body and their percentage of total body weight (Betts *et al.*, 2013; Brožek, 1965; Carlson, 2019; Lyer, 2009). Attribution: OpenStax.

Table 1.3: The most abundant elements found in the human body.

Element	O	C	H	N	Ca	P	K	S	Na	Cl	Mg
Wt.%	65.0	18.5	9.5	3.2	1.5	1.0	0.4	0.3	0.2	0.2	0.1
At.%	24.0	12.0	62.0	1.1	0.22	0.22	0.03	0.038	0.037	0.024	0.015

1.3 Body systems and functions

An organ system is a collection of all anatomical structures functioning together to achieve a specific purpose or task. There are 12 distinct human body systems namely lymphatic, digestive, cardiovascular, immune, endocrine, muscular, integumentary, reproductive, nervous, skeletal, respiratory, and urinary. Their major tissues and organs and their specific functions are presented in Table 1.4. Even though each system is a separate entity, their responsibilities are substantially overlapping, and the

Table 1.4:   Body systems, functions, and organs.

Organ system	Major tissues and organs	Function
Cardiovascular	Heart; veins; arteries; capillaries; red blood cells	Transports materials (oxygen and nutrients) to tissues and eliminates waste products
Digestive	Mouth; esophagus; stomach; small intestine; large intestine; pancreas; liver; gall bladder	Ingests food, digests food into smaller particles, and absorbs nutrients
Lymphatic	Spleen; lymph nodes; thymus; lymphatic vessels	Returns tissue fluid to blood and defends against foreign organisms
Endocrine	Glands; thymus; pancreas; gonads	Regulates body functions using hormones
Integumentary	Skin; hair; subcutaneous tissue	A barrier to invading organisms and chemicals; also acts as temperature control
Muscular	Muscles; tendons	Allows for movement by contraction and heat production
Nervous	Brain; spinal cord; nerves	Controls all other systems, gathers information and coordinates activities, and responds to sensations
Reproductive	Ovaries; uterus	Produces egg cells, and safeguards and sustains the offspring until birth
Respiratory	Lungs; trachea; larynx; pharynx	Responsible for taking in oxygen and expelling carbon dioxide

(Continued)

Table 1.4:   (*Continued*)

Organ system	Major tissues and organs	Function
Skeletal	Bones; cartilage; ligaments; bone marrow	Provides support, allows movement, and protects internal organs; also involved in mineral storage and blood formation
Urinary	Kidneys; urinary bladder; urethra	Eliminates waste and regulates pH and volume of blood
Immune	White blood cells	Fights off foreign invaders in the body

body does not operate without the cooperation of all of them. Indeed, only one organ system failure may be all it takes to result in serious impairment or even death. In order to completely understand the human body's anatomy and physiology, it is essential to recognize the functions and components of each system.

1.3.1 *Heart and blood*

The cardiovascular system, or the circulatory system, is a highly efficient transport system that keeps life flowing through the human body by its intricate network of blood vessels. This system consists of the heart (anatomical pump), blood, and a closed complex web of arteries, veins, and capillaries. The blood aids in carrying essential oxygen, nutrients, and hormones across the body, while eliminating metabolic waste. These also help protect the individual and control the temperature of the body.

1.3.1.1 *Heart*

The heart is a strong muscle that pumps blood through the network of arteries and veins (Figure 1.4). It is divided up into four chambers, two atria (upper chambers) and two ventricles (lower chambers). The two atria act as collection reservoirs of the blood, while the two ventricles act as pumps that discharge blood. A muscle wall known as the *septum* separates the left atrium and left ventricle from the right atrium and right ventricle. The four main valves of the heart, namely tricuspid valve, pulmonary valve, mitral valve, and aortic valve maintain unidirectional blood flow (Figure 1.4).

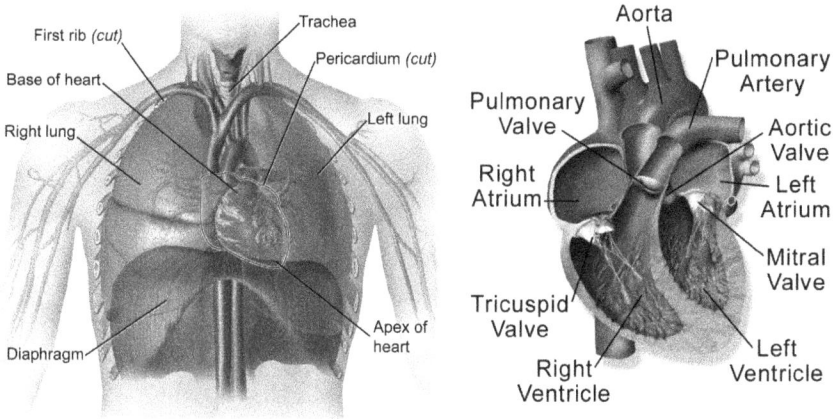

Figure 1.4:   Location and anatomy of the heart (Blaus, 2014; McConnell, 2013).

1.3.1.2 *Blood*

Blood consists of approximately 40–45% solids (cells) and 55–60% plasma fluids. The blood has cells such as white blood cells (monocytes, lymphocytes, neutrophils, eosinophils, basophils, and macrophages), red blood cells (erythrocytes), and platelets. The plasma comprises mainly water, proteins, nutrients, hormones, antibodies, and dissolved waste products. General types of blood cells are erythrocytes, leukocytes, and thrombocytes.

- **Erythrocytes:** Erythrocytes, or red blood cells, are made in the fetal liver or red bone marrow. These are found in the blood and have no nucleus (Figure 1.5). It is estimated that approximately 2.5×10^{11} new erythrocytes are released from the bone marrow into the bloodstream every day, and about the same number is discharged. They are typically biconcave disc-shaped structures with diameter and thickness of approximately 4–10 μm and 1.5–2.5 μm respectively. These cells are also believed to constitute approximately 25% of the body's total cells. Erythrocytes contain the red pigment known as haemoglobin, a substance necessary for oxygen transport. Haemoglobin is a protein molecule comprising four polypeptide chains with more than 140 amino acids each and iron. Their primary function is transporting oxygen from the lungs to all tissues.

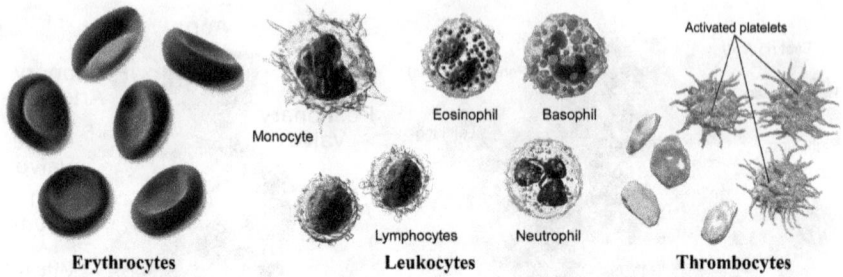

Figure 1.5:   Illustration of red blood cells, white blood cells, and platelets (Blaus, 2014).

- **Leukocytes:** Leukocytes, or white blood cells, are the backbone of the immune system (Figure 1.5). They help the body to fight against viruses, bacteria, and other foreign invaders by participating in immune and inflammatory processes. They are matured in the bone marrow before being released into circulation. They account for only about 1% of blood, but their impact is significant. There are five distinct classes of leukocytes:
  a. Neutrophils: Neutrophils are the most abundant type of white blood cells and the first responder to bacterial infection.
  b. Lymphocytes: Lymphocytes produce antibodies against bacteria, viruses, and other invaders. They are further divided into B cells (secrete antibodies) and T cells (recognize infected cells and destroy them).
  c. Monocytes: Monocytes are the largest of the leukocytes, averaging 15–18 μm in diameter.
  d. Eosinophils: Eosinophils are found very rarely in blood but are very noticeable at parasite infections.
  e. Basophils: Basophils make up the smallest amount of leukocytes in the body but are primarily responsible for triggering inflammatory responses by releasing histamine and heparin chemicals.
- **Thrombocytes:** Thrombocytes, also known as platelets, are the smallest cell fragments of the blood, averaging about 2–4 μm in diameter (Figure 1.5). These platelets circulate within the blood and aid in the formation of blood clots. Platelets are only about 20% of the

diameter of red blood cells and perform a crucial function in hemostasis, by stopping and repairing damaged blood vessels.

1.3.1.3 *Blood vessels*

- **Arteries:** Arteries make up the most important part of the circulatory system. They carry oxygen-rich blood (oxygenated blood) pumped away from the heart to the rest of the body.
- **Veins:** Veins carry blood low in oxygen (deoxygenated blood) from various regions of the body towards the heart.
- **Capillaries:** Capillaries are small blood-containing structures that connect the arteries and veins. They allow diffusion of gases and exchange of nutrients such as water and chemicals between the blood plasma and the interstitial fluid.

1.3.2 *Respiratory system*

The respiratory system is a network of organs and tissues involved in breathing, smelling, and creating sounds. To stay alive, cells need a steady supply of oxygen. Through inhalation and exhalation, this system facilitates the body to absorb oxygen from the air for cell metabolism and helps to clear cellular function waste product, i.e., carbon dioxide. It also supports controlling of blood pH. The human respiratory system (Figure 1.6) is generally separated into two sections: the upper and lower respiratory tracts. The upper respiratory tract includes parts lying outside of the thorax, namely nasal cavity, pharynx, larynx, and trachea. In comparison, the lower respiratory tract consists of bronchial tubes, diaphragm, lungs, and alveoli.

- **Nasal cavity:** Nasal cavity (nose) allows the outside air into the respiratory system. The air is warmed, moistened, and filtered by mucous secretions in the nose.
- **Pharynx:** Pharynx, a cone-shaped passageway, collects incoming air from the nose and passes it downward to the lungs through the larynx

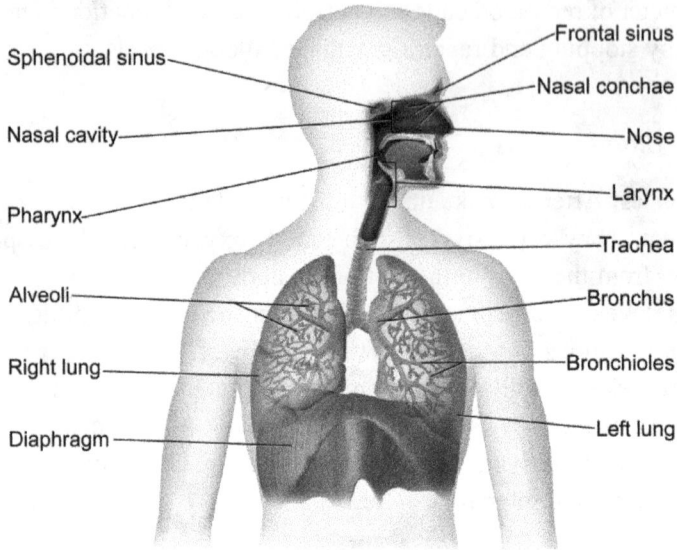

Figure 1.6:   The respiratory system (Blaus, 2014; Callard Preedy *et al.*, 2013).

and trachea. The pharynx chamber assists both respiratory and digestive functions.

- **Larynx:** The larynx, commonly referred to as the voice box, is a short 1.5-inch cartilaginous structure that connects the lower part of the pharynx with the trachea. It helps in the regulation of the amount of air that penetrates and leaves the lungs.
- **Trachea:** The trachea, commonly known as the windpipe, is a long 4-inch tube-like structure made up of cartilage and muscles. It begins just under the larynx. The primary function of the trachea is to transport air to and from the lungs.
- **Bronchial tubes:** The trachea splits into two bronchial tubes (left bronchus and right bronchus) in the lungs.
- **Alveoli:** The alveoli are tiny air sacs that allow oxygen to enter and CO_2 to leave.
- **Diaphragm:** The diaphragm is the primary dome-shaped muscle situated just below the lungs and heart. This muscle and fibrous tissue separate two large cavities, namely chest and abdomen. The

diaphragm plays an integral role in respiration, and its movement involuntarily helps the body to inhale and exhale.

- **Lungs:** The lungs are a pair of spongy cone-shaped organs positioned on each side of the chest (thorax) surrounded by a membrane known as the pleura. Movement of air into the lungs is known as inspiration, and movement out of it known as expiration.

1.3.3 *Skin*

The skin is the largest organ of the integumentary system, contributing between 15–20% of the total weight of adults. It consists of numerous cells and tissue layers that are connected by connective tissues to underlying structures. Anatomy of the skin is depicted in Figure 1.7. It is a fundamentally metabolically active organ that maintains the body's homeostasis, controls body temperature, receives sensory stimuli from

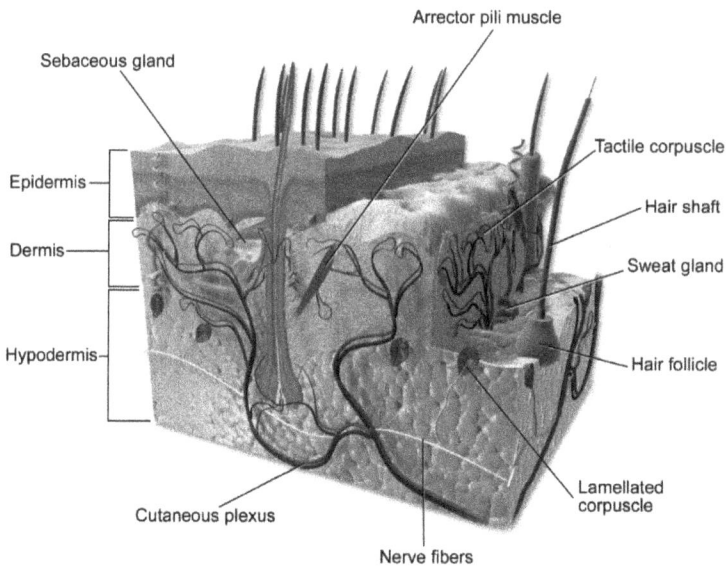

Figure 1.7: Anatomy of the skin (Blaus, 2014; Fenner *et al.*, 2016; Gilaberte *et al.*, 2016).

the external atmosphere, and serves as an external shield from foreign agents such as biological factors, microbes, UV radiation, as well as chemical, biological and physical agents. The skin primarily consists of three layers: the outermost thin epidermis, the underlying thick dermis, and a deeper subcutaneous hypodermis layer. The thickness of these layers differs significantly, depending on the physical location on the body.

1.3.3.1 *Epidermis*

The outermost layer, called the epidermis, contains the primary protective arrangement that functions as a blockade against environmental factors while controlling fluid loss for retention of hydration. It consists mostly of keratinocytes (the predominant cells of the epidermis), but also melanocytes (produce melanin, the pigment responsible for skin color), Langerhans cells (responsible for the immune system), and Merkel cells (sensory transduction touch). The epidermis layer itself is categorized into at least five separate parts from most superficial to deepest, as described below.

a. **Stratum corneum:** This is the outermost layer, also referred to as the "horny layer" generally composed of the many dead skin cells (dead keratinocytes). This sublayer is primarily responsible for all external functions of the skin that includes the prevention of microbe penetration and excessive dehydration.

b. **Stratum lucidum:** This layer is smooth, and a translucent layer of it is seen only on the palms of the hands, fingertips, and feet soles. It is responsible for the ability of the skin to stretch.

c. **Stratum granulosum:** It is a granular cell layer that is composed of 3–5 cell layers with a typical thickness of 7 μm. Cells begin to lose their nuclei and cytoplasmic organelles. In this sublayer, the keratinocyte differentiation programme (cornification) called keratinization gets initiated. The shape of these cells turns out significantly flatter after this process.

d. **Stratum spinosum:** It is the densest layer of the epidermis, and usually ranges from 50–150 μm. This prickle cell layer comprises approximately 10 layers of keratinocytes, created due to cell division in the stratum basale. This layer allows keratinocytes to mature and hosts the Langerhans' cells.

e. **Stratum basale:** Also known as stratum germinativum, it is the innermost epidermis sublayer that shares a boundary with the dermis layer. It contains a sole layer of basal cells (round cells). The predominant cells of the epidermis layer, keratinocytes, originate from here and push up to the surface of the epidermis. This layer also hosts melanocytes.

Because the epidermis has no direct blood supply, it depends on the underlying layer of skin, the dermis, for the delivery of nutrients and the disposal of wastes.

1.3.3.2 *Dermis*

The dermis is the middle layer, lying underneath the epidermis and above deeper subcutaneous tissue. It is essentially made up of the fibrillar structural protein known as collagen and elastic fibers (elastin). This layer is responsible for tensile strength (due to collagen) and elasticity (due to elastin). It has been observed that collagen takes up almost 70% of the skin's dry weight. There are numerous types of cells positioned inside the dermis connective tissues, such as fibroblasts, macrophages, adipocytes, and mast cells. This layer is responsible for most functions of the skin and contains all essential components such as blood capillaries, connective tissues, oil/sweat glands, unencapsulated nerve dendrites, and hair follicles. The dermis is home to two different sublayers: the papillary dermis layer and the reticular dermis layer.

a. **The papillary layer:** This layer lies directly underneath the epidermis and contains the projections of capillaries, lymph vessels, and sensory neurons. It provides support to the vascular epidermis with vital nutrients and a network for thermoregulation.

b. **The reticular layer:** This consists of dense (almost 80%) irregular connective tissues that constitute the bulk of the dermis. This layer of the dermis is responsible for providing the skin with its strength and elasticity.

1.3.3.3 *Hypodermis*

The innermost and thickest layer of subcutaneous tissue, the hypodermis is made of adipocytes (fat cells) and connective tissue. This layer is responsible for insulating the body from cold temperatures, providing shock absorption and buoyancy. It also acts as a repository for energy.

1.3.4 *Eyes*

The human eye is a sensory organ that is capable of obtaining visual images and relating them to the brain. It is responsible for approximately 40% of the total sensory input to the brain through the optic nerve. The eye consists of many sections, including the iris, pupil, cornea, and retina. Additionally, six distinct extraocular muscles regulate its mobility. The understanding and familiarity of the optical system have evolved quickly due to the collective effort of new experimental methodologies and advanced modeling. The structure of the eye and pathway of the vision system is illustrated in Figure 1.8.

- **Cornea:** It is the dome-shaped transparent protective layer that controls, refracts, and focuses the entry of light into the eye for vision. It also functions to cover the iris, pupil, and anterior chamber, and acts as an ultraviolet light filter. Unlike most of the tissues in the human body, the cornea does not contain blood vessels. It is just composed of proteins and cells.

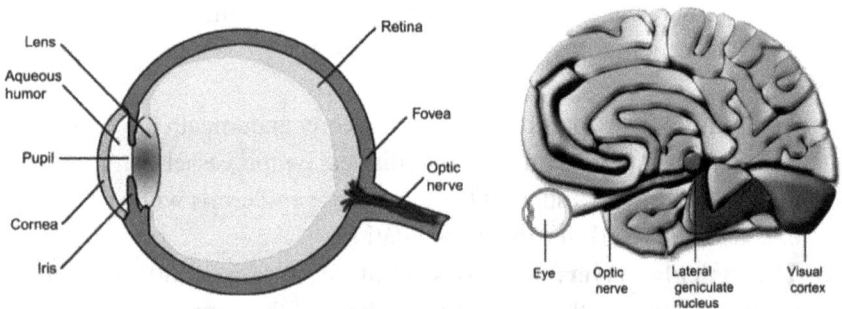

Figure 1.8: Structure of the eye and pathway of the vision system (Hejtmancik *et al.*, 2017; Rizzi *et al.*, 2017).

- **Iris:** It is a thin, circular structure that monitors the quantity of light entering the eye. It is the colorful part of the eye; if we say a person has blue eyes, it means the person has a blue iris. Eye color is established by the amount and type of pigment in the iris.
- **Pupil:** The pupil is the black circle in the center of the iris. It is the adjustable opening of the iris that defines the amount of light that is let into the eye. As light changes, the pupil's diameter (placed in front of the crystalline lens) fluctuates instinctually between 2–8 mm, which modulates the amount of light reaching the retina.
- **Lens:** It is a nearly transparent biconvex structure located behind the iris. The lens aids in transmitting light to the retina with minimal light scattering.
- **Retina:** It is the thin light-sensitive nerve tissue that lines the back of the eye. The 0.2 mm-thick retina gathers sensory information by absorbing light and generates electrical impulses to be processed and transmitted by the optic nerve into the brain. The retina processes light through a layer of light-sensing nerve cells and transforms the energy of photons into biochemical signals. The photoreceptors in the retina are called rods and cones. The retina is made up of nearly 200 million neurons.

1.3.5 *Ear*

The ear is an organ that is complex, sensitive, and delicate. It collects sound waves from the environment and transmits and transduce them to the brain through auditory nerves. It not only provides the ability to hear but also helps in maintaining balance. The anatomy of the human ear is demonstrated in Figure 1.9. It is made up of three parts: the outer, middle, and inner ear.

1.3.5.1 *The outer ear*

The main function of the outer ear is to harness the sound waves and guide them into the ear canal. The outer ear comprises the following parts.

- **Auricle:** Also called the pinna, it is a noticeable part of the ear that is outside the head. It is composed of elastic cartilage covered by the skin.

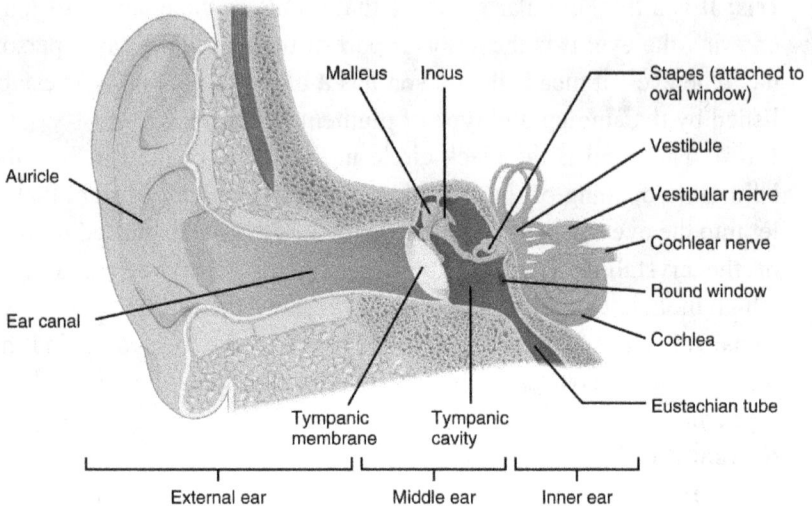

Figure 1.9: Anatomy of the human ear (Betts *et al.*, 2013; Coffin *et al.*, 2020). Attribution: OpenStax.

- **Auditory canal:** Also known as the ear canal, it is a passageway stretching from the outer ear to the middle ear.
- **Tympanic membrane:** Also known as eardrum or eardrum membrane. It is a thin cone-shaped layer of tissue membrane situated at the end of the auditory canal. The eardrum separates the ear canal from the middle ear.

1.3.5.2 *The middle ear*

The middle ear is the portion of the ear that lies in between the eardrum and the oval window, which aids in transmitting sound from the outer layer to the inner ear. It is an air-filled space that comprises three tiny bones known as malleus, incus, and stapes. Sound entering from the outer ear first reaches the tympanic membrane. The tympanic membrane causes the vibration, and the vibration generated is then communicated to the ossicles (tiny bones). The ossicles magnify or develop the sound and pass this amplified sound to the oval window. The oval window is a thin layer of tissue between the middle and inner ear. The eustachian tube is a narrow tube that links the middle ear to the back of the nose and throat.

1.3.5.3 *The inner ear*

The inner ear is the final part of the ear, which translates the sound waves to decipherable information and sent to the brain through nerves. It consists of the following.

* **Cochlea:** It is a spiral-shaped membrane (snail shell) that contains the nerves for hearing.
* **Vestibule:** This contains receptors for balance and posture. It also aids in maintaining equilibrium.
* **Semi-circular canals:** This also contains receptors for balance.

1.3.6 *Kidney*

The kidneys (Figure 1.10) are two bilateral bean-shaped organs, positioned on each side of the spine, which are accountable for purifying various minerals from the blood, sustaining total fluid balance, discharging waste products, and modulating blood volume. They are also accountable for water and electrolyte balance in the body. Each kidney has around a million tiny filters called nephrons, which are the functional units.

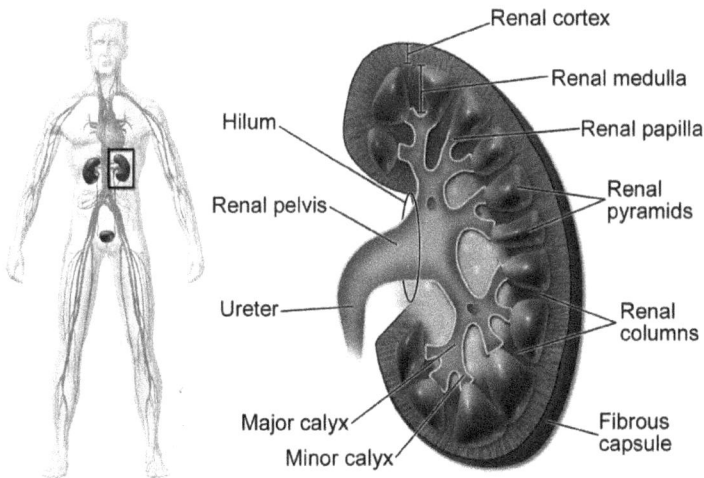

Figure 1.10: Anatomy of the kidney (Blaus, 2014; Feher, 2012; Moorthy *et al.*, 2009).

Each kidney weighs about 125–175 g in males and 115–155 g in females with dimensions of 11–14 × 6 × 4 (length × breadth × thickness). The kidneys accumulate and clear waste from the body in 3 steps.

- **Glomerular filtration:** It is the fundamental step of making urine, which is directly proportional to body weight and is sex-dependent. It is the renal procedure by which fluid in the blood is filtered across the capillaries in the nephrons called glomeruli.
- **Tubular reabsorption:** It is the passive process that pushes solutes and water out of the filtrate and back into the bloodstream.
- **Tubular secretion:** It is the opposite process of reabsorption. The filtrate transfers the materials through the tubules to the storing ducts and then the bladder.

1.3.7 *Brain*

The human brain, house for intelligence, memories, senses, body movement, and controller of behavior, is one of the most complex and key organs in the central nervous system (CNS). It monitors every function of the human body, deciphers information from sensory organs (sight, smell, touch, taste, and hearing), and outputs information to the muscles. Science associates the functioning brain and nervous system with the emergent mind. Those who believe in souls loosely associate it with the mind and body! The brain is akin to the central processing unit of a computer merged to a physical body (hardware) with the nervous system behaving as an operating system.

The brain is made up of dense greyish-pink nerve tissues (Figure 1.11), with approximately 100 billion neurons that broadcast in trillions of connections called *synapses*. Shielded by the skull, it comprises neurons, blood vessels, and supportive cells called glia. It is catagorized into three sections known as (i) cerebrum, (ii) cerebellum, and (iii) brainstem. The cerebrum is the major and uppermost portion of the brain structure. It is further divided into right and hemispheres. The hemispheres control opposite sides of the body, i.e., the right hemisphere regulates the left side of the body while the left hemisphere controls the right side of the body. Both are attached by a thick bundle of C-shaped nerve fibers called the corpus callosum. The cerebrum is further divided into four distinct lobes

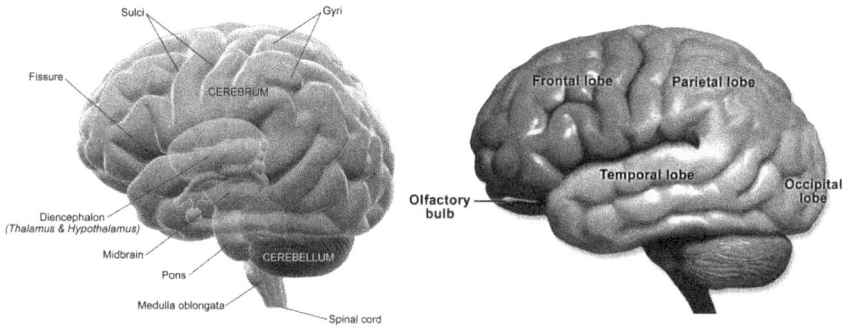

Figure 1.11:   Anatomy of the brain and different lobes present (Blaus, 2014; Carlson, 2019).

(Figure 1.11) that control senses, thoughts, and movements. They are named as frontal, parietal, temporal, and occipital lobes. As presented in Table 1.5, each lobe is identified by its own unique function.

The cerebellum is the second largest part of the brain, which is at the base and back of the brain. It is accountable for harmonization and balance. It subconsciously evaluates each movement and sends signals to the cerebrum. The cerebrum evaluates by indicating muscle movements. In a healthy body, all these sequences of events occur involuntarily.

1.3.7.1 *How the brain functions*

Information received through external stimuli is transmitted from the optic nerve to the brain and spinal cord through the brainstem. The brain is made up of two distinct types of cells: nerve cells (neurons) and glial cells. Neurons (Figure 1.12a) are highly polarized excitable cells of the brain and nervous system that form the fundamental blocks of the CNS. They are unique among cells in their large size, complexity, and the diversity of their form. They generate electric signals and spread them throughout their processes according to the information they receive. It is estimated that there are approximately 80–100 billion neurons in the human brain. Information is interpreted in the brain as electrical signals, which are conducted over the cell membranes of neurons and transmitted via an intersection between two nerve cells by diffusion of a neurotransmitter (Figure 1.12b).

Table 1.5:   Different lobes of the cerebrum and their functions.

Brain lobes		Functions	
Frontal		Controls important cognitive skills	Involved in abstract reasoning, creativity, decision making, problem solving, planning, etc.
Occipital		Visual processing and mapping center	Involved in analyzing contents such as shapes and colors
Parietal		Processes sensory information such as temperature, taste, touch, etc.	Involved in recognition, perception of stimuli, movement, and orientation
Temporal	Left Temporal	Mainly for recognizing, memorizing, and forming speech	Involved in the administering of verbal memories and the ability to recognize faces and objects
	Right Temporal	Mainly for learning and remembering non-verbal information (e.g. visuospatial material and music)	Involved in the processing of nonverbal memories and also deals with the ability to comprehend language in both spoken and written forms

1.3.7.2 *Mind*

The brain has physical form while the mind is non-physical. Diverse mental processes are collectively referred to as 'mind'. Generally speaking, the dynamics of diverse human behavior are underpinned by the combined acts of electrical processes of the nervous system and biochemical processes of the endocrine system. The mind is akin to computer software with several apps and data.

1.3.8 *Bone*

Bones in our body are highly vascularized dynamic tissues that protect the vital organs, provide structural support, and produce mineral homeostasis. They come in all shapes and sizes, such as long, short, flat, sesamoid, and irregular bones. During its entire lifetime, a bone continuously undergoes

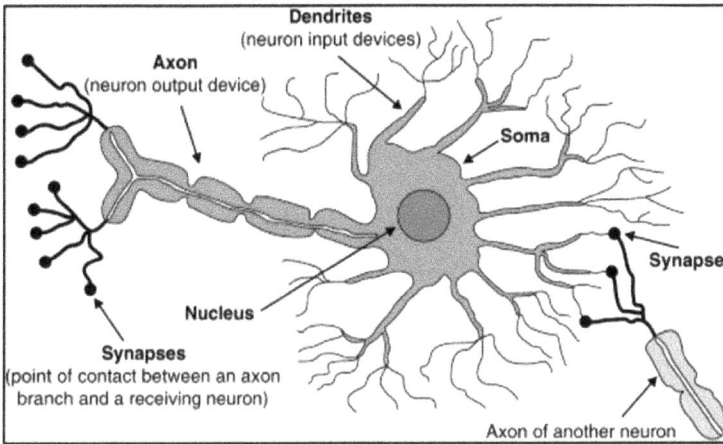

(a)

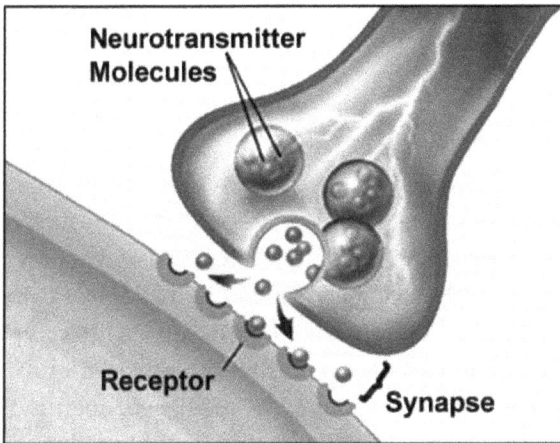

(b)

Figure 1.12: (a) Schematic of a biological neuron (Kalogirou, 2014); (b) Neurotransmitters mediate communication between adjacent neurons (Medpedia; Creative Commons).

remodeling, meaning it is endlessly being resorbed and rebuilt. A healthy human being is born with about 270–300 soft bones. Throughout childhood and adult phase, the cartilage matures and is gradually substituted with hard bones. Some of these bones later merge together, making it 206 in the adult skeleton, including bones of the skull, spine, chest, arms, hand, pelvis, legs, and feet.

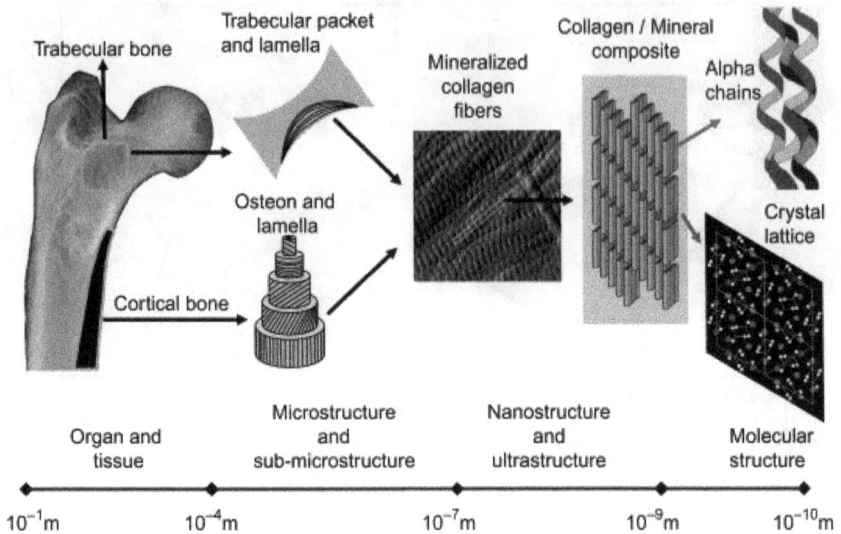

Figure 1.13: The chemical composition and multi-scale structure of natural bone (Burr *et al.*, 2014; Talal *et al.*, 2020).

As shown in Figure 1.13, a bone is well-organized in a hierarchical structure, from nanometer- to millimeter-sized. It is considered a composite, and at the nanostructural level, it is composed of a matrix phase type-I collagen and a mineral phase nanocrystalline biological carbonated apatite. The biological apatite is based on hydroxyapatite (HA, $Ca_{10}(PO_4)_6(OH)_2$), although the ionic sites are replaced by large amounts of CO_3^{2-} ions. The matrix phase imparts resilience, ductility, and viscoelasticity to the bone tissue, whereas the mineral phase is accountable for the strength, stiffness, mechanical rigidity, and homeostasis. Without these components, a bone can be twisted easily and would become very brittle. At the microstructural level, the dense outer hard layer of the bone is known as cortical or compact bone, which contains units called osteons and is responsible for nearly 80% of the mass of the human framework. The internal of the cortical bone is known as trabecular or spongy or cancellous bone, which forms the internal tissue of all bones. It does not contain osteons, but consists of trabeculae arranged as rods or plates lamellae in an irregular lattice. The density of the trabecular bone is much lighter when compared to the cortical bone, but it is very vital for producing blood cells. Bone is also an anisotropic material, which implies its properties differ in tension, compression, and shear.

1.3.8.1 *Bone composition*

The bone matrix has three main components, which contain 8–10% of water, 22–25% organic matrix, and 65–70% of inorganic matter in the form of small crystals. The organic matrix is made up of 90% type-I collagen fibres with some type-V, and 10% other proteins such as glycoprotein, osteocalcin, and proteoglycans. The chemical analysis of bone is shown in Figure 1.14.

1.3.8.2 *Bone cells*

As displayed in Figure 1.15, bone consists of four types of cells: (i) osteoblasts, (ii) osteocytes, (iii) osteoclasts, and (iv) osteogenic cells. Each bone cell type has a distinctive function and is found in different locations in a bone (Table 1.6).

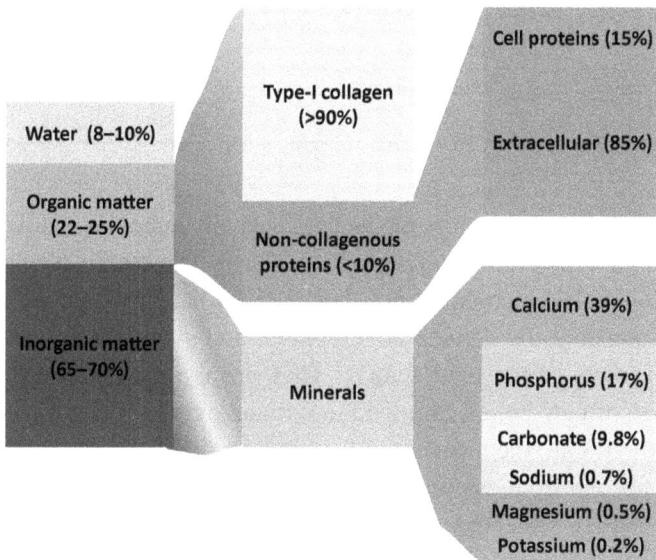

Figure 1.14:   The bone is composed of an organic matrix, minerals, and water.

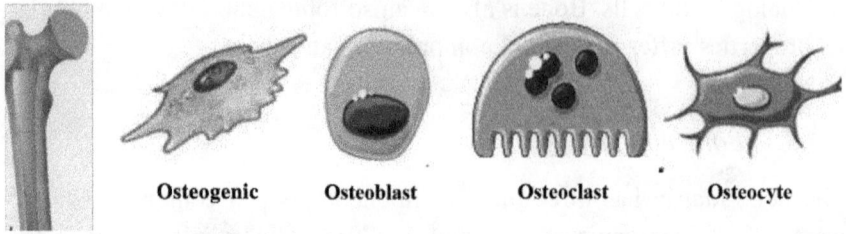

| | Osteogenic | Osteoblast | Osteoclast | Osteocyte |

Figure 1.15:   Illustration of human bone cell types.

Table 1.6:   Function and location of different bone cells.

Bone Cells		
Cell type	**Function**	**Location**
Osteoblasts	Cells that build bone tissue	Found in large numbers in the thin connective tissue layer on the outside surface of bones
Osteocytes	Cells that maintain bone tissue by maintaining mineral (Ca and P) concentration of the matrix	Entrapped within the mineralized bone matrix
Osteoclasts	Cells that degrade or break down bone tissue to initiate normal bone remodeling	Found in pits on the bone surface
Osteogenic cells	Develop into osteoblasts	Found in deep layers of the bone marrow

- **Osteoblasts** are the large active cells, usually cuboidal or low colum-nar in nature, with a diameter of 20–50 μm. These cells play a crucial role in the development of new bones. They have a single nucleus that is responsible for skeletal development and synthesizing the organic components of the bone matrix. They are typically located near the surface of new bones, arranged in a monolayer.
- **Osteocytes** are the most common, abundant, and mature type of bone cells formed from osteoblasts and located deep within the mineralized bone matrix. Osteocytes comprise almost 90–95% of total bone cells and help in maintaining local mineral deposition and chemistry of the bone matrix via secretion of enzymes. Osteocytes have numerous cell

outward projections which are understood to be engaged in interaction with other nearby bone cells.

- **Osteoclasts** are bone cells with more than one nucleus (approximately 10–20 nuclei) that degrade mineralized matrices of bone tissue and release them into the blood. In fact, it is the only type of bone cell capable of bone resorption. They are derived from the bone marrow and formed by the fusion of many cells. Osteoclasts are also responsible for keeping the balance of bone metabolism by cooperating with osteoblast cells.
- **Osteogenic cells** are the only bone cells that divide and are efficient in proliferating and then differentiating into bone-forming cells.

Key points

- Bones are vital to the human body by offering structural support and enabling movement.
- Ca is the essential mineral for bone health, and about 99% of the Ca in the body is found in bones and teeth.
- Collagen offers the structural framework on which Ca and other bone minerals are attached.
- Osteoblasts, osteocytes, osteoclasts, and osteogenic cells are the main cells of the bone.

1.3.9 *Teeth*

The human teeth function to mechanically break down food into smaller pieces and help in the process of digestion. The 32 teeth in the adult human body are divided into four quadrants, namely incisors, canines, premolars, and molars. Teeth develop from a process called odontogenesis. Each tooth, irrespective of the type, has two main sections: the crown and the root (Figure 1.16). The crown, visible top part of the tooth, is predominantly made up of extremely vascularized dental pulp enclosed by dentin and enamel on the outer surface. In comparison, the root is embedded in the gums and surrounded by the periodontal ligament. The teeth are composed of three layers, namely the hard outer layer enamel, the middle softer layer dentin, and a nerve-containing dental pulp. The

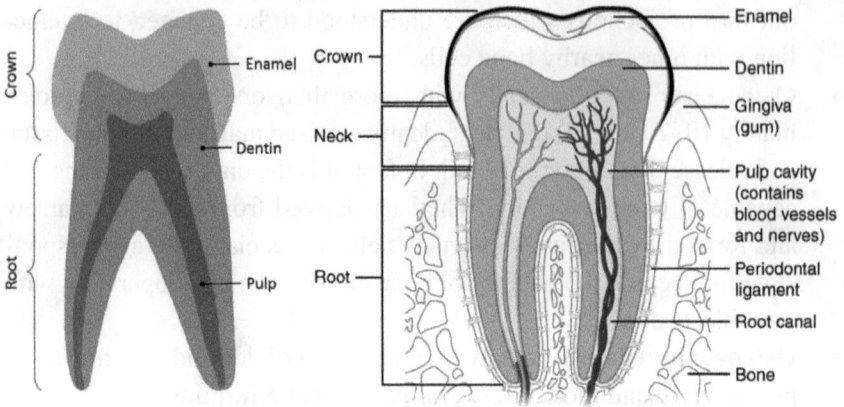

Figure 1.16:   Features and structure of the tooth (Betts *et al.*, 2013; Christensen *et al.*, 2019). Attribution: OpenStax.

enamel-covered crown is the exposed part of the tooth, whereas the root is the portion that is rooted in the jawbone.

1.3.9.1 *Enamel*

Enamel is the thin outer covering of a tooth and a highly mineralized substance with calcium salts. Due to high mineralization, it is harder and more rigid than dentin. The enamel is made up mostly of minerals with approximately 90% (by volume) of minerals, 4% of protein, and 6% of water. Its mechanical properties such as fracture toughness and ultimate tensile strength are much lower than those of dentin (Figure 1.16). This is because the enamel has more mineral content in the form of well-crystallized calcium and phosphate crystals, and the lowest organic matrix that is present is not in fibrous form but contains a mixture of proteins.

1.3.9.2 *Dentin*

Dentin is a calcified material that surrounds the pulp and lies immediately underneath the enamel. It is the largest dental tissue and a major component inside a tooth. The mineral calcium and phosphate ions (HA) make up approximately 70% of dentin, while 20% is organic matter (type-I collagen) and 10% water, which fills the pores within the tissue. Various non-collagenous proteins and lipids are also present in small percentages. Dentin acts as a shock absorber during biting and chewing. Odontoblast is the cell type that secretes and maintains the dentin. Like the bone matrix, a major part of the organic matrix of dentin consists of the fibrillar protein collagen. Due to the intricate arrangement of collagen fibres and the high amount of HA crystals, dentin shows high fracture toughness and elastic modulus (Figure 1.16). It also displays comparatively small variations with a change in direction, i.e., transverse and longitudinal. The intrafibrillar crystals are the reason for considerable stiffness in dentin.

1.3.9.3 *Pulp*

Pulp, the innermost part of the tooth, is a vascular, sensitive, soft connective tissue that forms the central chamber of the tooth. As it lies directly beneath the layer of dentin, it is often referred to as the *"dentin-pulp"* complex. It houses nerves, blood vessels, and has the ability to produce dentin.

1.3.10 *Hip and knee joints*

1.3.10.1 *Knee joints*

The knee is one of the major and most complicated synovial joints in the body. The distal end of the femur, the tibia, the patella, and the proximal part of the fibula are the four different bones that make the knee joint (Figure 1.17b). It is a complex hinge-type synovial joint that joins the femur (thigh bone) to the large tibia (shin bone). The flat-triangular convex-shaped patella is localized in front. Several layers in the knee work together to provide rotation, flexion, stability, and extension. Like any other joint, the knee joint also consists of dense, fibrous, connective tissues to aid in its movement. In order to ensure mechanical stability, four main ligaments guide the joint movement and reduce potential laxity.

1.3.10.2 *Hip joints*

The hip joint is one of the highly balanced joints in the human body that permits movement and provides stability needed to bear body weight. It is a structure of four bones, forming a ball and socket synovial joint

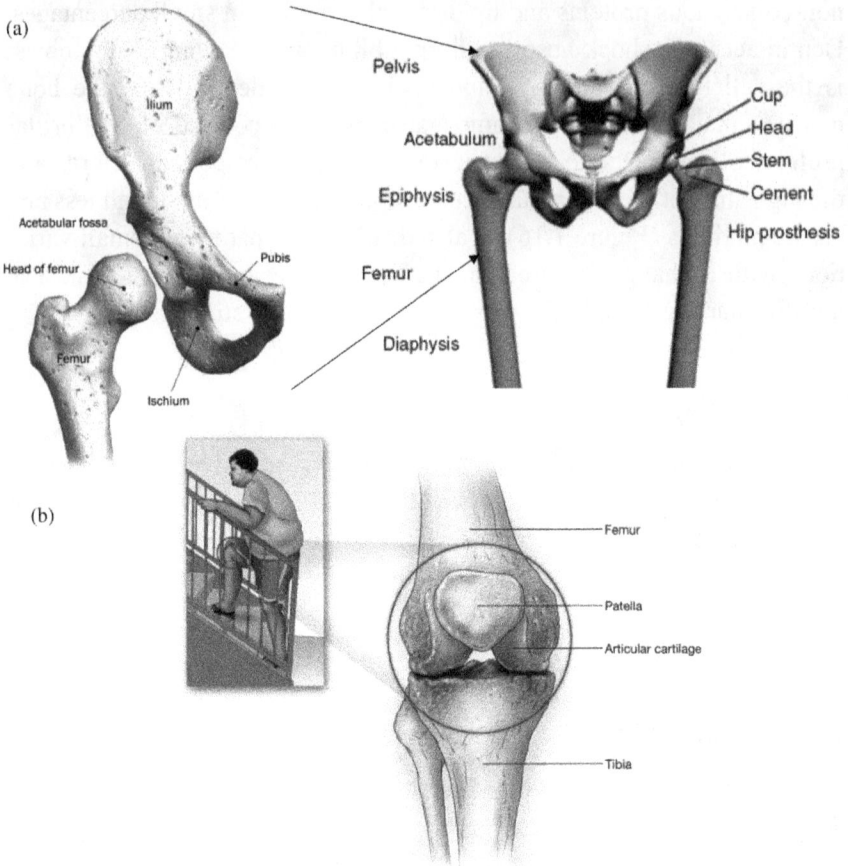

Figure 1.17:　(a) Anatomy of the human hip joint and (b) anatomy of the human knee joint (Affatato *et al.*, 2011; De Santis *et al.*, 2010; Waldman, 2019).

between the pelvis (the lower part between the abdomen and the thighs) and the femur. Anatomy of the human hip joint is displayed in Figure 1.17a. The ball (femoral head) at the top of the femur fits into the round cup-shaped structure of the pelvic bone known as acetabulum or socket. The rigid ball and socket configuration provides stabilization, whereas ligaments and muscles deliver momentum. The femoral bone's mechanical load is greatly affected by forces at the hip and knees. Extracellular matrix, e.g., collagen, apatite, and water, is the major component of the femoral bone.

1.4 Multiple choice questions

1. The term "cell" is not applicable for
   (a) algae
   (b) bacteria
   (c) virus
   (d) fungi

2. Which of the following about angiogenesis is TRUE?
   (a) it is the process of formation of new blood vessels
   (b) the endothelial cell is responsible for proliferation and migration
   (c) it involves matrix degradation and cell signaling
   (d) all of the above

3. The spherical defined organelle that comprises the genetic material is the
   (a) cell wall
   (b) ribosome
   (c) nucleus
   (d) mitochondria

4. What is the mechanism by which material absorption in cells takes place through the plasma membrane?
   (a) egestion
   (b) diffusion
   (c) mitosis
   (d) endocytosis

5. What portion of the human eye is implanted into a living person from a deceased donor?
   (a) cornea
   (b) retina
   (c) iris
   (d) sclera

6. Which of the following sequences about the human body is correct in increasing order?
   (a) chemicals, cells, tissues, organ, organ system, organism
   (b) organism, cells, chemicals, organ system, tissues, organ
   (c) organism, cells, organ, tissue, chemicals, organ system
   (d) tissues, cells, organism, chemicals, organ system, organ

7. Which of the following is NOT true?
   (a) the human body is composed of trillions of cells
   (b) cells contain the body's hereditary material
   (c) cells survive, grow, reproduce, and die on their own
   (d) a group of cells with similar structure and function is called an organ

8. What nutrient(s) become(s) part of the bone matrix?
   (a) only calcium
   (b) calcium and phosphorus
   (c) only phosphorus
   (d) calcium, phosphorus, vitamins A, B and D

9. An example of a ball and socket joint is found in between
   (a) femur and tibia
   (b) femur and pelvis
   (c) ankle bones
   (d) tibia and fibula

10. Which of the following is NOT true?
   (a) the ligaments of the hip joint act to increase stability
   (b) hip is the largest ball-and-socket joint in the human body
   (c) in the hip joint, the ball femoral head, and the socket is the acetabulum
   (d) the only weight-bearing bone in the lower leg is the femur

11. The receptors which detect movement of the body are located in the ___, and the first part of the eye that refracts light rays is the ___
   (a) vestibule; retina
   (b) semi-circular canals; cornea
   (c) middle ear; lens
   (d) organ of corti; optical nerve

12. Which part of the brain begins voluntary movement, and which neurons carry impulses from receptors to the central nervous system?
   (a) cerebellum; sensory
   (b) occipital lobes; mixed
   (c) temporal lobes; motor
   (d) frontal lobes; sensory

13. What are blood clots made up of, and which mineral is accountable for blood clotting?
    (a) fibrin; calcium
    (b) collagen; sodium
    (c) thrombin; phosphorus
    (d) albumin; magnesium

14. The mineral crystal found within the matrix of bone is called
    (a) calcium carbonate
    (b) hydroxyapatite
    (c) calcium phosphate hydrate
    (d) tricalcium ortho phosphate

15. The widening of blood vessels is known as
    (a) vasoconstriction
    (b) atherosclerosis
    (c) vasodilation
    (d) thrombosis

References & Further Reading

Affatato, S., & Traina, F. (2011). Chapter 6 — Bio and medical tribology. In J. P. Davim (Ed.), *Tribology for Engineers* (pp. 243–286): Woodhead Publishing.

Betts, J. G., Young, K. A., Wise, J. A., Johnson, E., *et al.* (2013). *Anatomy and Physiology*: OpenStax.

Blaus, B. (2014). Medical gallery of Blausen Medical 2014. *WikiJournal of Medicine, 1*(2). doi:10.15347/wjm/2014.010.

Brožek, J. (1965). Chapter 1 — Body composition and Human Biology. In J. Brožek (Ed.), *Human Body Composition* (pp. 287–301): Pergamon.

Burr, D. B., & Akkus, O. (2014). Chapter 1 — Bone Morphology and Organization. In D. B. Burr & M. R. Allen (Eds.), *Basic and Applied Bone Biology* (pp. 3–25): Academic Press.

Callard Preedy, E., & Prokopovich, P. (2013). Chapter 1 — Anatomy and patho-physiology of the respiratory system. In P. Prokopovich (Ed.), *Inhaler Devices* (pp. 3–12): Woodhead Publishing.

Carlson, B. M. (2019). Chapter 1 — Cells. In B. M. Carlson (Ed.), *The Human Body* (pp. 1–25): Academic Press.

Carlson, B. M. (2019). Chapter 6 — The Nervous System. In B. M. Carlson (Ed.), *The Human Body* (pp. 137–175): Academic Press.

Christensen, A. M., Passalacqua, N. V., & Bartelink, E. J. (2019). Chapter 2 — Human osteology and odontology. In A. M. Christensen, N. V. Passalacqua, & E. J. Bartelink (Eds.), *Forensic Anthropology (Second Edition)* (pp. 33–76): Academic Press.

Coffin, A. B., & Hudson, A. M. (2020). Chapter 23 — Inner Ear and Hearing. In S. C. Cartner, J. S. Eisen, S. C. Farmer, K. J. Guillemin, M. L. Kent, & G. E. Sanders (Eds.), *The Zebrafish in Biomedical Research* (pp. 255–260): Academic Press.

De Santis, R., Gloria, A., & Ambrosio, L. (2010). Chapter 12 — Composite materials for hip joint prostheses. In L. Ambrosio (Ed.), *Biomedical Composites* (pp. 276–295): Woodhead Publishing.

Feher, J. (2012). Chapter 7.2 — Functional Anatomy of the Kidneys and Overview of Kidney Function. In J. Feher (Ed.), *Quantitative Human Physiology* (pp. 626–632): Academic Press.

Fenner, J., & Clark, R. A. F. (2016). Chapter 1 — Anatomy, Physiology, Histology, and Immunohistochemistry of Human Skin. In M. Z. Albanna & J. H. Holmes Iv (Eds.), *Skin Tissue Engineering and Regenerative Medicine* (pp. 1–17): Academic Press.

Gilaberte, Y., Prieto-Torres, L., Pastushenko, I., & Juarranz, Á. (2016). Chapter 1 — Anatomy and Function of the Skin. In M. R. Hamblin, P. Avci, & T. W. Prow (Eds.), *Nanoscience in Dermatology* (pp. 1–14): Academic Press.

Hejtmancik, J. F., Cabrera, P., Chen, Y., M'Hamdi, O., *et al.* (2017). Chapter 19 — Vision. In P. M. Conn (Ed.), *Conn's Translational Neuroscience* (pp. 399–438): Academic Press.

Kalogirou, S. A. (2014). Chapter 11 — Designing and Modeling Solar Energy Systems. In S. A. Kalogirou (Ed.), *Solar Energy Engineering (Second Edition)* (pp. 583–699): Academic Press.

Lyer, S. (2009). Atoms and Life © Arizona Board of Regents, ASU — Ask A Biologist. https://askabiologist.asu.edu/content/atoms-life.

McConnell, A. (2013). Chapter 1 — Anatomy and physiology of the respiratory system. In A. McConnell (Ed.), *Respiratory Muscle Training* (pp. 3–36): Churchill Livingstone.

Moorthy, A. V., & Blichfeldt, T. C. (2009). Chapter 1 — Anatomy and Physiology of the Kidney. In A. V. Moorthy (Ed.), *Pathophysiology of Kidney Disease and Hypertension* (pp. 1–15): W.B. Saunders.

Rizzi, A., & Bonanomi, C. (2017). Chapter 2 — The human visual system described through visual illusions. In J. Best (Ed.), *Colour Design (Second Edition)* (pp. 23–41): Woodhead Publishing.

Talal, A., Hamid, S. K., Khan, M., & Khan, A. S. (2020). Chapter 1 — Structure of biological apatite: bone and tooth. In A. S. Khan & A. A. Chaudhry (Eds.), *Handbook of Ionic Substituted Hydroxyapatites* (pp. 1–19): Woodhead Publishing.

Waldman, S. D. (2019). Chapter 106 — Avascular Necrosis of the Knee Joint. In S. D. Waldman (Ed.), *Atlas of Common Pain Syndromes (Fourth Edition)* (pp. 415–419): Elsevier.

Chapter 2
Human disabilities and diseases

2.1 Introduction

A person with good physical health would probably have all organs, physical processes functioning at their best, and can carry out routine work effortlessly without any painful struggles. In deeper implication, the word "*health*" also refers to a state of complete emotional and mental well-being. However, the mechanisms in the body that regulate development and maintenance can be affected in various ways (Figure 2.1). These include genetic defects, developmental disorders or diseases that

---

Key points

Disease
- A disease is an abnormal medical condition negatively affecting a living organism in part or full, and is not due to any direct external injury.

Infectious disease
- It is triggered by many pathogenic microorganisms, such as bacteria, viruses, parasites or fungi. Examples include SARS, influenza, common cold, tuberculosis, COVID-19, etc.

Non-infectious disease
- These are non-communicable and non-contagious diseases that are not caused by pathogenic microorganisms. Examples include cancers, diabetes mellitus, obesity, and neurodegenerative diseases.

Disorder
- A disorder is a functional abnormality, disturbance or interruption to a normal physical or mental function.

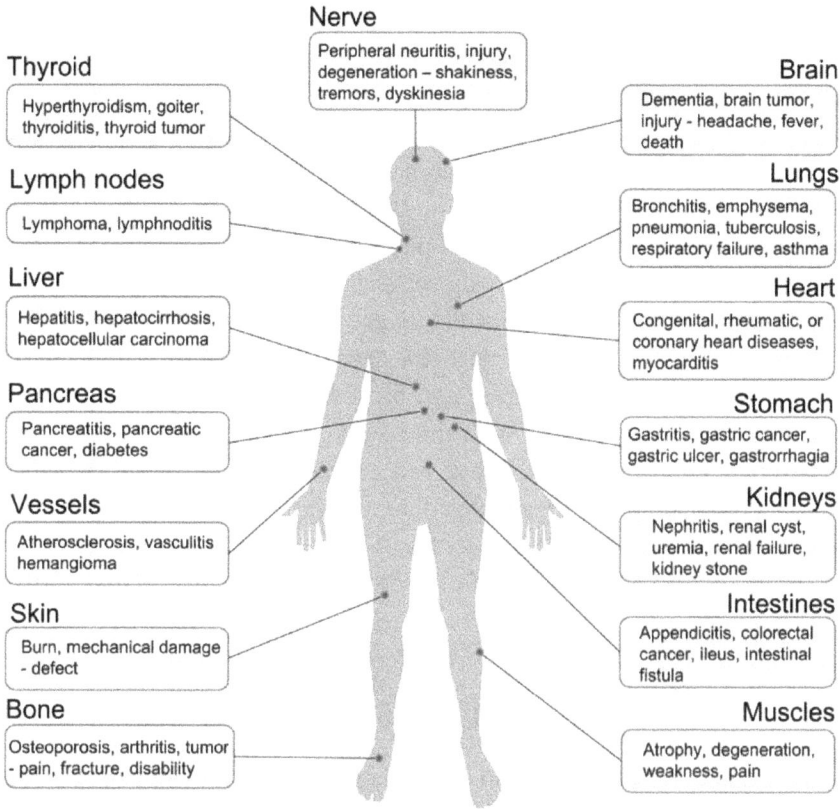

Figure 2.1:   Schematic of human anatomy and related diseases (Yi *et al.*, 2017).

may happen at or before birth. The term *"disease"* is defined as an abnormal condition affecting the proper function of the body or one of its parts, whereas the term *"disorder"* is a functional abnormality or disturbance that occurs in the body of an organism. There are probably thousands of diseases of different kinds existing in nature, with each having a specific set of indications and symptoms. In general, diseases are categorized as acute and chronic. The incidence of acute disease is quick; most of them are significantly shorter in duration with relatively mild to serious symptoms, such as fever and the common cold. In contrast, a chronic disease has a slow start but can last for many years and may never end. Type 2 diabetes is one such example.

Most infectious and non-infectious diseases are fought through the body's first line of defence. Details about the human cellular defensive system are discussed in Chapter 1. If not resolved, antibiotic therapy, such as infection-fighting drugs, is used to act in synchronicity with the body's immune system. Details about drug delivery systems are presented in Chapter 11. In order to substitute or sustain the diseased or inadequate biological structure, implantable medical devices are often inserted within or around the body surface. These devices may be placed temporarily or permanently to aid in diagnosing and treating diseases and disorder conditions. Over the past few decades, several workflows have been established for preparation and processing to increase quality and reliability of the treatments with minimally invasive manners either by drug delivery or implants. These procedures decrease tissue damage, reduce post-operation pain and swelling, increase the comfort of patients, and boost the overall health outcome. The sections below will give an overview of some of the specific disorders and diseases related to the human body.

2.2 Bone diseases and disorders

From Chapter 1, we understand that bones aid in movement and provide shape and support to the body. Like all other parts, bones are living tissues that rebuild continuously throughout life via a process called *"remodeling"*. It is a process where older bone tissue is slowly replaced by newly formed ones. We generally assess the strength of bones by their density or *"bone mass"*. For instance, an examination of bone mineral density will allow a physician to determine their calcium content and, therefore, measure their total strength.

Bone density peaks in adulthood, usually between the ages of 25 and 30 (Figure 2.2). However, as the individual continues to age, the bones progressively lose their density which leads to some common diseases or disorders. Bone tissue is an anisotropic material, which implies that its mechanical properties depend on the direction of force, i.e., compression, tension, and shear. The Young's modulus of bones at various places is tabulated in Table 2.1. External and internal stresses influencing bones and joints come in several ways, from a severe leg fracture to the progressively deteriorating arthritis of joints. Genetic abnormalities and

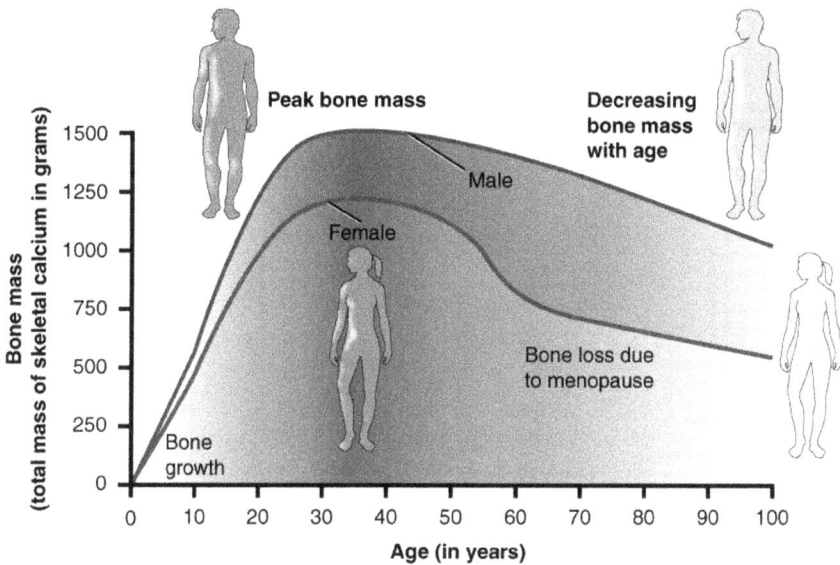

Figure 2.2: Illustrative diagram showing the connection between age and bone mass. Note that bone density is highest at about 30 years of age. Women suffer the loss of bone mass more quickly than men (Betts *et al.*, 2013). Attribution: OpenStax.

Table 2.1: Experimental values of human bones at different locations (Lakatos *et al.*, 2014).

Bone type	Preservation	Young's modulus (MPa)
Femur	Embalmed	20.68–965
	Frozen	423–1516
	Fresh	Avg 344.7
Tibia	Dried, defatted	1.4–79
	Frozen	4–430
Vertebra	Fresh	Avg 151.7
	Dried, defatted	1.1–139
	Frozen	15–30
Mandible	Frozen	3.5–125.6
	Embalmed	Avg 157

nutritional deficiencies (Vitamin D) can also generate weak, thin bones, or bones that are too dense. Abnormal conditions will result in chronic pain and impairment without proper care. The list of well-known bone diseases and disorders with their primary causes is presented in Table 2.2.

Table 2.2:   Common bone disorders/diseases and their primary causes.

Bone disorder / disease	Cause
Osteoporosis	It involves loss of the mineral part of the bone. Over a period, it causes bone fragility and increases the risk of fracture.
Osteonecrosis	It is also known as avascular necrosis. It is a disease where the bone starts to perish due to a lack of blood supply and collapses.
Osteopenia	It is a disorder of the bone which is characterized by bone loss that is not as serious as in osteoporosis. The bone density is lower than normal.
Osteomyelitis	It is a bacterial or fungal infection of bone tissue. It may occur if a bacterium or fungus enters the bloodstream during accidents, surgery, or infection.
Osteoarthritis	It is a degenerative joint disease (joint inflammation) commonly caused by cartilage loss in a joint.
Paget's disease	It is a chronic bone disorder that occurs when bone interferes with the body's normal remodeling process. It occurs most frequently in the spine, pelvis, long bones of the limbs, and skull.
Bone tumors	Forms a mass or lump of tissue when cells divide uncontrollably.
Rheumatoid arthritis	It is an autoimmune and inflammatory condition that causes pain, swelling, and loss of joint function.
Scoliosis	It is an abnormal curvature of the spine, causing an S- or C-shaped appearance when noticed from the person's back. It generally occurs in childhood or early adolescence.
Gout	It is a type of arthritis caused by additional uric acid in the bloodstream. It is characterized by severe pain, swelling, soreness, and inflammation in the joints.
Developmental skeletal disorders	These disorders can be developed genetically.

Among all bone diseases and disorders, knee osteoarthritis (Figure 2.3) is one of the joints' most common medical conditions, caused by progressive degeneration of the articular cartilage and results in decreased function and pain. The main reason for arthritis is unclear. However, ageing, high body mass index, diseases like diabetes, and genetic factors may chemically activate the molecular and biochemical differences and lead to unusual loading of the articular cartilage.

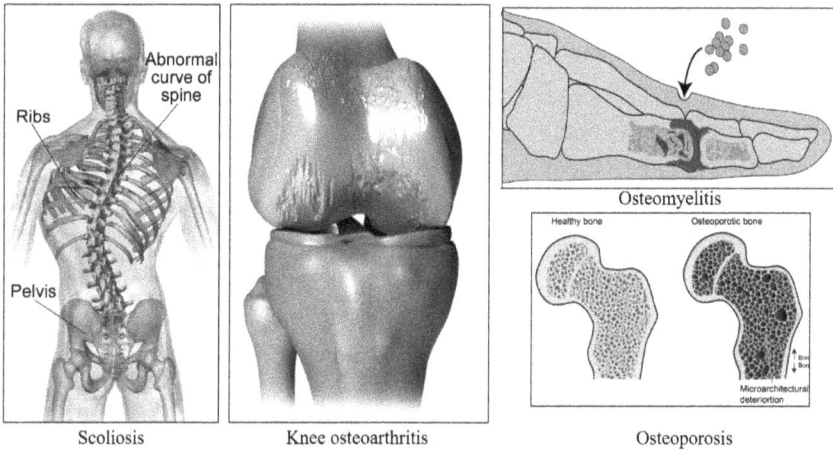

Scoliosis   Knee osteoarthritis   Osteoporosis

Figure 2.3: Illustrative images of common bone diseases and disorders (Birt *et al.*, 2017; Blaus, 2014; Salamanna *et al.*, 2020; Knee osteoarthritis picture attribution: www. MedicalGraphics.de under license CC BY-ND 4.0).

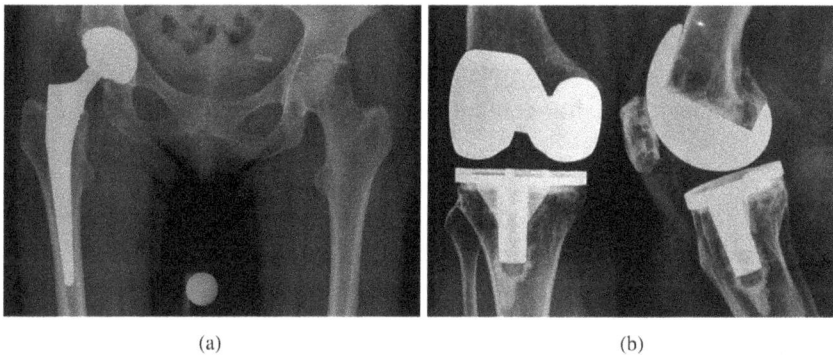

(a)   (b)

Figure 2.4: X-ray image of well-fixed (a) total hip replacement and (b) total knee replacement (Loughenbury *et al.*, 2018; Mullaji *et al.*, 2015).

Hip osteoporosis, hip fracture, and joint inflammation are also serious health issues facing the elderly. Knee replacement surgery (knee arthro-plasty) is now one of the extremely frequent and effective surgical proce-dures for knee arthritis, whereby a diseased knee joint is replaced with artificial material (Figure 2.4b). The procedure is known as total knee replacement (TKR). Total hip replacement (THR) is also probably the most successful, effective, and efficient surgery procedure performed for pain relief and restoration of mobility. In THR, worn-out or damaged bone and cartilage are removed and restored with prosthetic components. The main components of a well-fixed THR are depicted in Figure 2.4a.

Hip prosthesis is one of the main challenges for the design of biomaterials. This is due to the requirement of three separate primary parts, i.e., stem, head, and socket, with their extraordinary permutations of mechanical, chemical, and physical properties. In order to address the specifications of joint arthroplasty, properties such as high strength to toughness, long wearability, custom-made stiffness, resistance to impact, wear abrasion, corrosion resistance, and tolerable transparency of electromagnetic waves are critical for investigative purposes. Details about the different materials used are exclusively discussed in Chapter 4 (polymeric biomaterials), Chapter 5 (bioceramics), and Chapter 6 (metallic biomaterials).

2.3 Dental diseases and disorders

From Chapter 1, we have understood that teeth are made of hard, bone-like material. The four major tissues that make up teeth in humans are enamel, dentin, cementum, and pulp. The mechanical properties, mineral content, and organic content of all dental tissues are presented in Table 2.3.

- **Enamel:** This is the tooth's hard surface composed of calcium and phosphate ions. It provides the outer protective covering.

Table 2.3: Detailed composition of mineralized tissues of human teeth by volume (Berkovitz *et al.*, 2018).

Constituent	Enamel	Dentin	Cementum
Mineral (% v/v)	91.4	48.0	43.3
Organic material (protein + lipid) (% v/v)	5.0	30.6	34.3
Water (% v/v)	3.4	21.4	24.2
Elastic modulus (GPa)	80–105	20–25	8.6–20.8
Hardness (GPa)	3.4–4.6	0.5–1.0	0.48–1.1
Ultimate tensile strength (MPa)	12–42	34–62	—
Fracture toughness (MPa m$^{0.5}$)	0.5–1.3	1.97–2–3.4	—

- **Dentin:** The hard yellow part beneath enamel and cementum is the second mineralized tissue of the body.
- **Cementum:** It is the calcified or mineralized tissue layer covering the root of the tooth.
- **Pulp:** It is an unmineralized soft connective tissue area present within the center of the tooth. It contains nerves and blood vessels.

Dentistry and difficulties related to teeth have been associated with humans from as early as 5000 BC. Oral diseases represent a significant health issue for several nations and have a lifelong impact on people, triggering pain, discomfort, deformity, and even death. Dental caries, gingivitis, periodontitis, oral ulcers, and oral thrush are some very common oral and dental disorders or infections (Figure 2.5 and Table 2.4). The majority of these dental diseases are caused by bacteria, viruses, and fungi. Usually, a sticky layer called *plaque* flourishes with bacteria near the gum line. If not removed regularly, over a period plaque gradually builds up, hardens, and relocates down the length of the tooth. It can inflame the gums and induce several dental infections. Additionally, intensified inflammation causes the gums to develop a *pus*-like substance and leads to the most advanced stage of gum disease known as

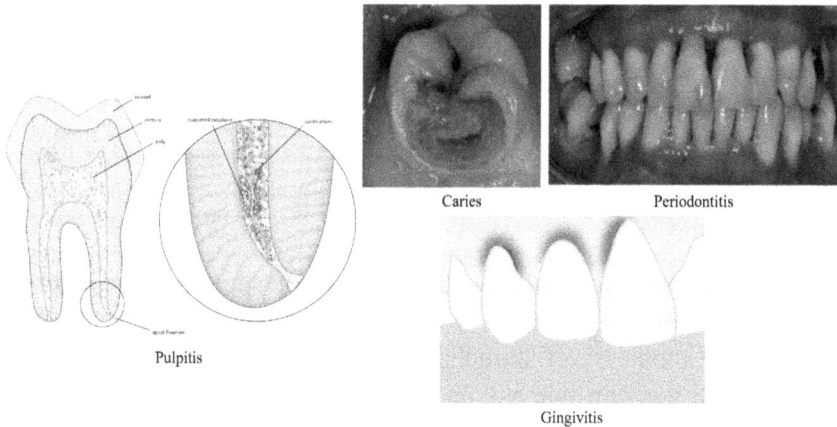

Figure 2.5: Illustrative images of common dental diseases and disorders (Aarabi *et al.*, 2018; Neuhaus, 2007; Gingivitis picture attribution: Die Zuckerschnute).

Table 2.4:   List of common dental diseases and disorders.

Dental disorder / disease	Cause
Cavities	Also known as tooth decay or caries. These are tiny holes in the hard surface of the teeth triggered by bacteria. It gradually grows to be larger if left untreated.
Gingivitis	It is an inflammation of the gums caused by bacteria infection. It is the mildest form of periodontal disease.
Periodontitis	It is a serious chronic inflammation of the gums that injures the tooth's supportive soft tissue and bone.
Pulpitis	It is inflammation of the dental pulp containing blood vessels, nerves, and connective tissue.
Oral cancer	Primarily caused by smoking and chewing tobacco.
Thrush	It is an yeast infection caused by the Candida Albicans fungus that develops on the mouth's mucous membranes and appears like a white film.
Cracked, broken or missing teeth	Generally due to an injury to the mouth or chewing hard foods.

Table 2.5:   Mechanical properties of parts of the jaw that hold the teeth (Li *et al.*, 2020).

Bone	Elastic modulus (GPa)	Hardness (GPa)
Maxilla (upper jaw)	16.52 ± 2.57	0.47 ± 0.08
Mandible (lower jaw)	21.36 ± 3.60	0.62 ± 0.09
Anterior (front teeth)	15.70 ± 2.30	0.53 ± 0.06
Posterior	17.50 ± 2.10	0.57 ± 0.06
Cortical (dense outer surface of bone)	15.85 ± 2.10	0.53 ± 0.06
Trabecular or cancellous bone	7.95 ± 2.10	0.55 ± 0.06

periodontitis. When this happens, the roots are damaged, start to weaken and lead to *bone resorption*.

A dental implant is a fixture that is surgically positioned into the jawbone beneath the gum line and enables bone fusion over a few months. The mechanical properties of parts of the jaw that hold the teeth are tabulated in Table 2.5. These orthodontic devices fulfil the role of the natural tooth root. The survival rate of dental implants usually exceeds 90% due to osseointegration. Osseointegration is a close approximation of bone to implant material. These fixtures are believed to be the model of care that revolutionized prosthetic dental replacements for trauma, accidents, dental diseases, dental disorders, and even poor oral hygiene. To restore function, dental implant surgery substitutes the tooth roots with artificial materials. Details about the different kinds of materials used for dental implants are discussed in Chapters 4–6.

Modern implant dentistry aims to restore the patient's teeth to normal contour, function, and comfort without losing the aesthetics. Implant dentistry has grown into an evidence-based, well-documented clinical science to affirm functional practices that were previously rejected. Recent developments made in dental implants and their associated components to replace or fix damaged or lost teeth have contributed progressively in developing implant dentistry (Figure 2.6). Significant studies focusing on implant dentistry biology and biomechanics have helped to improve and enhance clinical procedures based on the results evaluated by experts. The design, concept, and single-tooth or multi-tooth repair via dental implants and actual radiography image of the implanted tooth are presented in Figure 2.7.

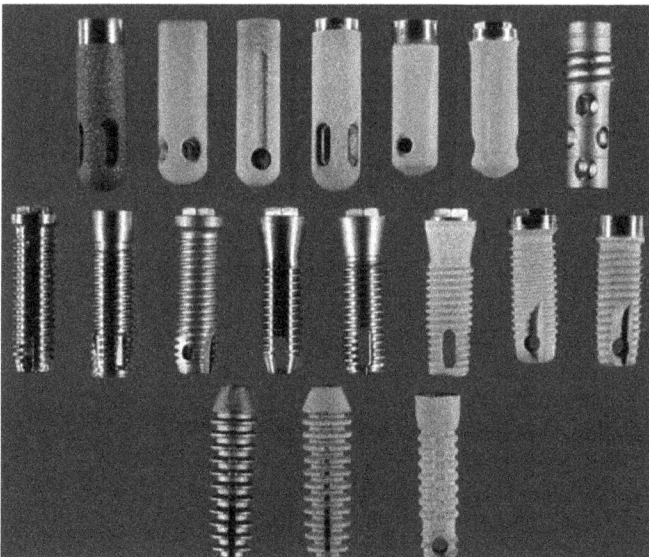

Figure 2.6:   Dental implants may be characterized by their design as cylinder-type (top row), screw-type (middle row), press-fit (bottom row), or a combination of features (upper row, far right) (Misch *et al.*, 2015).

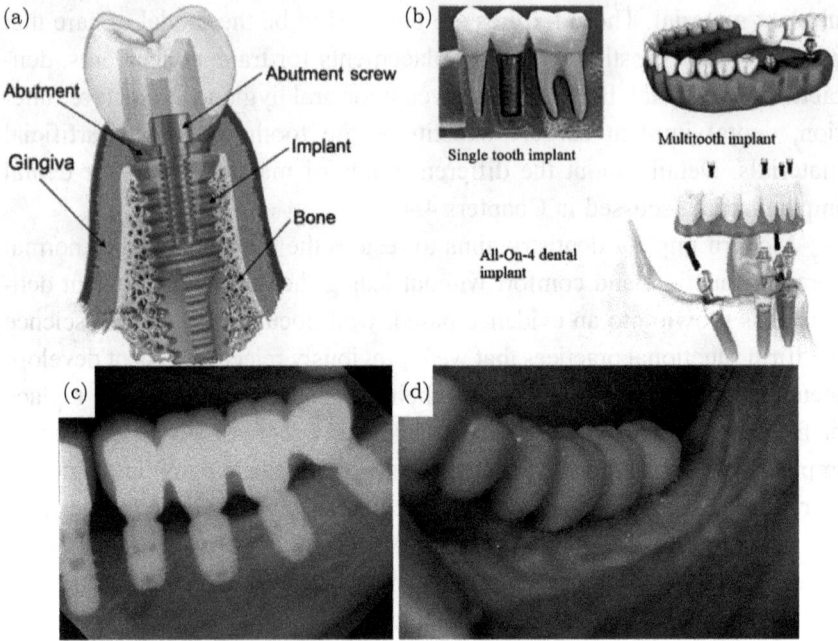

Figure 2.7:   (a) Schematic depiction of restoration of single-tooth functionality by means of a dental implant with abutment and retaining screw as a system to support the crown; (b) Illustrations of different types of dental implants; (c) One-year radiograph after restoration displaying exceptional bone stability; and (d) Clinical photograph of the fixed prosthesis splinted on these short implants (Block, 2018; Das *et al.*, 2019; Gubbi *et al.*, 2018).

2.4 Cardiovascular diseases and disorders

About one-quarter of the world's mortality is due to diseases involving the heart and circulatory system (cardiovascular diseases or CVDs). According to WHO, CVDs, including heart attack and ischemic heart disease, are the world's number one cause of death. The list of common types of heart and vascular diseases are tabulated in Table 2.6. CVDs are inherited sometimes or may arise due to lifestyle choices. Heart attacks and strokes are often acute and are caused by accumulation of deposits such as fat, cholesterol, calcium, and other substances on the internal walls of blood vessels which stop blood from moving into the heart or brain. Atherosclerosis (Figure 2.8) is one such heart disease where

Table 2.6: List of common heart and vascular diseases and disorders.

Heart disorder / disease	Cause
Atherosclerosis	It is narrowing of the arteries triggered by a gradual build-up of plaque (made up of fat, cholesterol, calcium, and other substances).
Cardiac arrhythmia	It is a coronary artery disease that occurs due to irregular heartbeat, i.e., too slowly or too quickly.
Heart valve disease	It occurs when one or more of the valves in the heart do not open and close as supposed to be. Most heart valve complications include the aortic and mitral valves.
Endocarditis	It is a case of heart infection due to bacteria, fungi, or other germs in the bloodstream. It mostly affects the inner lining of the heart and surface of its valves.
Congestive heart failure	It is a chronic progressive disorder that occurs when the heart muscle becomes incapable of pumping adequate blood and oxygen to meet the body's requirements.
Congenital heart defects	It is a heart abnormality that appears at the time of birth.
Rheumatic heart disease	It is a severe complication where heart valves are permanently damaged by rheumatic fever.

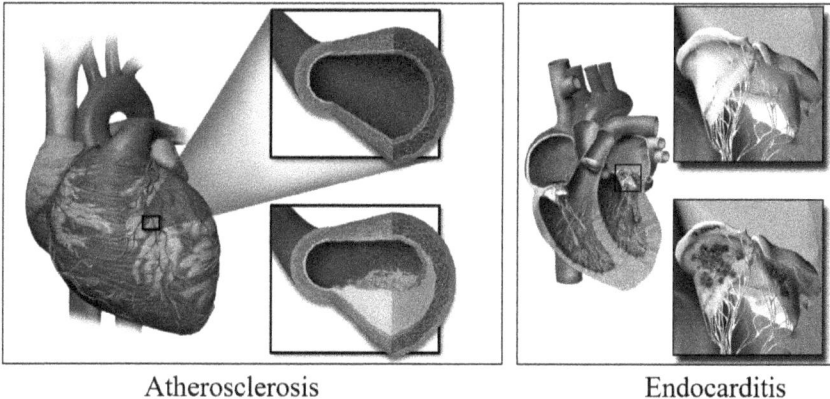

Atherosclerosis   Endocarditis

Figure 2.8: Schematic representation of atherosclerosis and endocarditis heart conditions (Author Attribution: Bruce Blaus; file licensed under CC-BY-SA-4.0).

thickening and hardening of arterial walls occur due to the build-up of deposits. Concerning heart valves, two common forms of heart valve defects occur: narrowing of valve (stenosis) and leakage in valve causing blood to return backward (regurgitation). Acute valve damage suggests the valve needs to be replaced and most often this involves replacing the aortic or mitral valve.

Unlike dental disease treatments, the treatments associated with heart disease are variable and highly dependent on the arteries, valves, and veins (Table 2.7). For any type of heart disease mentioned in Table 2.6, prescribed medication is followed initially unless the case is severe. Should improvements in the patient's lifestyle and prescription drugs fail to control the heart disease, other treatments such as surgery, special procedures, or medical devices may be followed. One of our most

Table 2.7:   Specialist-driven procedures to treat heart conditions.

Procedure	Summary
Coronary Artery Bypass Graft	It is a procedure used to treat coronary artery disease to increase the flow of blood to the heart. Usually, polymeric materials are used as graft materials.
Heart Valve Repair or Replacement	It is a procedure involving repairing or replacing the affected heart valves. Mechanical valves are usually made of carbon and metal.
Implantable Cardioverter-Defibrillator	A small battery-powered device is positioned in the chest to supervise any irregular heart rhythm and automatically delivers electric shocks to fix any abnormality. Outer case is usually made of metal.
Implantable Loop Recorder	It is a heart-monitoring device that is implanted underneath the chest skin to record the heart's electrical activity.
Heart Transplant	It is a surgical procedure to replace a diseased or failing heart with a healthy donor heart.
Ventricular Assist Devices	It is an electromechanical device that assists cardiac circulation in people with weak or failing hearts.
Percutaneous Coronary Intervention	Famously known as angioplasty with stent used to treat clogged or narrowed coronary arteries.
Pacemaker	It is a small electrical device implanted in the chest or abdomen to help abnormal heart rhythms and regulate heart function.

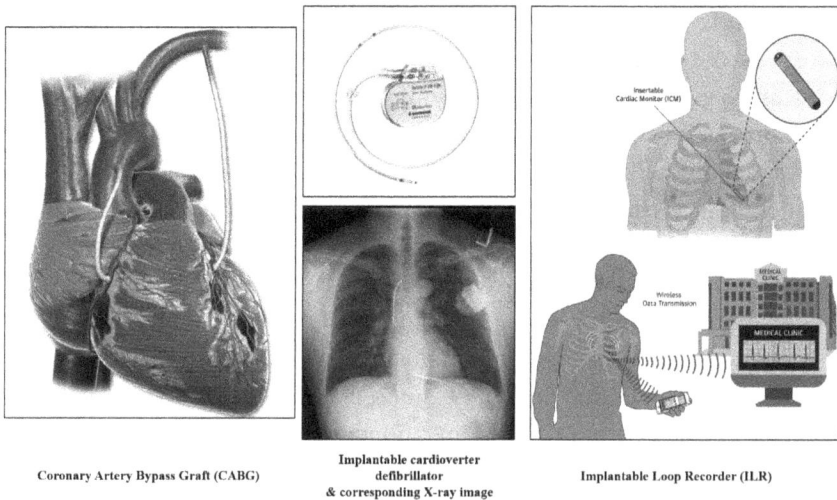

Coronary Artery Bypass Graft (CABG)

Implantable cardioverter defibrillator & corresponding X-ray image

Implantable Loop Recorder (ILR)

Figure 2.9: Illustrative images of various procedures to treat heart conditions (Blaus, 2014; Giancaterino *et al.*, 2018; Marcus, 2008; Biotronik Inc).

innovative and quickly embraced therapeutic methods is the diagnosis of coronary and peripheral artery diseases with artificial materials. Cardiovascular devices are commonly used in the diagnosis of CVDs and make a significant contribution to their care. Most of these devices are designed to regulate irregular heartbeat in people with rhythmic heart problems (Figure 2.9). For heart valve replacement, mechanical valves made from carbon and titanium are used. Vascular and cardiovascular implants such as vascular stents and vascular grafts are fabricated from various kinds of polymeric or biodegradable metals to treat cardiovascular diseases.

2.5 Disorders of the ears

2.5.1 *How do we hear sounds*

The ear is one of the body's most sophisticated and sensitive organs, and the human auditory system's anatomy is very complicated. Hearing relies on a variety of complicated steps that turn the waves of sound in the air into electrical signals, which are transferred by the auditory nerve to the brain. In brief, sound waves pass through the outer ear and travel through the ear canal to enter the eardrum. The eardrum detects the inbound vibrations and passes them through the middle ear bones or ossicles. These bones intensify or increase the sound vibrations and send them into the snail-shaped inner ear known as the cochlea. The cochlea is filled with liquid with thousands of small hair cells that convert the change in sensations or vibrations into electrical signals. The auditory nerve picks up these signals and sends them to the brain, where they are then translated into recognizable and meaningful sounds.

Ears are the most sensitive organs in the human body that can often have complications due to injury, microorganisms, or even noticeable changes in the environment. As mentioned in Table 2.8, ear infections, Ménière's disease, conductive hearing loss, and ear barotrauma are the most common illnesses associated with the ear. A cochlear implant is a neuroprosthetic electronic device (Figure 2.10) that partially restores

Table 2.8: List of the most common ear disorders.

Ear disease/ disorder	Summary
Otitis media	It is a type of contagious infection in the middle ear caused by virus or bacteria. This infection leads to a build-up of fluid at the rear of the eardrum.
Otosclerosis	It is a rare condition that is caused by abnormal remodeling or growth of bone in the middle ear.
Tinnitus	It is hearing of continuous ringing or buzzing sounds with no external source. Tinnitus is not considered as a disease.
Ménière's disease	It is an inner ear condition that can cause vertigo, tinnitus, hearing loss, etc. It is primarily due to irregularity in the inner ear structure or the fluid levels.
Presbycusis	It is a gradual loss of hearing caused by natural aging of the auditory system.
Ear barotrauma	It is pain or damage caused by rapid changes in pressure in the ear.
Acoustic trauma	It is damage to the inner ear that is frequently triggered by exposure to high-decibel noise.
Hearing loss	It is a partial or total inability to hear due to complications with the ear canal, eardrum, or middle ear.

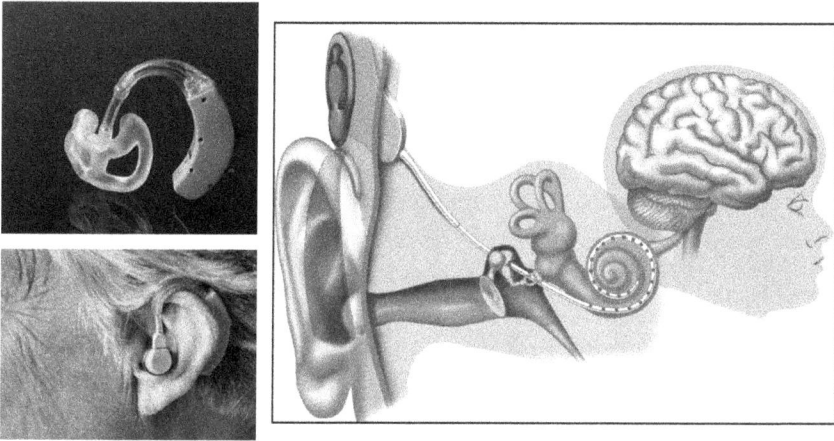

Figure 2.10: Schematic illustrations of hearing aids and the position of a cochlear implant (Kral, 2013; RawpixelCom, 2019; Matthijs/Flickr).

hearing for patients with critical to profound hearing loss. A cochlear implant functions differently from a traditional hearing aid (Figure 2.10). Listening aids usually enhance the incoming sound so that impaired ears can hear clearly, whereas cochlear implants bypass damaged areas of the ear and electrically stimulate the auditory nerve directly. Cochlear implants currently represent the standard for congenital surgery therapy in early childhood.

2.6 Disorders of the eyes

2.6.1 *Creation of vision*

The anatomy of the eye is complex and discussed briefly in Chapter 1. To understand human eye diseases and disorders, it is essential to know how vision is created and its interaction with the brain. Human vision involves the almost synchronized interaction between the two eyes and the brain *via* a network of neurons, receptors, and other cells. A schematic of the eye refraction process is presented in Figure 2.11. The very first stages in this sensory process are stimulating the light receptors in the eyes, converting visible light waves or images to electrical signals, and transmitting

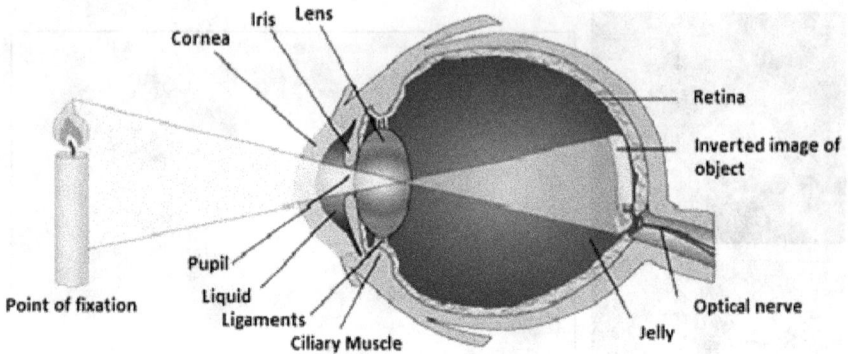

Figure 2.11:   Summary of eye anatomy and the refraction process (Hejtmancik *et al.*, 2017).

these electric signals to the brain *via* the optic nerves. This set of data or information is processed through several stages and eventually reaches the visual cortices of the brain. In a nutshell, the eye works a lot like a human-made camera where the pupil provides the f-stop (focal length), iris the aperture, and cornea the lens. The retina, through rod and cone photoreceptors, actively processes visual information, such as the location of edges and the identification of objects by neural processing through the neuronal network.

As found in the modern digital camera system, the retina acts as a digital image sensor with an analog-to-digital converter. Like a camera film, the light (meaning live image) passes through the cornea (the lens) and concentrates onto the retina. The retina then transforms these images into a neural signal, called transduction. The neuronal impulses come from the external retina and transfer to the inner retina. Neural signals are transmitted via optic nerves to the central structures, where more detailed sequencing is conducted, and data from other senses are assimilated to form visual pathways. The optic nerve should be thought of as the great messenger behind the eye, which serves as a high-speed telephone line linking the eye to the brain. The way the final visual image is formed is much like the way a convex lens forms an image. The image forms upside down, but the brain processes it and flips. Lastly, the oculomotive system, the effective limb of the visual system, maintains the location of the eye, and performs eye movements.

Table 2.9: List of the most common eye diseases and disorders.

Eye disease/disorder	Summary
Glaucoma	It is a progressive vision condition that can lead to permanent blindness due to damage of the optic nerve (Figure 2.12).
Refractive errors	It is a type of vision problem where the eye is incapable of bending and focusing light correctly onto the retina.
Age-related Macular Degeneration	It is a chronic degenerative retinal condition that affects the central vision.
Cataract	It is clouding of the lens in the eye or the surrounding fluid (Figure 2.12).
Diabetic retinopathy	It is triggered by damage to blood vessels in the back of the eye (retina) due to elevated blood sugar levels (type 1 or 2 diabetes).
Amblyopia	It is a disorder where the vision in one or both eyes does not grow correctly as the way it should.
Strabismus	It is a disorder in which both eyes do not look at the same object at the same time.

As discussed, many sections in the eye are required to work together to produce a clear vision. Eye disease and vision loss affect millions of people worldwide, including many older adults in the community. A list of the most common eye diseases and disorders is presented in Table 2.9.

Intraocular lens (IOLs) (Figure 2.13) are external artificial replacements inserted surgically into the eye to restore visual sharpness, particularly after the cataract is removed. The IOLs are also utilized for a kind of vision correction surgery known as *refractive lens exchange*. The material should be clear and suitable to the individual patient in the correct size, shape, and force. Most of the IOLs are fabricated from silicone and usually coated to protect eyes from UV rays.

2.7 Nervous system diseases

From Chapter 1, we have learned that the nervous system is a complex, sophisticated system of nerves and neurons regulating and coordinating body activities. Nervous system dysfunction is inclusive of

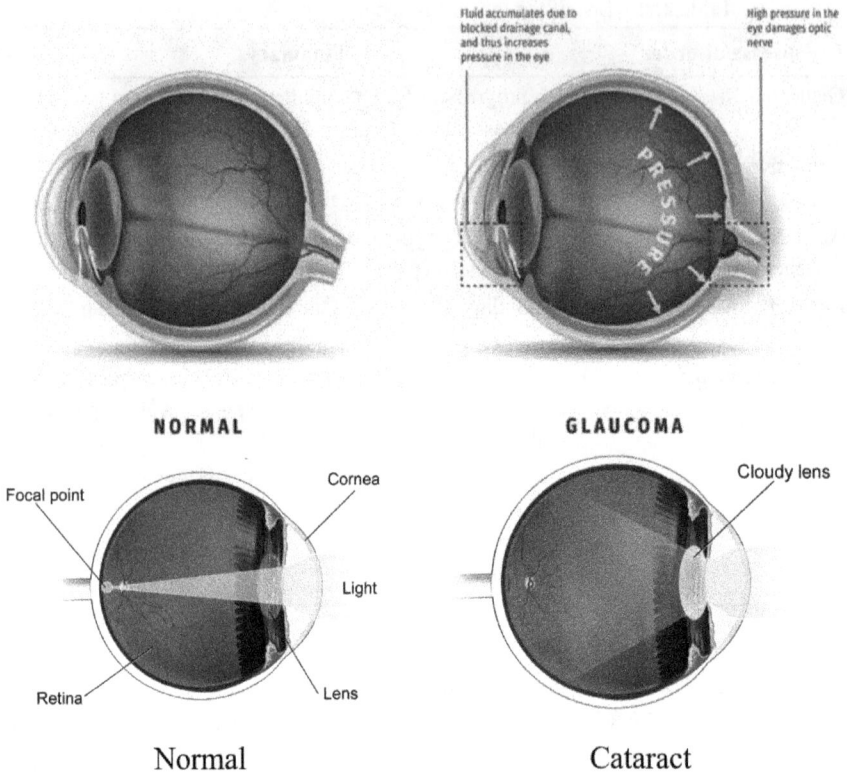

Fluid accumulates due to blocked drainage canal, and thus increases pressure in the eye

High pressure in the eye damages optic nerve

PRESSURE

NORMAL

GLAUCOMA

Focal point

Cornea

Light

Retina

Lens

Cloudy lens

Normal

Cataract

Figure 2.12: A medical illustration depicting glaucoma and cataracts (Blaus, 2014; Raghavendra *et al.*, 2018).

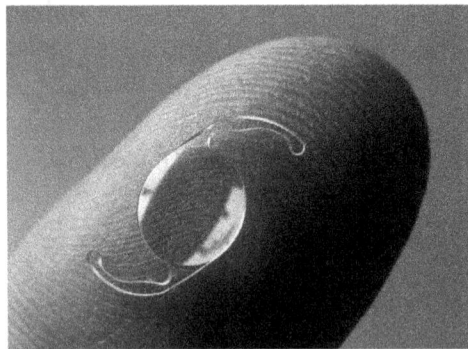

Figure 2.13: Intraocular lens (image licensed under CC-BY-SA-3.0).

disorders affecting any aspects of the central nervous system (CNS), such as the spine, backbone, and cranial nerves. Patients with nerve disorders suffer from functional difficulties, which result in conditions as tabulated in Table 2.10. The conditions may occur from many undetermined or multiple factors such as by inheritance, infection or a degenerative condition. Many nervous system complications may initially appear at a slow phase but cause a gradual loss of function over a long period. However, some diseases, such as cerebrovascular accident, may occur suddenly and cause life-threatening problems.

Table 2.10:   Nervous system disorders and diseases.

Type of disorder	Nervous system diseases	Summary
Degeneration	Alzheimer's disease	It is a chronic neurological disorder caused by the death of brain cells responsible for memory, thinking, and behaviour.
	Parkinson's disease	It is a progressive nervous system disorder that influences movement. It is caused when nerve cells in the brain do not produce enough dopamine.
	Huntington's disease	It is an inherited disease triggered by a defective gene and causes the progressive degeneration of nerve cells in the brain.
	Multiple sclerosis	It is an unpredictable long-term disease that disrupts the CNS, affecting flow of information to the brain, spinal cord, and optic nerves. It can cause difficulties with vision, balance, muscle control, and other basic body functions.
	Amyotrophic lateral sclerosis	It is a progressive motor neuron disease that disturbs nerve cells in the brain and spinal cord, affecting loss of muscle control.
Functional disorder	Epilepsy	It is a neurological disorder characterized by recurrent seizures due to repeated bursts of electrical activity in the brain.

(Continued)

Table 2.10:   (*Continued*)

Type of disorder	Nervous system diseases	Summary
Vascular disorder	Cerebrovascular accident	Also termed as "*stroke*" or "*brain attack*". It is caused by a sudden interruption in the flow of blood to cells in the brain.
Infections	Meningitis	It is a rare inflammation that affects the delicate membranes (meninges) of the brain and spinal cord.
	Encephalitis	It is a rare acute inflammation of the brain tissue caused by bacteria or through the immune system attack.
	Polio	It is an extremely infectious contagious disease instigated by a virus that damages the body's nervous system.
	Epidural abscess	It is caused by a pocket of pus that develops and causes swelling in the CNS.

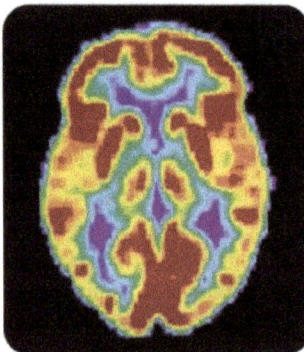

PET Scan of Normal Brain   PET Scan of Alzheimer's Disease Brain

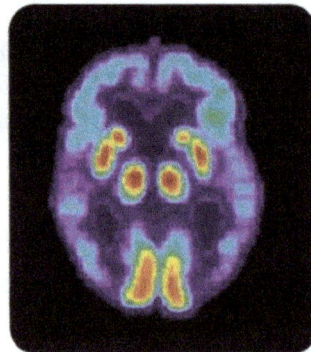

Figure 2.14:   Positron emission tomography (PET) scans illustrating the differences between a normal adult's brain and the brain of an adult who has Alzheimer's disease (User: 7mike5000 / Creative Commons / CC0 1.0).

CNS problems include movement disorders such as Parkinson's disease (Figure 2.14), dystonia, and severe tremor. The most common element in all these diseases is the loss of sufficient, intact nervous system circuits that operate as a voluntary motion. The majority of disorders associated with the CNS are not fully cured.

2.8 Age-related complications and diseases

In recent years, it has been noted that life expectancy has increased due to better medical treatments, vaccination, personal hygiene, and health awareness. The process of aging is dynamic and related to the progressive degeneration of tissues, which have a significant effect on vital structural organs and their functions. It is the prevalent risk factor for naturally occurring chronic diseases such as cancer, type 2 diabetes mellitus, Alzheimer's, Parkinson's, cardiovascular and neurodegenerative diseases that restrict a human's lifespan. The decline of physiological integrity, gradual decrease in homeostasis, and decreased capacity to respond to environmental stimuli lead to increased susceptibility and vulnerability to diseases. Ageing is also associated with several irreversible changes occurring at molecular, biophysical, and biochemical scales. Traditionally, aging has been regarded as a natural, inevitable process and consequently not considered as a disease by many.

The transitions that aging brings vary from person to person, though with some small variances among individuals. The list of alterations that occur in the body with age is remarkably long and is presented in detail in Figure 2.15. Some of the noticeable changes include wrinkled skin,

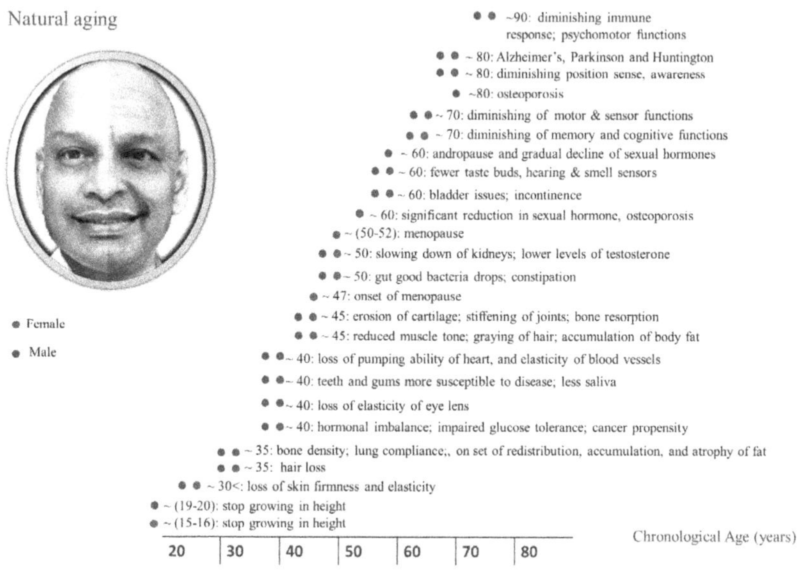

Figure 2.15: Age-related pathologies with comparison to males and females.

regular stopping of height, loss of weight as a result of the loss of muscle and bone mass, decrease in sexual activity (and menopause of women), and decline in function of most organ types such as the liver, lung, heart, and stomach. It is to be noted that natural aging is subjective of gender, genetics, lifestyle, and climate.

2.9 Multiple choice questions

1. Disease existing at or before birth is
   (a) congenital
   (b) communicable
   (c) non-communicable
   (d) none of the above

2. The immune system comprises
   (a) humoral and fibrous systems
   (b) humoral and cell-mediated systems
   (c) antigens
   (d) lymphocytes

3. Researchers believe that Paget disease may be caused by
   (a) virus
   (b) parasite
   (c) an abnormal gene
   (d) A and C

4. Gum disease is associated with
   (a) pregnancy
   (b) heart disease and stroke
   (c) diabetes
   (d) all of the above

5. Human Immunodeficiency Virus causes AIDS by attacking a type of white blood cell called
   (a) CD4
   (b) CD3
   (c) CD8
   (d) none of the above

6. Which of the following is a viral disease?
   (a) type 1 diabetes
   (b) type 2 diabetes
   (c) blood cancer
   (d) influenza

7. The hardest material in the human body is the
   (a) bone
   (b) enamel
   (c) dentin
   (d) skull

8. When the individual is unable to recognize everyday objects and name them correctly, this is known as
   (a) prosopagnosia
   (b) anomia
   (c) agnosia
   (d) aphosonomia

9. If the lens in the eye becomes opaque, the disease is called
   (a) myopia
   (b) astigmatism
   (c) glaucoma
   (d) cataract

10. Hypertension is the term used for
    (a) increase in heart rate
    (b) decrease in heart rate
    (c) decrease in blood pressure
    (d) increase in blood pressure

References & Further Reading

Aarabi, G., Schnabel, R. B., Heydecke, G., & Seedorf, U. (2018). Potential Impact of Oral Inflammations on Cardiac Functions and Atrial Fibrillation. *Biomolecules, 8*(3), 66. doi:10.3390/biom8030066.

Berkovitz, B., & Shellis, P. (2018). Chapter 2 — Mammalian Tooth Structure and Function. In B. Berkovitz & P. Shellis (Eds.), *The Teeth of Mammalian Vertebrates* (pp. 25–46): Academic Press.

Betts, J. G., Young, K. A., Wise, J. A., Johnson, E., *et al.* (2013). *Anatomy and Physiology*: OpenStax.

Birt, M. C., Anderson, D. W., Bruce Toby, E., & Wang, J. (2017). Osteomyelitis: Recent advances in pathophysiology and therapeutic strategies. *Journal of Orthopaedics, 14*(1), 45–52. doi:10.1016/j.jor.2016.10.004.

Blaus, B. (2014). Medical Gallery of Blausen Medical 2014. *WikiJournal of Medicine, 1*(2). doi:10.15347/wjm/2014.010.

Block, M. S. (2018). Dental Implants: The Last 100 Years. *Journal of Oral and Maxillofacial Surgery, 76*(1), 11–26. doi:10.1016/j.joms.2017.08.045.

Das, R., & Bhattacharjee, C. (2019). Chapter 16 — Titanium-based nanocomposite materials for dental implant systems. In A. M. Asiri, Inamuddin, & A. Mohammad (Eds.), *Applications of Nanocomposite Materials in Dentistry* (pp. 271–284): Woodhead Publishing.

Giancaterino, S., Lupercio, F., Nishimura, M., & Hsu, J. C. (2018). Current and Future Use of Insertable Cardiac Monitors. *JACC: Clinical Electrophysiology, 4*(11), 1383–1396. doi:10.1016/j.jacep.2018.06.001.

Gubbi, P., & Wojtisek, T. (2018). Chapter 5.2 — The role of titanium in implant dentistry. In F. H. Froes & M. Qian (Eds.), *Titanium in Medical and Dental Applications* (pp. 505–529): Woodhead Publishing.

Hejtmancik, J. F., Cabrera, P., Chen, Y., M'Hamdi, O., *et al.* (2017). Chapter 19 — Vision. In P. M. Conn (Ed.), *Conn's Translational Neuroscience* (pp. 399–438): Academic Press.

King, A., & Phillips, J. R. A. (2016). Total hip and knee replacement surgery. *Surgery (Oxford), 34*(9), 468–474. doi:10.1016/j.mpsur.2016.06.005.

Kral, A. (2013). Auditory critical periods: A review from system's perspective. *Neuroscience, 247*, 117–133. doi:10.1016/j.neuroscience.2013.05.021.

Lakatos, É., Magyar, L., & Bojtár, I. (2014). Material Properties of the Mandibular Trabecular Bone. *Journal of Medical Engineering, 2014*, 470539. doi:10.1155/2014/470539.

Li, J., Jansen, J. A., Walboomers, X. F., & van den Beucken, J. J. J. P. (2020). Mechanical aspects of dental implants and osseointegration: A narrative review. *Journal of the Mechanical Behavior of Biomedical Materials, 103*, 103574. doi:10.1016/j.jmbbm.2019.103574.

Loughenbury, F., McWilliams, A., Smith, M., Pandit, H., *et al.* (2018). Leg length inequality after primary total hip arthroplasty. *Orthopaedics and Trauma, 32*(1), 27–33. doi:10.1016/j.mporth.2017.11.006.

Marcus, G. (2008). A normal chest X-ray after placement of an ICD. *Creative Commons Attribution 3.0 Unported license.*

Misch, C. E., Strong, J. T., & Bidez, M. W. (2015). Chapter 15 — Scientific Rationale for Dental Implant Design. In C. E. Misch (Ed.), *Dental Implant Prosthetics (Second Edition)* (pp. 340–371): Mosby.

Mullaji, A., & Shetty, G. (2015). Cemented total knee arthroplasty remains the "gold standard". *Seminars in Arthroplasty, 26*(2), 62–64. doi:10.1053/j.sart.2015.08.006

Neuhaus, K. W. (2007). Teeth: Malignant neoplasms in the dental pulp? *The Lancet Oncology, 8*(1), 75–78. doi:10.1016/S1470-2045(06)71013-0.

Raghavendra, U., Fujita, H., Bhandary, S. V., Gudigar, A., *et al.* (2018). Deep convolution neural network for accurate diagnosis of glaucoma using digital fundus images. *Information Sciences, 441*, 41–49. doi:10.1016/j.ins.2018.01.051.

RawpixelCom. (2019). A senior citizen wearing a behind-the-ear hearing aid. *Creative Commons CC0 1.0 Universal Public Domain Dedication,* http://allfreephotos.net/.

Salamanna, F., Maglio, M., Sartori, M., Tschon, M., *et al.* (2020). Platelet features and derivatives in osteoporosis: a rational and systematic review on the best evidence. *International Journal of Molecular Sciences, 21*(5), 1762. doi:10.3390/ijms21051762.

Yi, L., & Liu, J. (2017). Liquid metal biomaterials: A newly emerging area to tackle modern biomedical challenges. *International Materials Reviews, 62*(7), 415–440. doi:10.1080/09506608.2016.1271090.

Chapter 3
Properties and microstructure
of tissues

3.1 Cellular aspects of tissues

3.1.1 *Cell source based on type: Primary cells*

3.1.1.1 *Autologous cells*

Autologous cells (Figure 3.1) are derived from the same person they are to be re-implanted into. As a result, they do not cause any immune response and have the least issues with rejection and disease/pathogen transmission. For some specific situations, cells may not be available (for example, genetic diseases) or may not yield a sufficient supply. Also, removing the cells does involve an extra surgical procedure that can

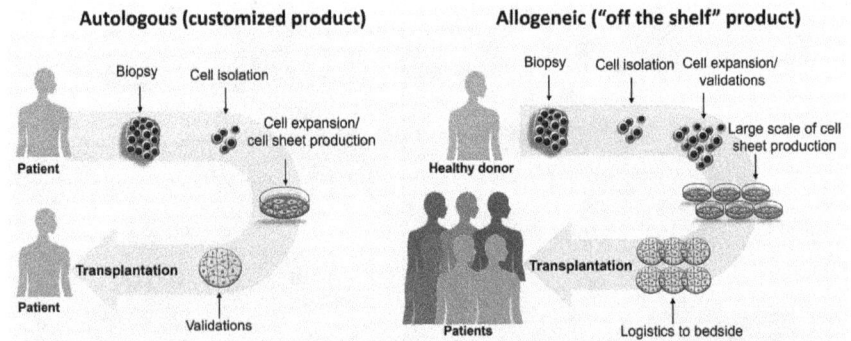

Figure 3.1: Example showing the cell sheet construction process utilizing autologous or allogeneic cell sources (Carlson, 2019; Kim *et al.*, 2019).

trigger/induce morbidity in the patient and increase the risk of illness and pain. However, autologous cells are not expensive, and are batch-operated for universal clinical usage.

3.1.1.2 *Allogeneic cells*

Allogeneic cells (Figure 3.1) come from the same species and can be used as a single prime source of cells to handle many patients. Cells are accumulated from a donor sample to establish a master cell bank (MCB). The MCB is then employed as the basis for generating cell populations according to the different treatment requirements. In contrast to autologous cells, allogeneic cells offer several advantages in terms of consistency, procedure regulations, quality control, and cost efficacy. In most cases, transplantation that involves allogeneic cells has usually been limited to younger patients with a decent general condition because of the potential risk of regimen-related toxicity. However, allogeneic transplants face immune rejection issues by the host.

3.1.1.3 *Xenogeneic cells*

Xenogeneic cells are isolated from individuals of a different species, for example, cells from animals. These are particularly effective in the formulation of common off-the-shelf engineered tissues. There are many risks connected with the use of xenogenic cells, such as immunological rejection, infectious disease transmission, ambiguity in long-term function, and long-term maintenance. Once all these jeopardies are taken into consideration, the extensive usage of xenogeneic cells is not very desirable compared to well established autologous or allogeneic cells. The main advantages of autologous, allogeneic, and xenogeneic cells are presented in Table 3.1.

3.1.2 *Cell source based on possible sources*

3.1.2.1 *Stem cells*

Several tissue techniques already available are highly dependent upon the availability of autologous tissue samples that isolate, expand, and seed a

Table 3.1:   Common differences between autologous, allogeneic, and xenogeneic cells.

Source	Pros	Cons
Autologous	No disease transmission	Inadequate availability; risk of infection and pain; delay in treatment
Allogeneic	Superior availability; less expensive	Disease transmission; immune reaction
Xenogeneic	Most abundant; least expensive	Disease transmission; immune rejection

particular cell type onto a matrix for re-implantation. Nevertheless, retrieval of normal cells is often challenging in cases of extreme end-organ failures or abnormality. In such cases, rather than using tissue-specific cells, the utilization of stem cells has become a possibility for tissue engineering applications due to their capability to self-renew, develop and become virtually any kind of cell in the body.

In simple terms, stem cells are the body's fundamental raw component cells from which all other cells with dedicated functions are created. Under ambient conditions (in body or laboratory), stem cells divide to create more cells called daughter cells. These newly formed daughter cells either become new stem cells (self-renewal) or more specifically functioned specialized cells (differentiation). Stem cell differentiation into various tissue types is shown in Figure 3.4. This unique capability to grow and differentiate into essential varieties makes them a desirable alternate source of cells for tissue engineering. It is critical to remember that stem cells are non-specialized cells that can divide indefinitely and regenerate for long periods, adding to their attractiveness. Their ability for differentiation allows stem cells to be classified into five principal categories: (i) totipotent stem cells, (ii) pluripotent stem cells, (iii) multipotent stem cells, (iv) unipotent stem cells, and (v) oligopotent stem cells. The distinction between totipotent, pluripotent, and multipotent stem cells is shown in Figure 3.2 and presented in Table 3.2. Pluripotent and multipotent stem cells are most studied.

- **Totipotent:** have unlimited capability and can differentiate into any cell type. Example: zygote.

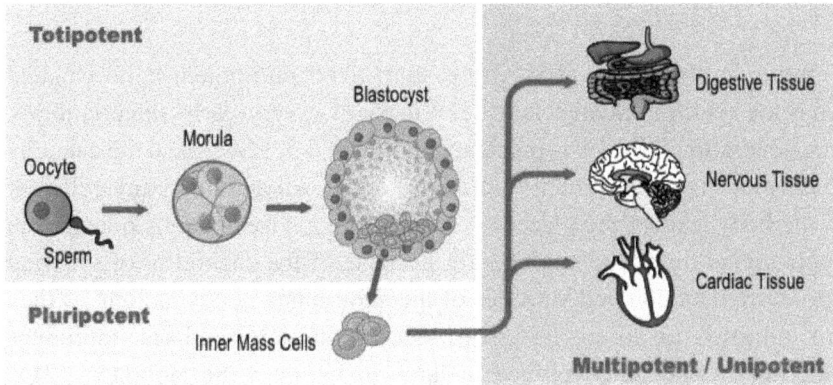

Figure 3.2: Difference between totipotent, pluripotent, and multipotent stem cells (Asal *et al.*, 2020; Jones, 2006).

Table 3.2: Common differences between totipotent, pluripotent, and multipotent stem cells.

	Totipotent	**Pluripotent**	**Multipotent**
Relative potency	High	Medium	Low
Cell types proficient of generating	Capable of giving rise to any cell type	Can give rise to all cell types of the body except the placenta	Can develop into more than one cell type, but have constrained range
Source	Cell embryos	Blastocyst, umbilical cord, iPSCs	Organs
Terminology	Toti = Whole	Pluri = Many	Multi = Several

- **Pluripotent:** competent of giving rise to all tissues of an organism, except the placenta. These are also known as master cells. Example: embryonic stem cells (ESCs) and induced pluripotent stem cells (iPSs).
- **Multipotent:** differentiate into a limited *range* of cell types and give rise to numerous types of mature cells. Example: adult stem cells.
- **Oligopotent:** differentiate into a limited *number* of cell types. Example: lymphoid and myeloid stem cells.
- **Unipotent:** differentiate into a single cell type. This implies that it is able to produce only its own type of cells. Example: muscle stem cells.

3.1.2.2 *Embryonic stem cells*

Embryonic stem cells (ESCs) are short-lived pluripotent cells isolated from the undifferentiated inner cell mass of a very early-stage embryo. The generation of ESCs is presented in Figure 3.3. ESCs have the capacity to develop (i.e., differentiate) into any sort of cell and build any cell type in the body, except the placenta. Such cells have tremendous potential in applications for tissue engineering because of the capability of growing into more than 200 cell varieties of the adult human body as long as they are indicated to do so. ESCs are usually immortal and can reproduce indefinitely and be developed in large numbers in the laboratory. Two distinctive properties distinguish the ESCs from others: their pluripotency and their ability to reproduce endlessly. But due to the destruction of an embryo, ESCs are challenging to regulate with respect to their differentiation.

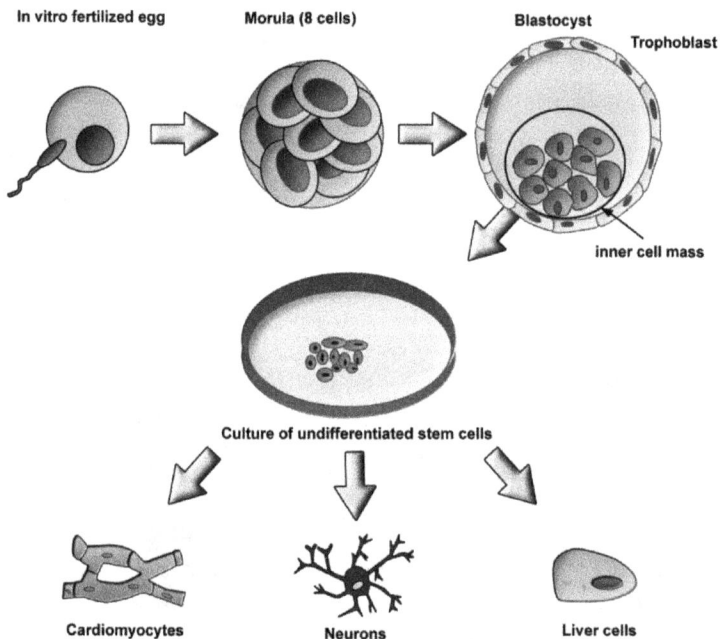

Figure 3.3: Generation of embryonic stem cells (Abou-Saleh *et al.*, 2018; Khademhosseini *et al.*, 2020; Tatullo *et al.*, 2020).

As ESCs are extracted from an early phase of embryos, i.e., a group of cells that develop when a woman's egg is fertilized in an *in vitro* fertilization clinic with a man's sperm, many questions and concerns regarding the ethics of using ESCs for research have been raised globally.

3.1.2.3 *Adult stem cells*

Adult stem cells (ASCs) are also undifferentiated cells located among the differentiated cells in a tissue or organ. They help sustain or rebuild the tissue when needed. ASCs are believed to be multipotent, meaning they can renew themselves and only differentiate into certain types of cells in the body, not to any kind of cell like ESCs. They give rise to cell types of one specific tissue in order to preserve and regenerate that specific organ or tissue feature. Hematopoietic (blood) stem cells, for example, can only substitute various blood cell forms, hepatic stem cells may rebuild liver tissues, muscle stem cells are able to regenerate muscular fibers, and epithelial (skin) stem cells can produce different cell types which compose the skin. As an organism grows, adult cells deliver new cells and replace the existing cells that are not functional. It is assumed that adult stem cells are buried deep within organs, surrounded by ordinary cells.

In several organs and tissues, ASCs are well-recognized in nervous tissue, bone marrow, synovium, skeletal muscle, adipose, cartilage, skin, dental pulp, heart, gut, pancreas, GI tract, and testis. They are assumed to live and work within a specific region or specialized vascular microenvironment of every tissue, known as *"stem cell niche"*. ASC can remain silent (non-divided) for prolonged periods until the need to generate more cells is triggered, tissue is injured or disease strikes. Hematopoietic stem cells (HSCs), mesenchymal stem cells (MSCs), adipose-derived stem cells, and epithelial stem cells are some of the ASCs that are widely used in cell therapy. Researchers often use the term *"somatic stem cell*s" as an alternative to ASCs, where *somatic* refers to body cells (not the germ cells, sperm, or eggs).

- **HSCs:** give rise to all types of blood cells
- **MSCs:** have been widely registered to be present in many tissues

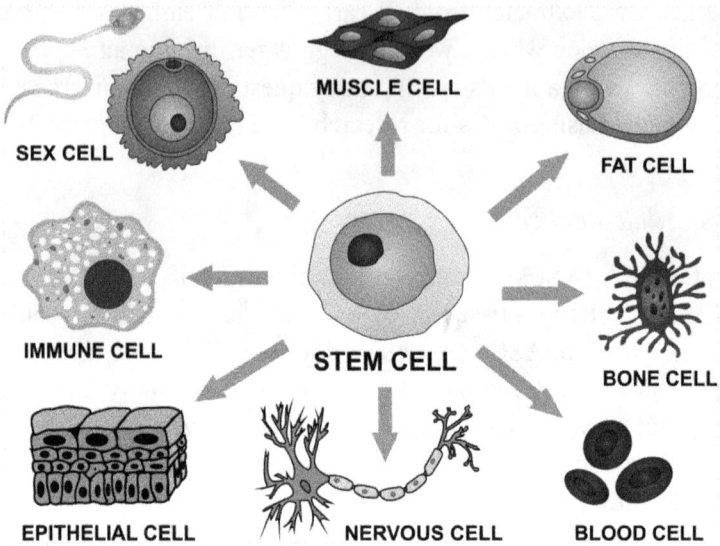

Figure 3.4:   Stem cell differentiation into various tissue types (Fournier, 2019).

3.1.2.4 *Induced pluripotent stem cells (iPS cells)*

Induced pluripotent stem cells, or iPS cells, are stem cells created *in vitro* using genetic reprogramming. The word "*induced*" generally means they are rendered in the laboratory by using typical adult cells, such as the skin or blood cells, and transforming them into stem cells. By carefully altering the genes in adult cells, scientists are able to reprogram them to act very equally to ESCs. The procedure for establishing iPSCs with reprogramming aspects and differentiating them into other cell categories is shown in Figure 3.5. As these kinds of cells display a high resemblance to ESCs, they also inherit the ability to develop into every type of cell (except the placenta). These iPS cells are derived from various somatic cell types and animal species. It is crucial to note that reprogramming such cells to become iPS cells requires certain genetic modifications. This may trigger certain variations that are not existing in usual ESCs.

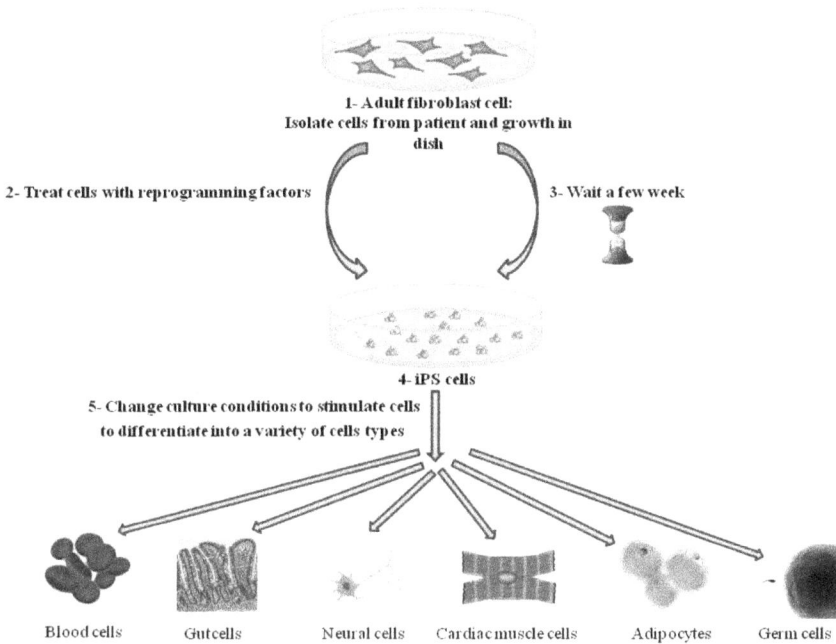

Figure 3.5: Creating iPSCs with reprogramming factors and differentiating them into other cell modes (Amini Mahabadi *et al.*, 2018; Cakir *et al.*, 2020).

3.2 Extracellular matrix

By nature, the extracellular micro-environment / matrix (ECM) is a complex network made up of a wide range of multi-domain macromolecules formed in a cell/tissue-specific manner. ECM has the most essential active and indispensable components that glue together all cells, tissues, and organs by reflecting their activities in the cell/tissue surroundings. This three-dimensional architectural molecular ECM network is critical in supporting tissues with structural and mechanical integrity, and facilitates repair and reconstruction of tissues after injury. In addition to providing mechanical support for neighbouring cells to sustain the basic structure of tissues and organs, this unique and extracellular network also serves as a storehouse for growth factors, hormones, and other biochemical signalling compounds. It provides a mechanism through which nutrients and chemical messengers can spread. Apart from the mentioned biophysical and biochemical properties, through cell-ECM interactions, the ECM establishes and aids in retaining basic cell structure, survival, proliferation, migration, and differentiation.

The ECM composition and structure are not fixed but are highly dependent on the location within the tissues and organs, the age of the host, and the tissue's physiological conditions. But the underlying three-dimensional ECM structure consists of a complex network of fibrous proteins that provide tensile strength and recoil, highly viscous proteoglycans (PGs) that provide flexibility and lubrication, and adhesion proteins that connect the matrix elements to one another and cells. All these are arranged in a particular distinct tissue-specific structure. The typical structure and components of the ECM are shown in Figure 3.6 and Table 3.4. The main fibrous ECM proteins are collagen, elastin, fibrillin, and fibulin.

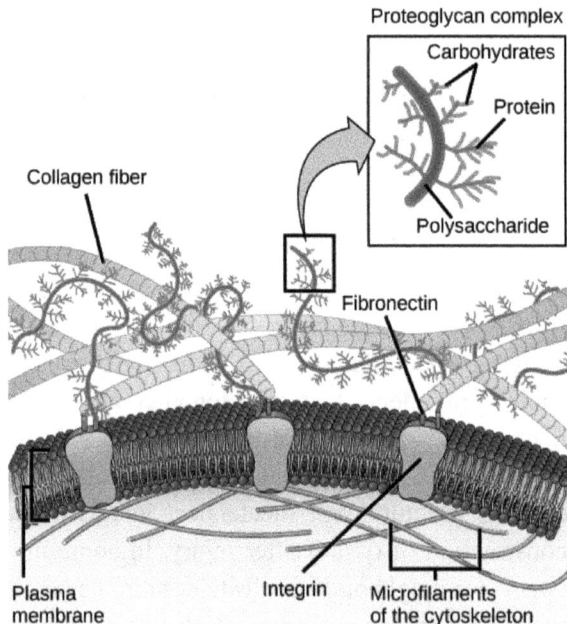

Figure 3.6: Graphical representation of the extracellular matrix (ECM). Typical elements include collagen, proteoglycans (with hydration shell depicted around sugars), fibronectin, and laminin. The cellular receptors for a number of these ECM components are integrins (Zedalis *et al.*, 2018). Attribution: OpenStax.

PGs have a broad array of functions reflecting their special properties of buffering, hydration, binding, and strength resistance. They often occupy most of the interstitial extracellular space inside the tissue in the form of a hydrated gel.

a. **Collagen:** This is the main component of ECM which models the framework of connective tissues. It is the richest protein in the human body and represents up to 30% of the total protein mass. Collagen aids ECM in maintaining structural integrity, regulating cell adhesion and preserving its molecular architecture. It also helps in the maintenance of the strength, flexibility, and hemostasis throughout the body. There are 30 types of collagen, but 80–90% of the collagen in the body comprises types I, II, and III. The most important collagen types and their distribution are presented in Table 3.3.

b. **Elastin:** Collagen collaborates with elastin, another key ECM fiber protein that is essential to elasticity, compliance, and resilience. Elastin is approximately 1000 times more flexible than collagen. It is responsible for imparting elastic properties by offering recoil to tissues that undergo repeated stretch such as vascular vessels, skin, and the lungs.

c. **Fibronectin:** Fibronectin is a huge adhesive glycoprotein (approximate molecular weight: 250,000 Da), one of the major elements of ECM, and second only to collagen in quantity. Termed as "biological glue", fibronectin is involved in diverse functions and has a crucial role in attachment, migration, and mediating adhesion and function of many cell types, thereby promoting host biocompatibility.

Table 3.3: Most important collagen types and their distribution in the human body.

Type	Location in the body
I	Found in connective tissues including skin, tendon, and bone tissue.
II	Found primarily in cartilage, inner ear and in the gel that fills the eyeball
III	Found in hollow organs such as large blood vessels, uterus, and bowel
IV	Found in the basal lamina
V	Found in the interstitial tissue matrix

Table 3.4:   Elements of the ECM, their structure, and main purpose.

ECM component	Structure	Main purpose in ECM
Collagens	Developed as fibrils within the ECM.	Provide mechanical integrity (tensile strength) and influence.
Elastin	The soluble monomer of elastin is tropoelastin. In its polymerized form, elastin comprises more than 90% of the mature elastic fibers and is constructed by the hierarchical assembly and cross-linking of many tropoelastin monomers.	Provides elasticity and is responsible for compliance and resilience of tissues.
Fibronectin	It is a large glycoprotein that forms a fibrillar network comprising units of three types of repeating homologous amino acid sequences.	Responsible for a large number of cellular functions, including initial cell adhesion, cell migration, cytoskeletal organization, oncogenic transformation, ingestion of other cells, response to blood vessel injury and bleeding, and embryonic differentiation.
Laminins	These are cross-shaped high molecular weight proteins consisting of three heterotrimer subunits of alpha, beta, and gamma chains.	Responsible for cell binding with other proteins and aids in enhancing cell adhesion and migration.
Tenascins	Exist as TN-C, TN-R, TN-W, TN-X, and TN-Y.	Do not promote but modulate cell adhesion, migration, and growth.
Glycosaminoglycans (GAGs)	GAGs consist of multiple copies of basic disaccharide repeat monomers, which are normally linked to a protein core.	GAGs involve a variety of ligand recognition and cell signaling processes.

d. **Laminins:** These are found in vault membranes and exploited by many cell types as a substratum for cell adhesion and movement. They are web-like assemblies that oppose tensile forces in the basal lamina. Many laminins auto-assemble to form networks that maintain close connection with cells via cell surface receptor interactions. It is interesting to note that laminins share several properties with fibronectin.

e. **Tenascin, thrombospondin, and osteonectin:** These proteins are all modulators of cell adhesion, migration, and growth.

f. **Glycosaminoglycans (GAGs):** GAGs are unbranched linear chains of anionic polysaccharides that offer the ECM additional physical properties not provided by structural proteins alone. They are highly negatively-charged essential components of ECM, which play a key role in binding growth factors and cytokines, water retention, and the ECM gel properties.

3.3 Tissues

The tissue, after the cell, is the next organizational level within the human body. In a complex organism, cells with similar functions are linked together to form a tissue. There are four fundamental types of human tissues (Figure 3.7) that comprise all organs, namely connective, epithelial, muscle, and nervous.

Each tissue is an arrangement of similarly specialized cells assembled to serve a specific purpose.

3.3.1 *Connective tissues*

Connective tissues are the richest and most extensively distributed primary tissues in the human body. As the name suggests, they provide a connecting function and help the body to hold itself together. They serve many roles, but notably, they support, protect, connect, and insulate tissues and organs. They also store reserve fuel and allow diffusion of water, salts, and various nutrients. The ECM, made up of cells, protein fibers,

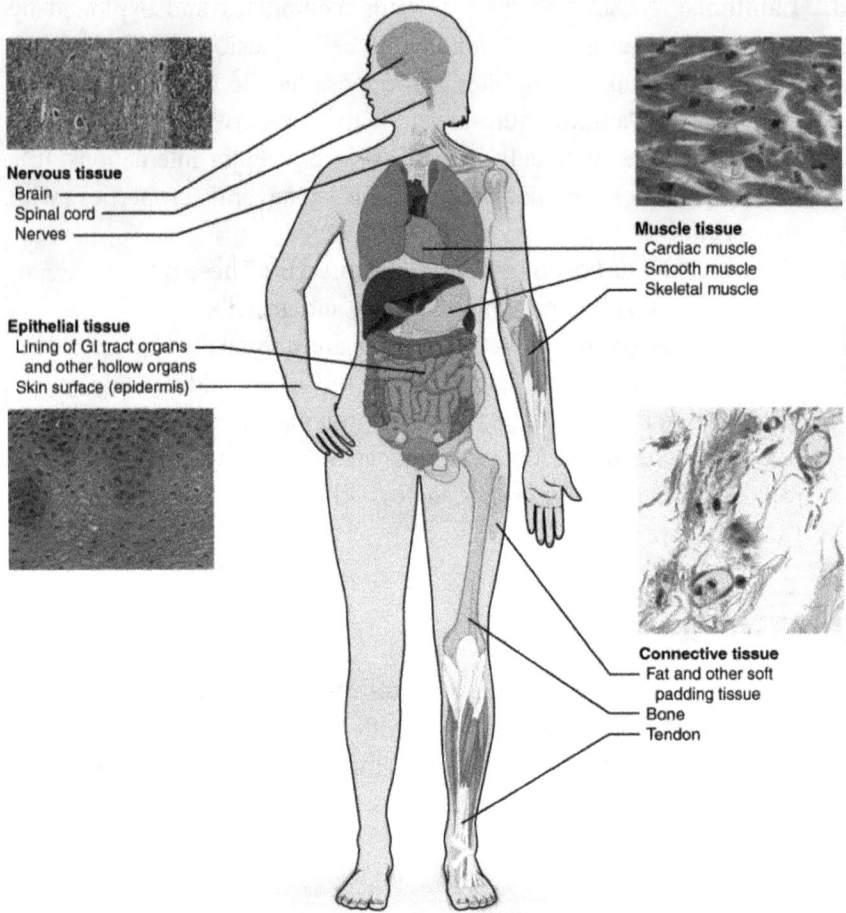

Nervous tissue
Brain
Spinal cord
Nerves

Muscle tissue
Cardiac muscle
Smooth muscle
Skeletal muscle

Epithelial tissue
Lining of GI tract organs
and other hollow organs
Skin surface (epidermis)

Connective tissue
Fat and other soft
padding tissue
Bone
Tendon

Figure 3.7:   Four major types of tissues in the human body (Betts *et al.*, 2013; Love, 2017). Attribution: OpenStax.

and an amorphous matrix (ground substance), is the major component of most connective tissues. The principal cell type of connective tissues is the fibroblast, a fiber-producing cell. Connective tissues are further categorized into loose, dense, and specialized.

- **Loose connective tissue:** this tissue form comprises cells with a loose fiber structure and a moderately viscous fluid matrix. It is primarily found between many organs to provide support and connect epithelial tissue to other underlying tissues.

- **Dense connective tissue:** this is also termed as dense fibrous tissue due to the predominant amount of fibers, especially type I collagen. When compared, it is much thicker and arranged irregularly. Ligaments (connect bone to bone to form joints), tendons (connect muscle to bone), and cartilage are examples of dense connective tissues.
- **Specialized connective tissue:** specialized connective tissues have various specialized cell tissues such as adipose, cartilage, bone, blood, and lymph.

3.3.2 *Epithelial tissues*

Epithelial tissues are avascular, meaning without blood vessels. They spread extensively like a large sheet of cells either as a single layer or multiple layers covering all the surfaces of the body and lines of all cavities, organs, and vessels. They are primarily responsible for a variety of functions that includes protection of the underlying tissues, secretion, regulation, and transportation of chemicals between the tissues. The shapes and sizes of epithelial cells are variable, and the cells in epithelial tissues are closely packed with a very thin intercellular matrix.

3.3.3 *Muscle tissues*

Muscle tissues are distinguished by their movement-generating properties. Muscle cells, commonly known as myocytes, are excitable which means they act in response to a stimulus. Muscle tissues are categorized into three distinct types, namely cardiac, smooth, and skeletal. The structures of native muscle tissues are shown in Figure 3.8. Each type of muscle tissue in the human body has a distinctive structure and a specialized role.

Skeletal muscle tissues occupy close to 40% of body mass and aid in the movement of bones and other hard structures. Most skeletal muscles are affixed to bones by bundles of collagen fibers known as tendons. Cardiac muscle tissues, found in the heart, contract the heart to pump blood involuntarily throughout the body. The highly coordinated heart muscle contractions pump blood through the circulatory system vessels. Smooth muscle tissues, composed of sheets or strands of smooth muscle

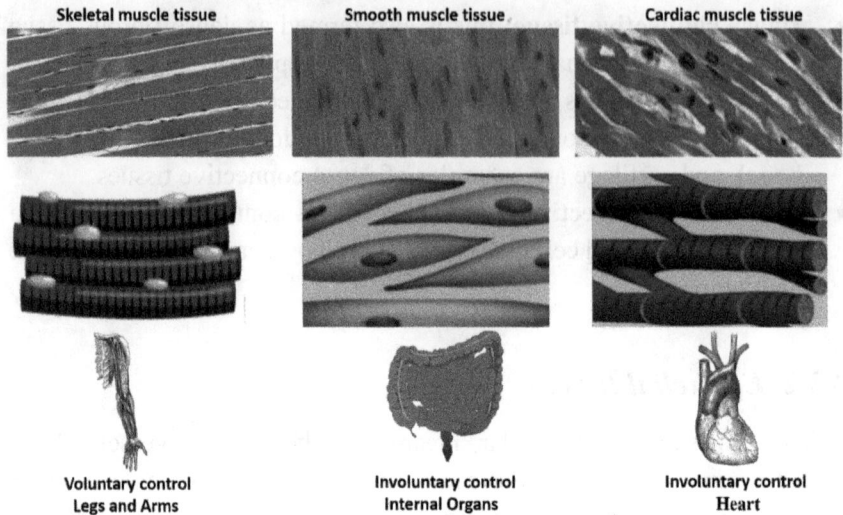

Skeletal muscle tissue	Smooth muscle tissue	Cardiac muscle tissue

Voluntary control Legs and Arms	Involuntary control Internal Organs	Involuntary control Heart

Figure 3.8:   Different kinds of muscle tissues (Betts *et al.*, 2013). Attribution: OpenStax; Author Attribution for organ images: Mikael Häggström.

cells, are generally located in the walls of hollow organs such as the esophagus, small intestine, colon (large intestine), and stomach.

3.3.4 *Nervous tissues*

Nervous tissues, also called neural tissues, are found in the central nervous system (brain and spinal cord) and the peripheral nervous system (peripheral nerves and ganglia). They receive stimuli, conduct impulses, regulate the body's movements, and control many body activities. Integration and communication are the two major functions of nervous tissues. They are composed of two principal types of cells, neurons and glial cells. Neurons are the structural and functional unit of the nervous system, which are *"conducting"* cells that transmit electrochemical impulses called action potentials. As presented in Figure 1.12, neurons display distinctive morphology, which consist of a cell body, dendrites, and axons. The specifics about the brain and neurons are discussed in detail in Chapter 1. The other type, glial cell or neuroglia, is a non-conducting cell which provides a supportive and protective system for neurons.

Key points

Tissues
- Tissues consist of cells with comparable structure and function grouped to form an organ.
- The four basic tissue types are epithelial, muscle, connective, and nervous.
- Connective tissues give shape and hold everything in place. Muscle tissues produce force and generate motion.
- Nervous tissues form the communication network. Epithelial tissues cover the external parts of organs.

3.4 Multiple choice questions

1. Which of the following is TRUE?
   (a) collagen fibers in the ECM have higher Young's modulus than elastin
   (b) collagen is protein fiber found in the minimum amount throughout our body
   (c) fibrin is responsible for strength and cushioning in the human body
   (d) collagen is arranged as simple bundles and has a limited length

2. Which of the following is NOT true?
   (a) ECM is a molecule network composed of various proteins, glycosaminoglycan, and glycoconjugate
   (b) ECM is a structural scaffold that aids in enhancing cellular properties
   (c) ECM is as it is, does not undergo any remodeling
   (d) ECM controls communication between cells

3. Which of the following tissues cannot be formed from embryonic stem cells?
   (a) connective tissue
   (b) epithelial tissue
   (c) endodermal tissue
   (d) none of the above

4. What is the least invasive source of stem cells from the human body?
   (a) adipose tissue
   (b) bone marrow
   (c) umbilical cord blood
   (d) liver

5. A stem cell has the ability to
   I. produce daughter cells that are an exact replica of itself
   II. develop only into certain cell types
   III. produce daughter cells that are dedicated to differentiation
   IV. develop into many cell types
      (a) only I and II
      (b) only I and III
      (c) only I, III and IV
      (d) none of the above

6. Which of the following proteins are abundant in the ECM, and which of the cells do not reside in the ECM?
   (a) actin; mesenchymal stem cells
   (b) elastin; fibroblasts
   (c) collagen; hepatocytes
   (d) laminin; adipose cells

7. Which of the following is/are TRUE about integrins?
   I. integrins are the principal receptors
   II. integrins regulate the interaction between a cell and its microenvironment to control cell fate
      (a) only I
      (b) all of the above
      (c) none of the above
      (d) only II

8. In a developing embryo, stem cells differentiate into
   (a) ectoderm
   (b) endoderm
   (c) mesoderm
   (d) all of the above
   (e) none of the above

9. What is the role of adult stem cells in the human body?
   (a) always offer the source of cells for diagnosing diseases
   (b) play a role as a repair system for the body
   (c) regulate the functioning of an organ
   (d) all of the above

10. Which of the following is correct for ESCs?
    (a) they are multipotent
    (b) they are already differentiated inner mass cells of a human embryo
    (c) they have the potential for self-renewal
    (d) they have the ability to become any type of cell in the body

11. Which of the following is NOT true regarding growth factors?
    (a) growth factors are naturally occurring substances and can also be produced by genetic engineering
    (b) growth factors typically act as signaling molecules between cells
    (c) cytokines and hormones are growth factors
    (d) growth factors do not have binding capacity

12. Which adult cells can be transformed into iPSs cells?
    (a) bone cells
    (b) nerve cells
    (c) no cells can convert themselves into iPS cells
    (d) any adult cell which has a capability of dividing

13. Which of the following techniques is facing bioethical issues?
    (a) embryonic stem cell therapy
    (b) cell therapy
    (c) DNA microarray
    (d) all of the above

14. Which term describes grafts from other humans?
    (a) allografts
    (b) allogeneic
    (c) xenogeneic
    (d) none of the above

References & Further Reading

Abou-Saleh, H., Zouein, F. A., El-Yazbi, A., Sanoudou, D., *et al.* (2018). The march of pluripotent stem cells in cardiovascular regenerative medicine. *Stem Cell Research & Therapy, 9*(1), 201. doi:10.1186/s13287-018-0947-5.

Amini Mahabadi, J., Sabzalipoor, H., Kehtari, M., Enderami, S. E., *et al.* (2018). Derivation of male germ cells from induced pluripotent stem cells by inducers: A review. *Cytotherapy, 20*(3), 279–290. doi:10.1016/j.jcyt.2018.01.002.

Asal, M., & Güven, S. (2020). Chapter 7 — Stem cells: Sources, properties, and cell types. In N. E. Vrana, H. Knopf-Marques, & J. Barthes (Eds.), *Biomaterials for Organ and Tissue Regeneration* (pp. 177–196): Woodhead Publishing.

Belleghem, S. M. V., Mahadik, B., Snodderly, K. L., & Fisher, J. P. (2020). Chapter 2.6.2 — Overview of Tissue Engineering Concepts and Applications. In W. R. Wagner, S. E. Sakiyama-Elbert, G. Zhang, & M. J. Yaszemski (Eds.), *Biomaterials Science (Fourth Edition)* (pp. 1289–1316): Academic Press.

Betts, J. G., Young, K. A., Wise, J. A., Johnson, E., *et al.* (2013). *Anatomy and Physiology*: OpenStax.

Cakir, O. O., Fabio, C., & Edoardo, P. (2020). Chapter 16 — Stem cell and future treatments. In G. I. Russo & A. Cocci (Eds.), *Peyronie's Disease: Pathophysiology and Treatment* (pp. 247–255): Academic Press.

Carlson, B. M. (2019). Chapter 2 — Tissues. In B. M. Carlson (Ed.), *The Human Body* (pp. 27–63): Academic Press.

Fournier, H. (2019). Cellular differentiation. *Wikimedia Commons, Creative Commons Attribution-Share Alike 4.0 International license.*

Jones, M. (2006). The source of pluripotent stems cells from developing embryos. *Wikimedia Commons, Creative Commons Attribution-Share Alike 2.5 Generic license.*

Khademhosseini, A., Ashammakhi, N., Karp, J. M., Gerecht, S., *et al.* (2020). Chapter 27 — Embryonic stem cells as a cell source for tissue engineering. In R. Lanza, R. Langer, J. P. Vacanti, & A. Atala (Eds.), *Principles of Tissue Engineering (Fifth Edition)* (pp. 467–490): Academic Press.

Khan, I., Neumann, C., & Sinha, M. (2020). Chapter 24 — Tissue regeneration and reprogramming. In D. Bagchi, A. Das, & S. Roy (Eds.), *Wound Healing, Tissue Repair, and Regeneration in Diabetes* (pp. 515–534): Academic Press.

Kim, K., Grainger, D. W., & Okano, T. (2019). Utah's cell sheet tissue engineering center. *Regenerative Therapy, 11*, 2-4. doi:10.1016/j.reth.2019.03.003.

Love, B. (2017). Chapter 4 — Connective and Soft Tissues. In B. Love (Ed.), *Biomaterials* (pp. 67–95): Academic Press.

Tatullo, M., Gargiulo, I. C., Dipalma, G., Ballini, A*., et al.* (2020). Chapter 17 — Stem cells and regenerative medicine. In S. T. Sonis & A. Villa (Eds.), *Translational Systems Medicine and Oral Disease* (pp. 387–407): Academic Press.

Wong, E. V. (2009). *Cells — Molecules and Mechanisms*: Axolotl Academica Publishing.

Zedalis, J., & Eggebrecht, J. (2018). Biology for AP® Courses: OpenStax.

Chapter 4
Biomaterials: Basic principles

4.1 Introduction

Human tissues and organs sometimes fail to perform their regular actions due to genetic defects, age, illness, trauma, degeneration, or injuries. Some of these conditions are handled with the use of day-to-day medication, i.e., drugs. However, some cannot be repaired/rectified by providing medicines and require the use of unique materials and devices. These then bring about the inevitability of surgical repair, which encompasses anatomical sections such as knee joints, elbow joints, vertebrae, teeth, and other crucial organs such as heart, skin, kidney, etc. In the broadest sense, the unique materials (other than drugs) or combinations of materials that are primarily expected to be used inside a mammal or human to treat, repair, augment or replace any tissue is referred to as biomaterials. These biomaterials can either be formed from nature or physically manufactured by utilizing a wide range of physical and chemical methods.

The field of biomaterials is multidisciplinary (Figure 4.1). The design of a simple biomaterial (for example, a bone screw or bone plate) necessitates knowledge and ideas from multiple disciplines. It needs the synergistic integration of materials, biology, medicine, mechanical sciences, and chemistry. The number of medical devices used annually by humans is significant, estimated at 1.5 million by the World Health Organization, with around 10,000 forms of standardized device classes available worldwide.

The term *"biomaterials"* is often described as any material that comes into contact with humans or animals to fulfil their intended function without causing any toxic reaction. This is the single most crucial aspect that differentiates a biomaterial from any other material, i.e., its capacity to be in

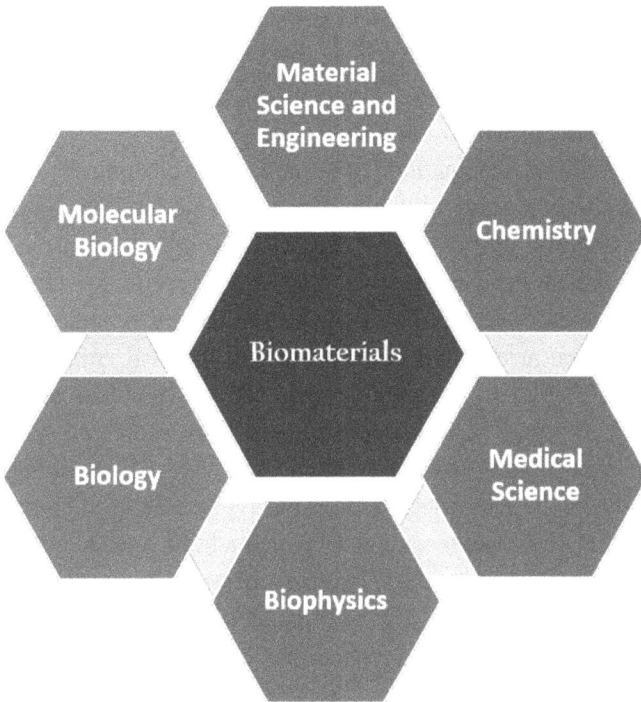

Figure 4.1: Interdisciplinary system of biomaterials (Cooke *et al.*, 1996; Marin *et al.*, 2020; Ramakrishna *et al.*, 2010; Ratner, 1996).

contact with human body tissues without instigating an undesirable degree of response. For thousands of years, humans have inevitably used or at least attempted to use materials to make devices and instruments of practical value by converting basic available substances into materials. Biomaterials have a long history of medical use, and at various times they were seen in a different way. Based on the development and its uses, the broad definition has evolved over the years and could be further expanded as new applications in medicine emerge. Nevertheless, the meaning of biomaterials attained a harmony of opinion by scientists worldwide and is now defined now as "*a material designed to take a form that can direct, through interactions with living systems, the course of any therapeutic or diagnostic procedure.*" In most cases, a biomaterial is any natural or synthetic *biocompatible* material that is used to replace or assist part of an organ or a tissue while maintaining close contact with living tissue. They may be produced from materials including solid, liquid, and gel substances (metallic components, polymers, ceramics or composite materials). It should be noted that the *bio* prefix of biomaterials applies to biocompatible, rather than *biological* or *biomedical*, as many would intuitively assume.

Biomaterials, a fascinating and highly interdisciplinary area, have grown to become an integral component in the modern-day improvement of human condition and quality of life. It is accomplished by addressing numerous health-related issues that come from several sources. Over the past few decades, biomaterials have broadened their applications from diagnostics (gene arrays and biosensors) and medical equipment (blood bags, surgical tools) to therapeutic medications (medical implants and devices) and emerging regenerative drugs (tissue-engineered skin and cartilage), and more. Many uses of synthetic and naturally occurring medicinal materials can be classified by their place and role in the human body: skeletal system (joint replacements, bone fractures and defects, artificial tendons and ligaments, dental implants), cardiovascular system (blood vessel prosthesis, heart valves), organs (artificial heart, skin repair), etc. The vital applications are presented in Figure 4.2 and tabulated in Table 4.1.

Impact of Biomaterials

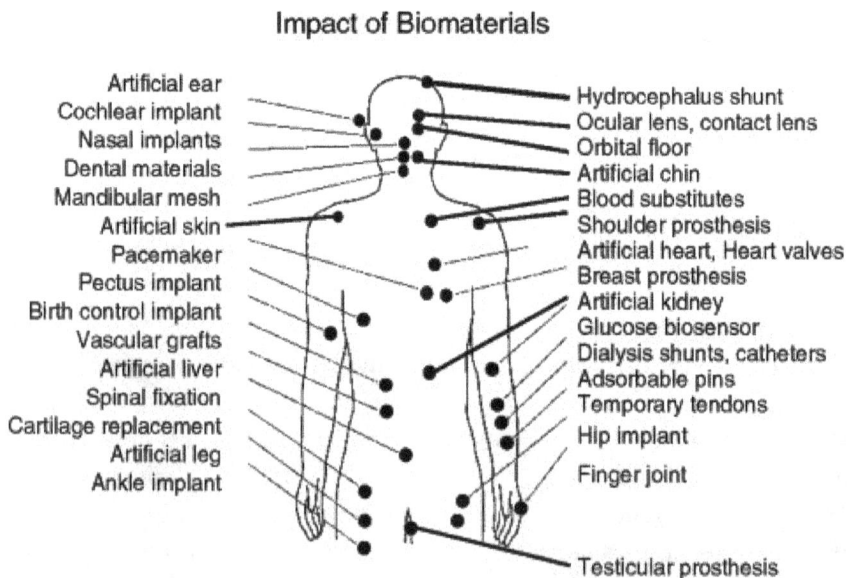

Artificial ear	Hydrocephalus shunt
Cochlear implant	Ocular lens, contact lens
Nasal implants	Orbital floor
Dental materials	Artificial chin
Mandibular mesh	Blood substitutes
Artificial skin	Shoulder prosthesis
Pacemaker	Artificial heart, Heart valves
Pectus implant	Breast prosthesis
Birth control implant	Artificial kidney
Vascular grafts	Glucose biosensor
Artificial liver	Dialysis shunts, catheters
Spinal fixation	Adsorbable pins
Cartilage replacement	Temporary tendons
Artificial leg	Hip implant
Ankle implant	Finger joint
	Testicular prosthesis

Figure 4.2: Biomaterials have made an enormous impact on the treatment of injury and disease and are used throughout the body (Cooke *et al.*, 1996; Kuhn, 2005; Ratner *et al.*, 2020).

Table 4.1: Applications of biomaterials.

Organ/Tissue	Examples
Heart	Biventricular pacemakers, artificial valves, artificial heart
Eye	Contact lens, artificial intraocular lens
Ear	Hair-clip artificial stapes, cochlear implants
Muscle	Sutures
Kidney	Dialysis machines
Skin	Skin wound repair, burn dressings, skin substitutes, artificial skin
Circulation	Synthetic blood vessels
Bone	Bone screws, plates, pins, intramedullary rods, bone cement to repair defects
Teeth	Fillings and replacements

4.2 Desired properties of biomaterials

As discussed earlier, the ultimate goal of biomaterials in medicine is to treat, improve, or substitute tissue organs (e.g., bone, muscle, skin) or body function. Such goals can be accomplished by integrating the properties of materials, nature of the system, device architecture, and physiological specifications. The biomaterial application method must combine the chemical and mechanical features of the biological system in order to achieve the required functional results (Figure 4.3). For the processing of biomaterials and related medical items, different elements from science and social parameters are also considered.

4.2.1 *Biocompatibility*

From a biological point of view, biocompatibility is nothing but the acceptability of non-living materials (synthetic or natural) in a living body (mammal/human). This acceptance is broadly defined as the *"ability of a material to perform its desired functions with respect to a medical therapy, to induce an appropriate host response in a specific application and to interact with living systems without having any risk of injury, toxicity, or rejection by the immune system and undesirable or inappropriate local or systemic effects"*. Since a biomaterial is intended to be used in intimate contact with living tissues, it is important that the implanted material does

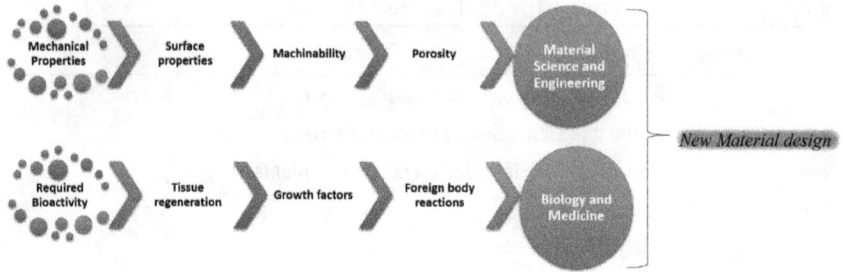

Figure 4.3: Primary requirements of new material design.

not cause any undesired reactions to the surrounding tissues and host organs. Apart from that, the implanted material is expected not to subdue the activity of normal cells or provoke any unwanted local or systemic reactions in the recipient, but is encouraged to generate positive cellular or tissue response.

Usually, the criteria for this biocompatibility are dynamic and detailed and differ with individual specific medical applications. For example, a specially designed material (screw or plate) may possibly be biocompatible in bone implant surgery, but the same components may not be biocompatible in skin applications.

4.2.2 *Host response*

Host response is defined as the *"response of the host organism (local and systemic) to the implanted material or device"*. Most of the materials are never inert, and a biomaterial's clinical success depends significantly on the host tissue's reaction with the foreign material. For material establishment-host tissue interaction, these reactions depend heavily on the time-length, purpose, and site of implantation.

4.2.3 *Non-toxicity*

Toxicity of biomaterials deals with elements that migrate out of the biomaterials. A carefully designed biomaterial should serve its purpose in the living body's environment without negatively influencing other cells, organs, or the whole organism. It is logical to assume that, unless specifically designed to do so, a biomaterial should not release or generate anything from its bulk.

4.2.4 *Mechanical properties*

In addition to biocompatibility, mechanical properties are embedded in biomaterial design prior to implementation and will majorly contribute to the outcome. Materials undergo several forces which are primarily stress, strain, shear, and a mixture of these. The tensile strength, yield strength, elastic modulus, corrosion, creep, and hardness are some of the most important properties of biomaterials that should be carefully studied and evaluated before implantation. For hard tissue applications, the mechanical properties are of top priority.

4.2.5 *Corrosion, wear, and fatigue properties*

Wear is often considered as one of the leading causes of implant failure. In some cases, wear has also been shown to accelerate the corrosion of biomedical devices and implants. The fatigue resistance is related to the material's reaction to repeated cyclic loads.

4.2.6 *Design and manufacturability*

Appropriate material design is also one of the critical factors to consider for biomaterials. For example, in the early 1900s, bone plates were utilized to assist in fixing long bone fractures. Many of these experimental plates broke because of their primitive mechanical design where they were too narrow and had a stress-focusing corner. Manufacturability is the ability to manufacture the item with relative ease that is ideal for its intended use at minimal cost and high reliability. Concerning biomaterials, the manufacturability, in a broader sense, incorporates the potential of the material to be sterilized by a validated sterilization technique which is deemed appropriate for biomedical applications. The material is expected to not get impaired by standard sterilizing techniques such as autoclaving, dry heat, radiation, ethylene oxide, etc. (see Chapter 8 for more details).

In summary, for any material to qualify as a biomaterial, it should

- Be biocompatible, i.e., non-toxic, non-carcinogenic, non-allergenic, etc.
- Have required/suitable physical and chemical properties
- Have suitable mechanical properties
- Have stable durability for the period it is intended for, i.e., hours to years
- Be easy to process with the available techniques
- Be sterilizable with current facilities without any difficulty
- Be cost-effective and accessible

4.3 Types of biomaterials

Depending on the chemical bonding, materials can be categorized into three broad groups. These are (i) polymers, (ii) ceramics, and (iii) metals. Because these material structures vary by their nature of bonding (covalent, ionic or metallic), they have different properties, and hence different uses in the body (Table 4.2). Different kinds of biomaterials and chemical bonds associated with it are shown in Figure 4.4. Metals and ceramics are differentiated in the field of materials engineering, although they are both

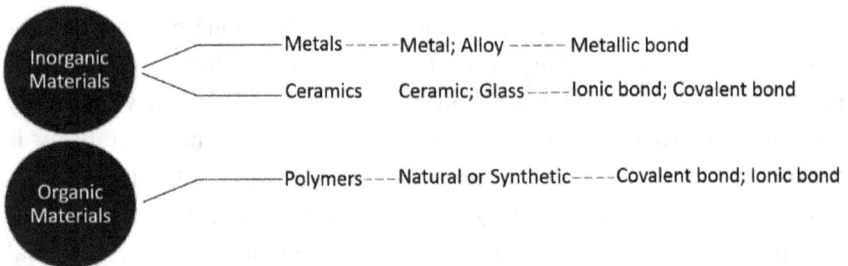

Figure 4.4:   Different kinds of biomaterials and chemical bonds associated with them (Gul *et al.*, 2020; He *et al.*, 2017; Zindani *et al.*, 2019).

Table 4.2: Classification of biomaterials and typical properties associated with them (Wagner, 2020).

Attributes	Polymers	Metals & Alloys	Ceramics
Type of bonds present	Covalent & van der Waals forces	Metallic	Ionic/Covalent
Melting point	Low	Intermediate	High
Chemical stability	Poor	Good	Very high
Electrical conductivity	Very low	High	Very low, but varies
Thermal conductivity	Very low to intermediate	High	Low
Properties and advantages	Degradable, inert, similar density to soft tissues and ease of processing	High strength and hardness	Non-conductive and inert; closely mimic biological properties of bone
Mechanical deformation	Very high, plastic (can be easily shaped and processed)	High (ductile)	Low (brittle)
Major issues	Thermally unstable; low strength	Wear and corrosion	High density and brittle
Biomedical applications	Soft tissue implants; drug delivery systems; tissue engineering	Hard tissue applications (Orthopedic and dental implants)	Tissue engineering

inorganic compounds. Each material has its own benefits and drawbacks, and its biomedical applications are decided according to its individual properties and intended place substitution.

4.3.1 *Metals*

Metals are the most widely known biomedical materials and are indispensable in the medical field. Nearly all of the metal biomaterials are crystalline in nature, i.e., with regular atomic arrangements. Metals have great strength, resistance to fracture toughness, better elasticity, and rigidity compared with ceramics and polymers. Their outstanding mechanical reliability properties are controlled by dislocation and crystallization. For this reason, metals are extensively employed for load-bearing implant applications such as orthopaedic, dental, and maxillofacial surgery. Apart from these, metals are also used in making stents and stent-grafts for cardiovascular surgeries. The most common metals and alloys used for biomedical applications are stainless steel, titanium, titanium-based alloys, cobalt-based alloys, magnesium-based alloys, and tantalum-based alloys.

4.3.2 Ceramics

Ceramics are inorganic solid materials consisting of metallic and non-metallic elements that are predominantly bound together by ionic bonds. They exist as both crystalline and non-crystalline (amorphous) compounds. Ceramics are typically characterized by excellent biocompatibility, high corrosion resistance, high wear, high strength, extremely high stiffness, and hardness. The advancement of ceramic material applications in the biomedical industry has focused mostly on orthopaedics and dentistry. Bioinert ceramics such as alumina (Al_2O_3), zirconia (Zr_2O_3) and pyrolytic carbon, and bioresorbable ceramics such as calcium phosphates are some of the widely employed bioceramics.

4.3.3 Polymers

Polymers are macromolecules and they represent a major and versatile class of biomaterials being widely applied in biomedical applications due to their low toxicity in biological fluids, easy pre/post-processing, sterilization, better shelf life, lightweight nature, and remarkable physical and chemical properties.

Biomaterial use is primarily dependent on the need, function, and environment of the intended application. In a variety of implants, metal, polymers, ceramics, and composites are being used. The specific material or material combinations for use in a device will significantly affect both its patient performance and marketing potential. The next three chapters will discuss in detail each of the material types.

4.4 Multiple choice questions

1. Biomaterials
   (a) are always synthetic materials; natural materials are not employed
   (b) are always natural materials; synthetic materials are not employed
   (c) can be natural or synthetic materials
   (d) are always polymeric materials

2. Select the statement which correctly relates to biocompatibility.
   (a) a biocompatible material should provide healing characters
   (b) a biocompatible material should have therapeutic characteristics
   (c) a material is considered as a biocompatible material as long as it causes no harm to the host body
   (d) a biocompatible material should have the exact dimensions as the damaged tissue or part

3. Select the option(s) which do(es) NOT come under the class of biocompatible materials.
   (a) eyeglasses; wheelchair
   (b) contact lenses; dental implants
   (c) orthopedic implant; stents
   (d) external hip prosthesis; massage footwear

4. Which of the following has the best osteointegration properties?
   (a) SS316
   (b) porous titanium
   (c) Co-Cr alloys
   (d) all of the above

5. Which of the following is/are biomaterial(s)?
   I. materials used for tooth filling
   II. materials used for cardiovascular repairs
   III. glucose meters and stethoscopes
   IV. materials used for hip implants
      (a) only I
      (b) only I, II and IV
      (c) only I, III and IV
      (d) only III

6. Select the option(s) which is/are TRUE about biodegradation.
    (a) it depends on the molecular architecture
    (b) it is a precise breakdown of the material over time
    (c) metals biodegrade faster than polymeric materials
    (d) all of the above

7. Which class of biomaterials has chemical structures similar to bone?
    (a) polymeric biomaterials
    (b) ceramic biomaterials
    (c) metallic biomaterials
    (d) all of the above

8. Which class of biomaterials encourages bonding with surrounding tissues and stimulates new bone growth?
    (a) bioinert ceramics
    (b) bioactive ceramics
    (c) Co-Cr alloys
    (d) all of the above

9. Which of the following is TRUE?
    (a) ceramics possess excellent wear and friction properties
    (b) SS316, Co-Cr and Ti alloys form a protective oxide layer on their surfaces
    (c) bioceramics are more reactive then certain metallic implants
    (d) all of the above

References & Further Reading

Cooke, F. W., Lemons, J. E., & Ratner, B. D. (1996). Chapter 1 — Properties of Materials. In B. D. Ratner, A. S. Hoffman, F. J. Schoen, & J. E. Lemons (Eds.), *Biomaterials Science* (pp. 11–35): Academic Press.

Ghasemi-Mobarakeh, L., Kolahreez, D., Ramakrishna, S., & Williams, D. (2019). Key terminology in biomaterials and biocompatibility. *Current Opinion in Biomedical Engineering, 10*, 45–50. doi:10.1016/j.cobme.2019.02.004.

Gul, H., Khan, M., & Khan, A. S. (2020). Chapter 3 — Bioceramics: Types and clinical applications. In A. S. Khan & A. A. Chaudhry (Eds.), *Handbook of Ionic Substituted Hydroxyapatites* (pp. 53–83): Woodhead Publishing.

He, W., & Benson, R. (2017). Chapter 8 — Polymeric Biomaterials. In M. Kutz (Ed.), *Applied Plastics Engineering Handbook (Second Edition)* (pp. 145–164): William Andrew Publishing.

Kuhn, L. T. (2005). Chapter 6 — Biomaterials. In J. D. Enderle, S. M. Blanchard, & J. D. Bronzino (Eds.), *Introduction to Biomedical Engineering (Second Edition)* (pp. 255–312): Academic Press.

Marin, E., Boschetto, F., & Pezzotti, G. (2020). Biomaterials and biocompatibility: A historical overview. *Journal of Biomedical Materials Research Part A, 108*(8), 1617–1633. doi:10.1002/jbm.a.36930.

Ramakrishna, S., Ramalingam, M., Kumar, T. S. S., & Soboyejo, W. O. (2010). *Biomaterials: A Nano Approach*: CRC Press Taylor & Francis.

Ratner, B. D. (1996). Biomaterials Science: An Interdisciplinary Endeavor. In B. D. Ratner, A. S. Hoffman, F. J. Schoen, & J. E. Lemons (Eds.), *Biomaterials Science* (pp. 1–8): Academic Press.

Ratner, B. D., & Zhang, G. (2020). Chapter 1.1.2 — A History of Biomaterials. In W. R. Wagner, S. E. Sakiyama-Elbert, G. Zhang, & M. J. Yaszemski (Eds.), *Biomaterials Science (Fourth Edition)* (pp. 21–34): Academic Press.

Wagner, W. R. (2020). Chapter 1.3.1 — The Materials Side of the Biomaterials Relationship. In W. R. Wagner, S. E. Sakiyama-Elbert, G. Zhang, & M. J. Yaszemski (Eds.), *Biomaterials Science (Fourth Edition)* (pp. 83–84): Academic Press.

Zindani, D., Kumar, K., & Paulo Davim, J. (2019). Chapter 4 — Metallic biomaterials — A review. In J. P. Davim (Ed.), *Mechanical Behaviour of Biomaterials* (pp. 83–99): Woodhead Publishing.

Chapter 5
Polymeric biomaterials

5.1 Polymers

Polymers or plastics are everywhere and touch almost every aspect of modern life, be it water bottles, grocery bags, soda cans, food packaging materials, toys or phones. The phrases polymer and polymeric material comprise very broad groups of natural and synthetic, organic (mostly) and inorganic with an exceptional variety of properties. The simplest definition of a polymer is a large three-dimensional or two-dimensional network of long, repeating chemically linked molecular chains. Such units consist primarily of hydrocarbons (carbon and hydrogen) and, occasionally, oxygen, nitrogen, sulfur, chlorine, fluorine, as well as phosphorous and silicon. Based on the attachment of other molecules, polymers may possess exceptional properties for applications such as solution casting, injection molding, melt molding, or machining.

To appreciate and understand polymers, it is crucial to know about the term *monomer* first. A monomer is a low molecular weight single molecule capable of connecting to at least two other monomers. The process of joining together monomer molecules of the same or different type through a chemical reaction is known as polymerization. There are four essential structures of polymers that appear in Figure 5.1. However, in reality some polymers can contain a mixture of different fundamental structures. These polymeric materials are formed via polymerization and polycondensation processes and can be linear, branched, networked, or cross-linked.

- **Linear polymers:** Linear polymers are polymers in which monomeric units are linked together in a long continuous chain of carbon-carbon bonds. These polymers often experience a high melting point,

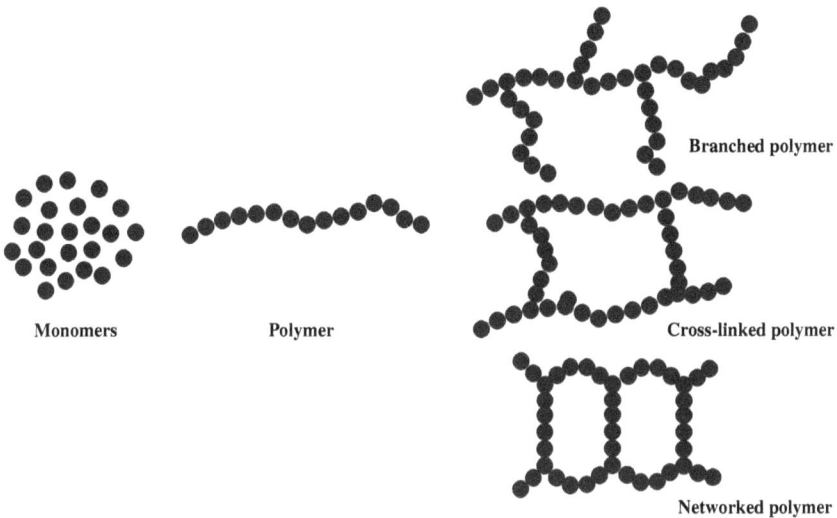

Figure 5.1: Skeletal structures of polymers: linear, branched, cross-linked, and networked.

density, and tensile strength due to the high magnitude of intermo-lecular forces of attraction arising from close packing of the chains. Examples include polyethylene, Teflon, nylons, polyesters, and polystyrene.

- **Branched polymers:** Branched polymers have secondary polymer chains or branches that are the same repeating units linked to a primary backbone. These polymers often have low melting/boiling point, low density, and low tensile strength due to lower packing efficiency of the branched chains. Some example includes low-density polyethylene, starch, and glycogen.

- **Crosslinked polymers:** Cross-linking refers to the joining of polymer chains with covalent bonds. Compared to the same polymers without cross-linking, cross-linked polymers have high rigidity, hardness, and a higher melting point. Some elastomers, binders, and hydrogels are loosely cross-linked polymers.

- **Networked polymers:** Networked polymers are heavily complex polymers that are chemically cross-linked to form a network of three-dimensional linkages.

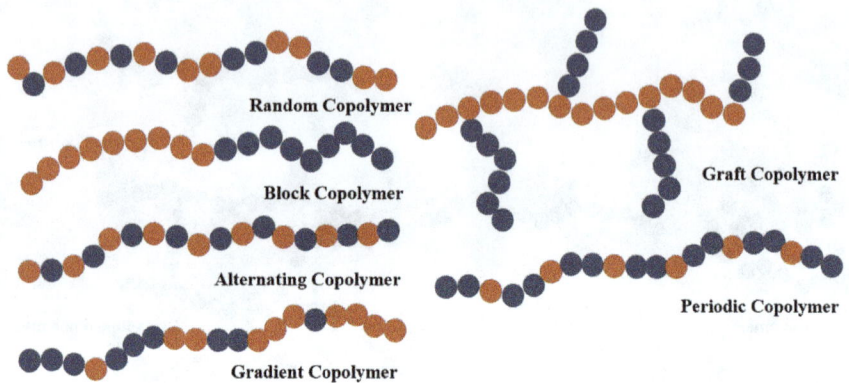

Figure 5.2:   Overview of various forms of copolymers.

Copolymers are made up of two or more types of monomers. Examples include polyethylene-vinyl acetate (PEVA), nitrile rubber, and acrylonitrile butadiene styrene (ABS). Copolymers are categorized based on the way the two different monomers are arranged along the polymer chain, namely random, block, alternating, periodic, and graft. The schematic of such copolymers is shown in Figure 5.2.

- **Random copolymers:** monomers are randomly arranged
- **Alternate copolymers:** monomers are arranged alternately
- **Block copolymers:** two different polymers linked together
- **Periodic copolymers:** monomers are arranged in a repeating sequence
- **Graft copolymers:** host polymer is made up of one type of monomer, and side chains another type

5.2 Molecular weight

Polymer molecular weight defines a variety of physical properties including mechanical (tensile strength, toughness), thermal (melting point, boiling point), and chemical (chemical resistance). Above-average molecular weights are generally linked with superior physical properties, whereas lower molecular weights are related to poorer properties. Unlike small molecules or other elements, polymers are typically a mixture of differently sized monomers. Therefore usually, polymers do not have a single value for molecular weight, and only an average can be defined. There are several ways to measure the average molecular weight of a polymer, such as size exclusion chromatography, light scattering measurements, and viscosity measurements. Weight average molecular weight (M_w), number average molecular weight (M_n), and viscosity average molecular weight (M_v) are the three ways to define a polymer's average molecular weight.

a. Number average molecular weight (M_n)

M_n is defined as the total weight of all chains in a polymer divided by the total number of molecular chains. It does not take the shape or size of a single molecule into account and considers all molecules equally.

$$\langle M_n \rangle = \frac{\sum n_i M_i}{\sum n_i}$$

b. Weight average molecular weight (M_w)

Unlike M_n, M_w is a little more complex to determine as it accounts for the molecular size rather than simply the numbers. M_w is based on the fact that a larger molecule contributes more weight to the polymer sample than the smaller molecules. It is important to note that M_w depends not only on the number of molecules present but also on each molecule's weight. M_w is always greater than M_n (Figure 5.3).

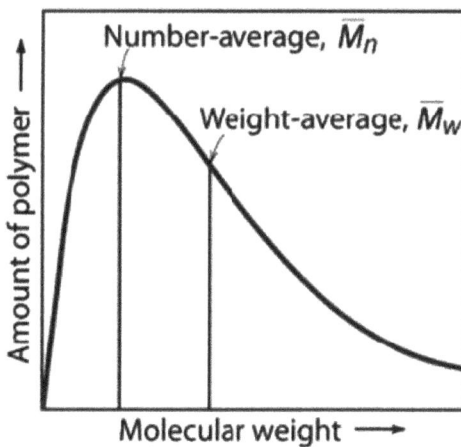

Figure 5.3: Molecular weights M_n and M_w distribution.

$$\langle M_w \rangle = \frac{\sum w_i M_i}{\sum w_i} = \frac{\sum n_i M_i^2}{\sum n_i M_i}$$

w_i is the weight fraction of polymer
M_i is the molecular weight of a chain
n_i is the number of chains of that molecular weight
i is the number of polymer molecules

c. Polydispersity index

The polydispersity index (PDI) is defined as the ratio of M_w to M_n. Based on the size, it is a measurement of heterogeneity of a sample, i.e., the broadness of molecular weight distribution within a sample is given. The greater the PDI, the broader the molecular weight. PDI value is greater than or equal to one. The value of 1 is only for monodisperse molecules, i.e., the weight of all molecules is equal.

$$PDI = \frac{\langle M_w \rangle}{\langle M_n \rangle}$$

5.3 Polymeric biomaterials

As discussed, polymers are high molecular weight molecules built from chains of repetitive units (monomers) threaded together in a sequence that are held via covalent bonds or secondary forces (van der Waals or hydrogen bonds). Polymer materials are considered for biomaterials for their versatility and biocompatibility, and in particular, for their suitable mechanical, chemical, thermal, and electrical properties. Polymeric biomaterials represent the largest use of organic and natural materials in medicine today. They are synthetic or natural materials meant to interact with biological systems for the regeneration, augmentation/repair, and treatment of any form of an organ tissue or human body function.

The important advantages of polymeric biomaterials over other classes are:

- lack of difficulty in manufacturing,
- ease of secondary processability,

- availability with required chemical, physical and mechanical properties,
- compatibility with other polymers, and
- acceptable cost structure.

Polymers are usually characterized by their thermal properties, particularly their reaction against temperature. There are two major transition temperatures for polymers: glass transition temperature (T_g) and melting point (T_m). In general, applications of amorphous polymeric biomaterials (Figure 5.4) are related to their T_g values, and T_m is generally associated with crystalline regions (Figure 5.4) of polymers (where $T_m > T_g$) (Bass *et al.*, 2020).

- **Temperature > T_g:** Polymers soften and become more stretchable and easier to deform.
- **Temperature < T_g:** Polymer chains are incapable of moving and become hard and brittle.
- **Temperature > T_m:** Polymers are in a melt liquid state.
- **Temperature < T_m:** Polymers are ordered crystalline solids.

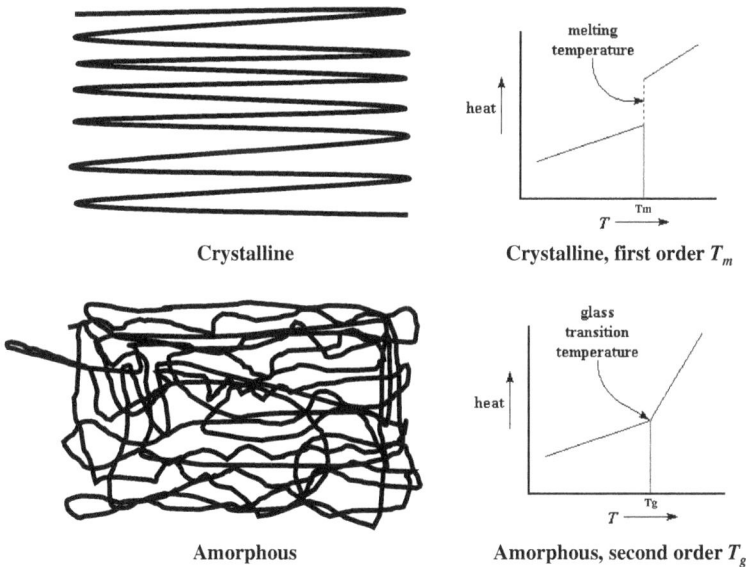

Figure 5.4:   Example of amorphous and crystalline polymeric structures, and behaviour at the glass transition temperature and melting temperature.

Thermoplastics, commonly referred to as "*plastics*", are linear or branched (not cross-linked) polymers which can become flexible or moldable above a specific temperature and return to a solid state when cooled. They can be formed or re-formed from previous forms, and can be shaped more than once. Thermoplastic polymers can also be further altered according to their density and graded into their constituents of copolymers and homopolymers. These materials are usually used as replacements for blood vessels. Thermosets, on the other hand, are intensely cross-connected rigid polymers due to their severely restricted cross-linking chain motion. These polymers do not melt but degrade on heating. What distinguishes thermoplastics from thermosets is the bonds: bonds are usually reversible in thermoplastics while irreversible in thermosets. Occasionally polymers can also be grouped according to their origin, stable chain structures, chemical properties, mechanical properties, etc. Classification of polymers based on the backbone, origin, and degradable properties is presented in Figure 5.5.

- **Response against temperature:** thermoplastics, thermosets
- **Mechanical properties:** elastomers or rubbers
- **Chemical properties:** Hydrogels
- **Origin:** Natural (plants or animals) and synthetic
- **Stability:** Biodegradable and non-biodegradable

While polymers are inherently softer compounds (compared to metals and ceramics), they have the fundamental structure-derived capacity to model biomaterials with a mechanical behavior appropriate for restorative and regenerative applications of hard and soft tissues. Even though polymers are mainly classified as thermoplastics, thermosets and elastomers, for biomedical applications degradability properties are crucial. They can thus also be classified according to their biostability, i.e., biodegradable and non-biodegradable polymers (Table 5.1).

5.3.1 *Biodegradable polymers*

Biodegradable polymers are an extensive class of polymers that contains any polymer that degrades hydrolytically and enzymatically after its

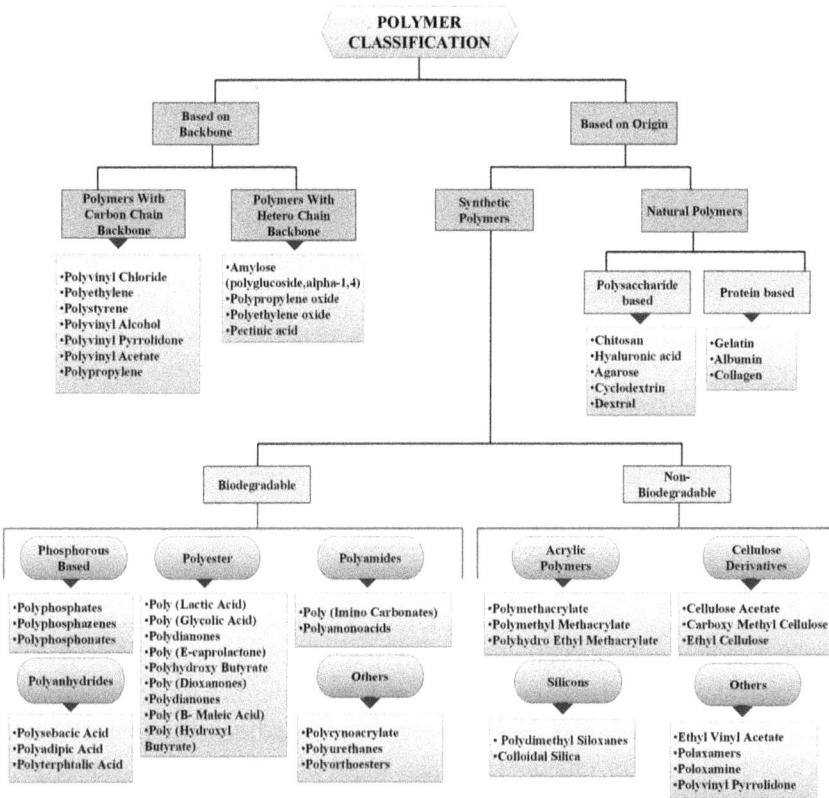

Figure 5.5: Classification of polymers based on the backbone, origin, and degradable properties (He *et al.*, 2017; Prajapati *et al.*, 2019).

Table 5.1: List of commonly used biodegradable and non-biodegradable polymers for biomedical applications.

	Polymer	Biomedical applications
Non-biodegradable polymers	Polymethyl methacrylate (PMMA)	Bone, dental cements; rigid contact lens; intraocular lens
	Polyethylene (PE)	Joint replacement devices, total hip arthroplasty
	Polyether ether ketone (PEEK)	Hard tissue engineering (partial replacement of skull)
	Polyurethane (PU)	Breast implants, catheter coatings, blood/device interfaces

(Continued)

Table 5.1:   *(Continued)*

	Polymer	Biomedical applications
	Polypropylene (PP)	Heart valve structures, surgical mesh, sutures
Biodegradable polymers	Polyglycolic acid (PGA)	Sutures; scaffolds
	Polylactic acid (PLA)	Sutures; scaffolds
	Polycaprolactone (PCL)	Coatings; drug delivery
	Polylactic-co-glycolic acid (PLGA)	Tissue engineering; wound dressing
	Polyhydroxybutyrate (PHB)	Drug delivery
	Collagen	Tissue engineering; wound dressing
	Gelatin	Membranes; tissue engineering
	Chitosan	Bone grafting; tissue engineering; wound healing

intended function over time. Biodegradable polymers are primarily categorized as natural and synthetic. Synthetic-based polymers can be manufactured under regulated conditions and have the ability to modify or adjust the material properties for certain applications by altering their molecular weight or chemistry. Since these are artificially produced in laboratories, the properties are generally anticipated and reproducible. Mechanical and physical properties such as tensile strength, elastic modulus, and degradation rate can be tailored by altering the polymer chains. Polysaccharides (starch, chitin/chitosan, hyaluronic acid derivatives, etc.), proteins (collagen, fibrin, silk, etc.), and polyesters originated/developed from plants or animals represent the family of natural biodegradable polymers. These polymers are vital to daily life as our human forms are based on them. The applications of biodegradable polymers are presented in Figure 5.7.

5.3.1.1 *Polyglycolic acid*

Polyglycolic acid (PGA), also known as polyglycolide, is an aliphatic polyester (Figure 5.6) and was one of the early degradable polymers investigated for biomedical applications (absorbable sutures). PGA, in

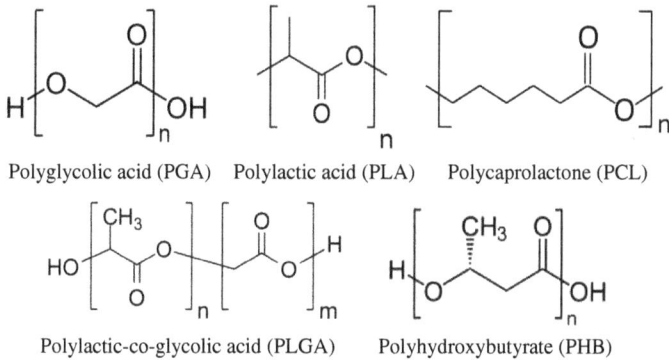

Polyglycolic acid (PGA)   Polylactic acid (PLA)   Polycaprolactone (PCL)

Polylactic-co-glycolic acid (PLGA)   Polyhydroxybutyrate (PHB)

Figure 5.6: Chemical structures of various biodegradable polymers (Balakrishnan *et al.*, 2018).

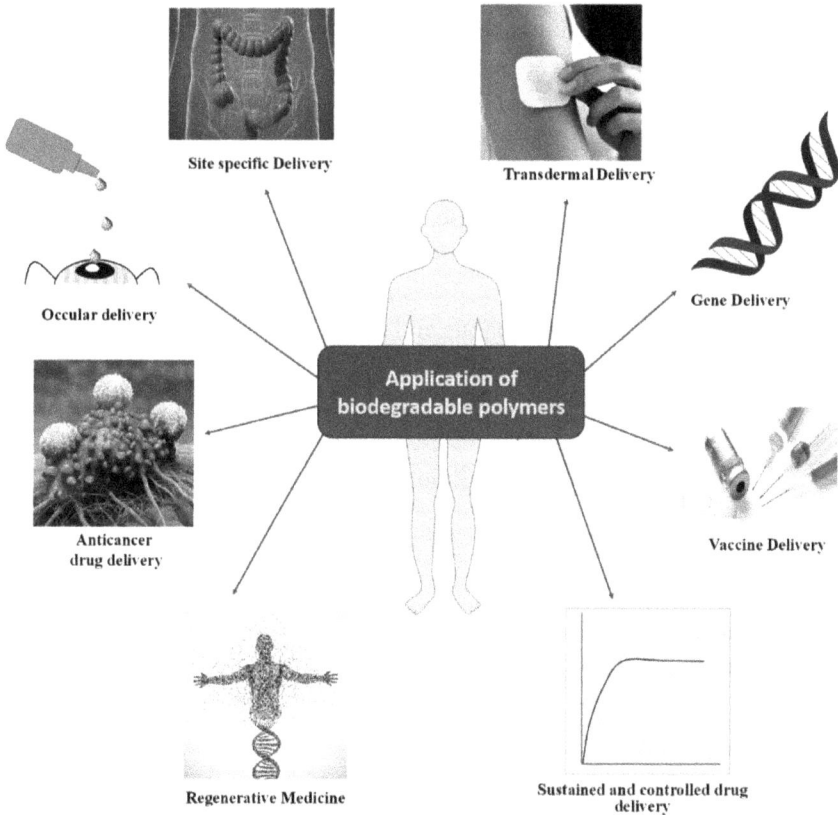

Figure 5.7: Applications of biodegradable polymers (Love, 2017; Prajapati *et al.*, 2019).

general, is a highly crystalline polymer (46–55% crystallinity) with T_m greater than 200°C, and T_g in the range of 35–40°C. The high crystallinity of PGA provides great mechanical properties (high tensile modulus) and low dissolvability in natural solvents. PGA is usually degraded by bulk hydrolysis in the body and has a resistance of about 60% at 14 days; complete absorption is completed between 60 and 90 days.

5.3.1.2 *Polylactic acid*

Polylactic acid (PLA) is one of the most essential aliphatic biodegradable thermoplastic polyesters made from renewable sources including corn starch or sugar cane. This semi-crystalline polymer has a T_m of about 174°C and a T_g of 57°C. Although similar in structure to PGA, due to the occurrence of an additional methyl group in its repeating unit (Figure 5.6), PLA demonstrates different chemical, physical, and mechanical properties. Owing to its longer resorption time and degradation via simple hydrolysis, PLA is being used in the biomedical field for various applications like wound dressings, removable prosthetic implants, bone tissue engineering, and controlled drug release systems. PLA exists in three forms: (i) L-PLA, (ii) D-PLA, and (iii) a racemic mixture of D- and L-PLA.

- ᴅ,ʟ-**PLA (PDLLA):** amorphous and low T_g; thus mostly explored used for drug delivery applications
- ʟ-**PLA (PLLA):** semi-crystalline; due to its improved mechanical properties it is explored for sutures or orthopaedic devices
- ᴅ-**PLA (PDLA):** semi-crystalline

5.3.1.3 *Polycaprolactone*

Polycaprolactone (PCL), a synthetic semi-crystalline versatile polymer (Figure 5.6), has been implemented into various biomedical research studies due to its slow degradation rate. The complete hydrolytic degradation of PCL ($M_w \sim 50,000$ Da), under physiological conditions usually takes approximately 2–3 years. It is a hydrophobic polymer with a T_m of around 60°C and a very low T_g of about –60°C. Due to the long degradation rates, tailorable degradation kinetics, high drug permeability, and processability (ease of shaping), PCL is being used mainly for long-term implantable medical devices and drug delivery systems. Furthermore, PCL is one of the very few biodegradable polymers that have been qualified as FDA-approved (Food and Drug Administration, USA) and CE-registered (European Community) for usage in a huge number of controlled drug delivery systems and long-term implantable medical devices.

5.3.1.4 *Polylactic-co-glycolic acid*

Polylactic-co-glycolic acid (PLGA or PLG), a copolymer of PLA and PGA, is one of the most successful FDA-approved biodegradable and biocompatible polymers (Figure 5.6) for sutures, wound healing, drug delivery devices, and tissue engineering scaffolds. PLGA is also largely used for preparing nanoparticles to encapsulate many biologically active compounds and for improving the therapeutic efficacy of drug delivery. In water, PLGA biodegrades by hydrolysis of its ester linkages.

5.3.1.5 *Polyhydroxybutyrate*

Bacterial polyester and its copolymers are plastic biodegradable polymers of biological origin produced by bacteria or engineered plants and have the potential to replace fossil-derived polymers. Polyhydroxybutyrate (PHB) (Figure 5.6) is such a highly crystalline polymer made by the bacteria *Bacillus megaterium*. PHB is a member of the family of polyesters known as polyhydroxyalkanoates (PHAs). It is water-insoluble and relatively resistant to hydrolytic degradation.

5.3.1.6 *Collagen*

Collagen is the human body's richest protein and the main structural component of connective tissues of bone, skin, ligament, cartilage, and tendon. It provides the fundamental structure for certain tissues, including blood vessels. Collagen is made up of specific polypeptides, namely the glycine, proline, and hydroxyproline repeating chain. At least 30 unique types of collagen have been detected so far in the human body. However, collagen types I, II, III, and IV are the most thoroughly studied ones.

- Type I collagen (~80 and 160 nm) is the most abundant fibrillar-type collagen. It builds into fibers that form the structural and mechanical scaffold of almost all connective tissues such as tendons, ligaments, and blood vessel walls. It is also a major structural protein of bones.
- Type II collagen (80 nm) is also fibrillar-type, and is present in articular cartilage and intervertebral disks. In this type of collagen, all three chains are indistinguishable.
- Type III collagen is a fibrillar-forming collagen type and a major element of the ECM. It is an important component of hollow internal organs (intestines and uterus), blood vessels, and skin. It is a major protein that attempts to repair and work in wound healing of the skin.
- Type IV is an extremely specialized form of collagen and is the major structural component of all basement membranes.

5.3.1.7 *Chitosan and Chitin*

Chitin is the most abundant biopolymer made of N-acetylglucosamine and N-glucosamine monomers. The monomer components in chitin can be either randomly allocated or block-distributed. It is mainly found in skeletal structures and outer shells of invertebrates such as arthropods, mollusks, and annelids. Nevertheless, the industrial source of chitin is found mainly in crustaceans. After cellulose, chitin is the second richest natural polymer. Its biodegradation occurs by enzymes such as lysozyme and chitinase. Both chitin/chitosan's structure strongly resembles that of cellulose, except the hydroxyl units in position two have been substituted by acetylamino groups.

Chitosan is a well-known naturally occurring linear polysaccharide, composed of a long biopolymer chain of N-acetylglucosamine. It is the second most abundant biopolymer after cellulose. The commercial forms are derived primarily from extensive deacetylation of chitin. It is a semicrystalline polymer, and the degree of crystallinity hangs on the degree of acetylation. The main difference between chitin and chitosan is the beta linkage and D-glucosamine.

5.3.2 *Non-biodegradable polymers*

5.3.2.1 *Polyethylene*

Polyethylene (PE), having the basic structure of any polymer (a repetition of CH_2 units), is the highest volume global plastic available today. PE is generally classified by its molecular weight: (i) low-density polyethylene (LDPE), (ii) high-density polyethylene (HDPE), and (iii) Ultrahigh-molecular-weight polyethylene (UHMWPE), which could be used according to their properties in different applications.

- **LDPE:** The most common PE type is LDPE, which was first developed in the presence of catalysts through the reaction of ethylene gas under high pressure (100–300 MPa).
- **HDPE:** this is a linear polymer with a molecular weight of up to 0.2×10^6 g/mol and is used mainly for bone and cartilage substitutes.
- **UHMWPE:** It is a linear polyethylene form with an extremely high molecular weight, usually between 3×10^6 g/mol and 6×10^6 g/mol. These values are opposed to 20,000 and 300,000 for standard polyethylene LDPE and HDPE, respectively. In addition to biocompatibility, UHMWPE has many desirable mechanical properties, including high resistance to abrasion, low friction, exceptional machinability, and quick processing. These properties make it especially suitable for use in the manufacture of bearing surfaces in arthroplasties. UHMWPE is extensively used in orthopedic total joint implants. It is also the only material currently used to produce the acetabular cup liner in total hip arthroplasties, and the tibial insert and patellar portion in total knee arthroplasties. The issue associated with using UHMWPE is the wear debris, which will cause a variety of undesirable effects.

5.3.2.2 *Polyurethanes*

Polyurethanes and poly(ether-urethanes) are the most flexible and commonly recognized polymers in biomedical applications. Polyurethanes are especially used as blood-contacting material in cardiovascular devices, catheters, heart valves, and artificial blood vessels. They are considered the most significant biocompatible polymer with remarkable mechanical properties such as durability, elasticity, fatigue resistance, and compliance. However, polyurethanes are vulnerable to bacterial colonization and have a higher risk of infection.

5.3.2.3 *Polymethyl methacrylate*

Polymethyl methacrylate or PMMA is an essential material in medicine and dentistry. PMMA is a hard, inflexible, glassy but brittle polymer with a T_g of about 100°C. It is famously known by many different names, including the commercial name Plexiglas® and acrylic resin. Interestingly PMMA has both thermoplastic and thermosetting polymer plastic properties, depending upon the form in which it is used. Due to these properties, PMMA is extensively used in ocular implants, contact lenses, bone cements, and tooth replicates.

Polymeric biomaterials and tissue engineering scaffolds as structural templates with specific morphologies play a crucial role in addressing many critical issues in biomedical engineering. When combined with ceramic derivatives, known as composites or hybrid materials, polymers have become known as viable alternatives for many tissue engineering applications. The development of appropriate polymeric materials for tissue engineering scaffolds is the focus of continuing discovery and innovation. In view of this, many research efforts are dedicated to developing materials with biodegradable polymers and bioactive ceramics such as calcium phosphates for tissue engineering applications.

5.3.3 *Hydrogels*

Hydrogels are two- or multi-component interconnected three-dimensional network of polymers made from chemical cross-linking of hydrophilic (or amphiphilic) polymeric chains. Apart from covalent bonds, physical interactions such as secondary forces, crystallite formation, and chain entanglements also contribute to a hydrogel's unique behavior. Under a neutral environment, the hydrophilic groups or parts of the polymer network are hydrated to form a gel-like structure. The schematic representations of the preparation process of polymer hydrogels using different methods are presented in Figure 5.8. Hydrogels have the capacity to absorb and retain

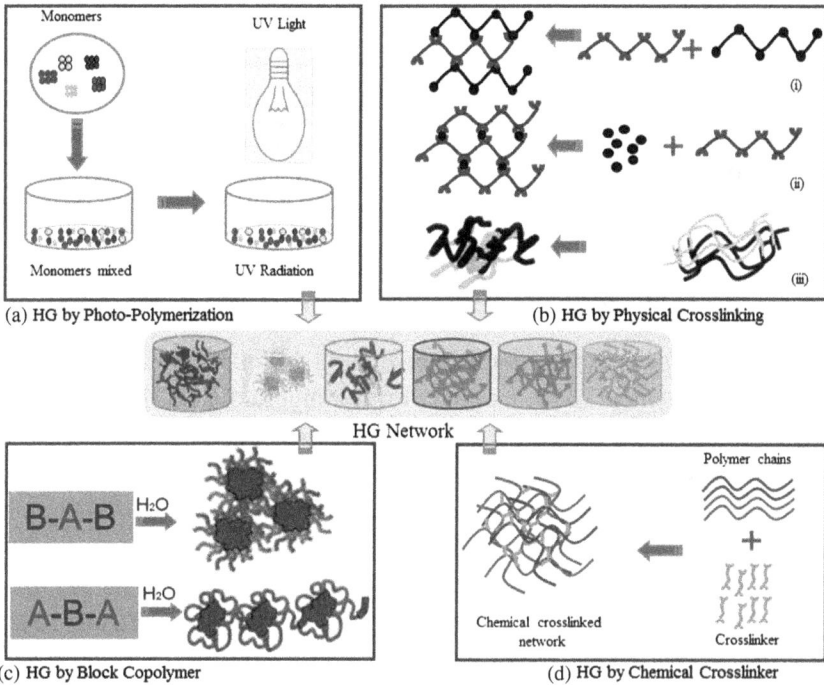

Figure 5.8: Schematic representations of the preparation process of polymer hydrogels using different methods (Khan *et al.*, 2015).

huge amounts of water or biological fluids in the interstitial space of the networks while maintaining their structural integrity. This superabsorbent property is primarily due to their network configuration and differs as per the conditions of the network.

The core capacity to absorb aqueous fluids is due to the hydrophilic functional groups affixed to the polymeric backbone. At the same time, their dissolution resistance comes from cross-links between network chains or segments. The dissolution of hydrogels can be stimulated by varying external and internal parameters such as temperature, pH, and ionic strength. Hydrogels can be designed to be impenetrable in any high concentration solvent due to the inherent covalent bond cross-links or physical interactions. Interestingly, highly cross-linked hydrogels have rheological properties with extremely high viscosity ($>10^5$ Pa s) and elastic properties almost similar to solids, i.e., the shear yield stress is greater than

2000 Pa. Also, high water affinity offers hydrogels close resemblances to the extracellular matrix, and as a result they are exceptionally appropriate for a wide range of biomedical applications (Figure 5.11). Due to these unique properties, hydrogels are extensively found in pharmaceutical applications, drug delivery, personal care products, masks in cosmetics, self-healing materials, and hemostasis bandages.

5.3.3.1 *Swelling ratio*

A typical characterization method of hydrogels for biomedical applications is measurement of the amount of water ingested inside the hydrogel, often termed "*swelling ratio*". The swelling ratio is directly proportional to the volume of water absorbed in the hydrogel. This ratio determines the diffusion properties of a solute inside the hydrogel. The swelling properties of hydrogels can be evaluated by comparison of weights of the hydrogel before (W_{dry}) and after (W_{wet}) water or solution uptake. The swelling ability of the hydrogel can be studied in phosphate-buffered saline (pH 7.4) or hydrochloric acid buffer (pH 1.2). The hydrogel is immersed in acidic or basic solutions at different time durations. Depending on the hydrogel and its stability, the time durations to calculate swelling ratio can be varied and studied at regular intervals of minutes (10, 20, 30, 60, 120) to days (1, 3, 7, 14). Thereafter, the hydrogel is gently pulled out from the solution, and the water absorbed onto the surface is slowly stained onto a filter paper, and the wet weight is documented as W_{wet}. The ratio of swelling is calculated by applying the following equation:

$$\text{Swelling ratio} = \frac{W_{wet} - W_{dry}}{W_{dry}}$$

5.3.3.2 *Classification of hydrogels*

Hydrogels can be classified based on source (natural or synthetic) or synthesis method. The classification of hydrogels based on different properties is illustrated in Figure 5.9. Due to advancements in applications, they are also being classified based on the degradation rate and responses towards internal and external environments. Numerous polymers are

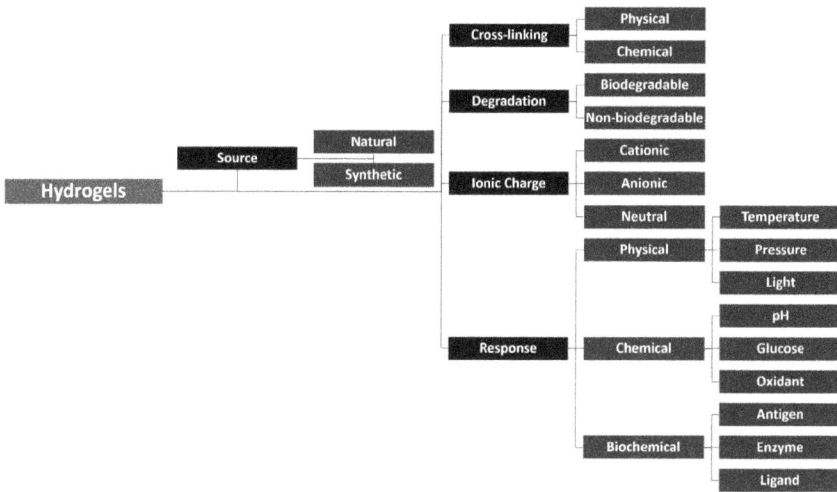

Figure 5.9: Classification of hydrogels based on different properties.

competent enough to form hydrogels from both natural and synthetic sources. Naturally occurring hydrogels are being progressively replaced by synthetic hydrogels for tenable mechanical properties, long service life, high water absorption ability, and high gel resistance.

Natural polymer hydrogels designed from collagen, gelatin, hyaluronic acid, fibrin, etc., have inadequate mechanical properties. However, they have active and reactive sites that are suitable for ligand conjugation, cross-linking, and other adaptations which provide certain potential advantages including biodegradability, biocompatibility, and biologically recognizable molecules that assist cellular activity. Synthetic polymer hydrogels possess considerably low bioactive properties when compared to natural hydrogels but have excellent mechanical properties and can be modified accordingly to provide tailored degradability and functionality. Examples include polyacrylic acid, PVA, PEG and its copolymers, PVP, etc. Currently, among all classifications, stimuli-responsive hydrogels and ionic charge-responsive hydrogels are extensively studied and utilized.

5.3.3.3 *Stimuli-responsive hydrogels*

Stimuli-responsive hydrogels "*sense and react*" and alter their characteristics reversibly in reaction to the internal and external environments.

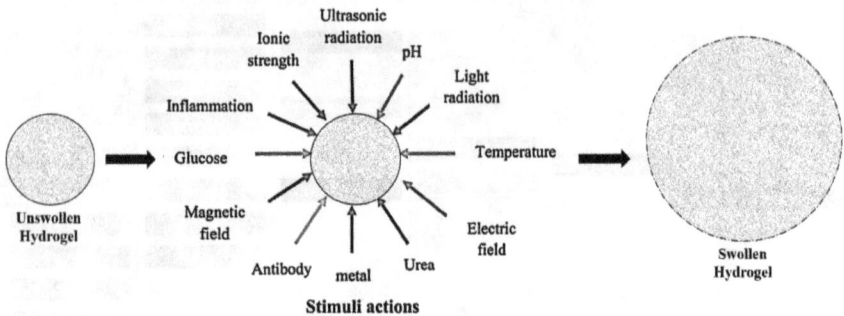

Figure 5.10:   Stimuli responsible for swelling of hydrogels.

Temperature, pH, ionic strength, magnetic fields, and electric currents are some of the acknowledged parameters in stimuli-responsive hydrogels (Figure 5.10).

a. Thermoresponsive hydrogels

Thermoresponsive hydrogels modulate their gelation and changes in swelling with a change in temperature. The critical solution temperature (CST) is the temperature at which the polymer aqueous solution endures a phase transition between liquid and solid phases. Many thermoresponsive polymers exploited in biomedical applications exhibit lower critical solution temperature (LCST), i.e., they are soluble below LCST and form a gel-like structure when heated above LCST. The cycle is reversible, meaning that when the temperature is dropped below LCST, the polymers return to the solution. In contrast, for polymers with upper critical solution temperature (UCST), hydrogels are formed upon cooling and become soluble upon heating.

b. pH-responsive hydrogels

pH-sensitive systems are hydrogels that include ionic monomers in their polymeric backbone and exhibit pre-programmed physical and chemical changes at specific pH ranges. The polymer chains are generally bonded to acidic or basic groups. When immersed in an appropriate solvent, the chains in the network interact with solute ions or molecules. Cross-links prohibit the complete mixing of the polymer chain. For hydrogels containing acidic groups, the acidic groups lose H^+ at high pH (basic conditions) and combine with OH^- ions to form H_2O molecules.

Similarly, when the basic groups accept the addition of a proton at low pH (acidic solutions), charge neutrality is preserved. However, the enhanced cationic (for acidic groups) and anionic (for basic groups) binding of several ions to polymer chains gives rise to an osmotic pressure that causes swelling of a hydrogel aqueous solution.

c. Light-responsive hydrogels
Upon light irradiation, photo-responsive hydrogels exhibit volumetric changes, phase changes, or color changes by swelling or shrinking due to water absorption. The swelling ratio is calculated primarily by the hydrophilicity and cross-linking density of the network, controlled with light. Hydrogel photo-responsiveness largely occurs from functional groups integrated into the polymer backbone, and is not a characteristic feature of the polymers that occur naturally. For light-responsive hydrogels, choosing an effective light source is as important as choosing photoactive groups to suit the respective application needs.

5.3.3.4 *Ionic charge-responsive hydrogels*

The major factors that influence hydrogels are the degree of swelling, the polymer (ionic concentration, pK_a, density), and the medium in which the hydrogel is present. The influence of these on positively charged, negatively charged, and neutral hydrogels are discussed in a very concise manner with one example each.

a. Positively charged (cationic) hydrogels
Cationic hydrogels are best known for creating hydrated space for the diffusion of nutrients. They are less sensitive to degradation, thus giving an advantage for cells (fibroblasts and osteoblasts) to attach and spread better. These hydrogels are famously studied for drug delivery applications due to their capability for controlled release of drugs. They are also studied to develop a self-regulated insulin delivery system, which releases insulin in response to fluctuating glucose concentrations. Examples include N-isopropyl acrylamide (NIPAM), 3-acrylamidopropyl trimethyl ammonium chloride (AAPTAC), chitosan, and polylysine.

b. Negative charged (anionic) hydrogels

In an anionic polymeric system comprising carboxylic or sulphonic acid groups, ionization occurs as the pH of the external swelling medium increases beyond the pK_a of that ionizable moiety. The charge density of the anionic gel can be exploited in designing site-specific drug delivery of therapeutic proteins to the large intestine where the drug can be slowly released in acidic medium while at a faster rate in basic medium. Examples include hyaluronic acid and dextran sulphate.

c. Neutral hydrogels

The unique quality of pH-neutral chitosan helps in minimal surgical destruction to a patient by becoming a scaffold after injection. This

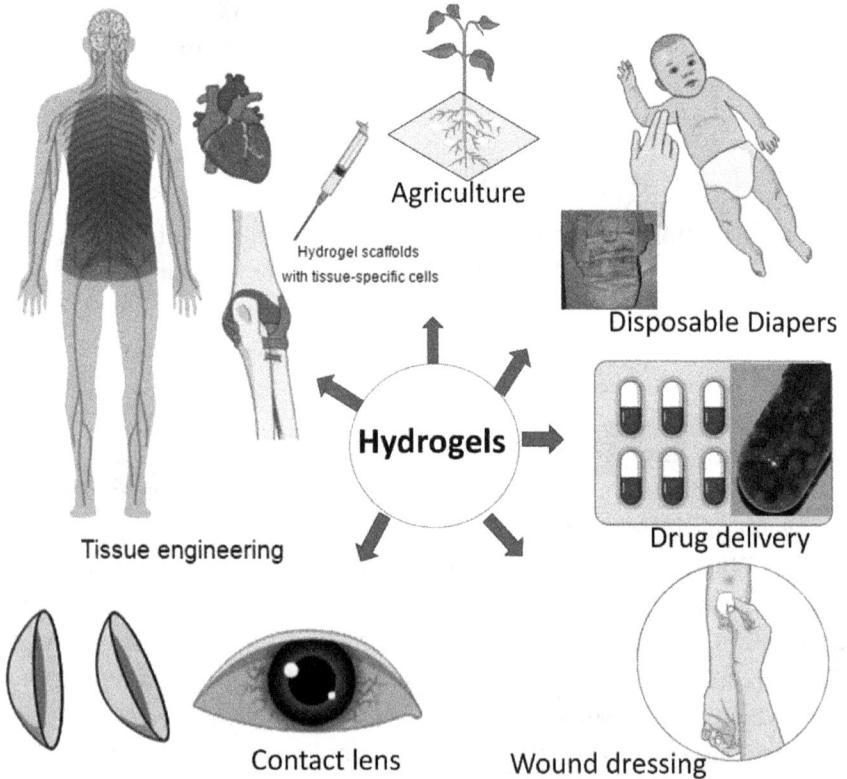

Figure 5.11: Hydrogels and their importance in their distinctive fields of application (Varaprasad *et al.*, 2017).

hydrogel remains in a liquid form at 27°C, but when the temperature rises above 37°C it instantaneously transforms into a macroporous gel. Other examples are polyacrylamide, chitin, dextran, and polyvinyl alcohol. These neutral hydrogels swell to stability when the solvent's pressure is stabilized with the chain stretching energy.

5.4 Multiple choice questions

1. Increasing molecular weight of a polymer usually
   (a) increases the strength of the polymer
   (b) decreases the strength of the polymer
   (c) has no effect on the strength of the polymer
   (d) none of the above

2. Which of these polymers cannot be recycled, and which is the strongest polymer group?
   (a) thermoplasts; thermosets
   (b) thermosets; thermosets
   (c) elastomers; thermoplasts
   (d) all polymers; elastomers

3. Which of the following is/are NOT true about polymers?
   I. high mechanical strength
   II. high-temperature stability on par with ceramics
   III. high elongation with viscoelastic behaviour
   (a) only I and II
   (b) only II
   (c) only I and III
   (d) all of the above

4. Which compound is made up of many monomers joined in long chains, and which pattern is not a copolymer?
   (a) ethanol; BBAABBAABBAABB
   (b) methanol; ABCABCABCABC
   (c) cellulose; CCCCCCCCCCC
   (d) fibrin; AACAACAACAA

5. Which of the following is/are TRUE?
   I. a thermosetting polymer will not melt
   II. a thermoplastic will melt and be malleable into any desired shape
   (a) only I
   (b) only II
   (c) all of the above
   (d) none of the above

6. Which is the best method to store degradable hydrogels?
   (a) storing in a refrigerator at 4°C or under alcohol
   (b) storing in a beaker at 20°C
   (c) physicochemical properties of hydrogels are not dependent on storage
   (d) all of the above

7. Composite materials are classified based on
   (a) type of matrix
   (b) size and shape of reinforcement
   (c) melting points
   (d) mechanical and biological properties

8. The calculation of number average (M_n) and weight average (M_w) depends, respectively, on
   (a) total weight of all polymer chains; molecular weight of each molecule
   (b) molecular weight of each molecule; total weight of all polymer chains
   (c) individual weight of each polymer chain; total weight of all polymer chains
   (d) none of the above

9. Which of the following is NOT a polymeric biomaterial?
   (a) chitosan
   (b) hydroxyapatite
   (c) Polylactic-co-glycolic acid
   (d) Polymethyl methacrylate

10. Which of the following is TRUE?
    (a) degradation rate of PCL is very fast
    (b) PCL is an amorphous polymer
    (c) crystallinity of a polymer affects the degradation rate
    (d) all of the above

References & Further Reading

Balakrishnan, P., Geethamma, V. G., Sreekala, M. S., & Thomas, S. (2018). Chapter 1 — Polymeric biomaterials: State-of-the-art and new challenges. In S. Thomas, P. Balakrishnan, & M. S. Sreekala (Eds.), *Fundamental Biomaterials: Polymers* (pp. 1–20): Woodhead Publishing.

Bass, G., Becker, M. L., Heath, D. E., & Cooper, S. L. (2020). Chapter 1.3.2 — Polymers: Basic Principles. In W. R. Wagner, S. E. Sakiyama-Elbert, G. Zhang, & M. J. Yaszemski (Eds.), *Biomaterials Science (Fourth Edition)* (pp. 85–102): Academic Press.

He, W., & Benson, R. (2017). Chapter 8 — Polymeric Biomaterials. In M. Kutz (Ed.), *Applied Plastics Engineering Handbook (Second Edition)* (pp. 145–164): William Andrew Publishing.

Khan, F., Tanaka, M., & Ahmad, S. R. (2015). Fabrication of polymeric biomaterials: a strategy for tissue engineering and medical devices. *Journal of Materials Chemistry B, 3*(42), 8224–8249. doi:10.1039/C5TB01370D.

Love, B. (2017). Chapter 9 — Polymeric Biomaterials. In B. Love (Ed.), *Biomaterials* (pp. 205–238): Academic Press.

Prajapati, S. K., Jain, A., Jain, A., & Jain, S. (2019). Biodegradable polymers and constructs: A novel approach in drug delivery. *European Polymer Journal, 120*, 109191. doi:10.1016/j.eurpolymj.2019.08.018.

Varaprasad, K., Raghavendra, G. M., Jayaramudu, T., Yallapu, M. M., *et al.* (2017). A mini review on hydrogels classification and recent developments in miscellaneous applications. *Materials Science and Engineering: C, 79*, 958–971. doi:10.1016/j.msec.2017.05.096.

Chapter 6
Bioceramics

6.1 Ceramics

Ceramic materials such as tiles, bricks, plates, crockery, pottery kiln, glass, etc., have been part of our day-to-day life for thousands of years. Ceramics are inorganic solid materials composed of metallic and non-metallic elements that are predominantly bound together by ionic bonds. These materials occur as both crystalline and non-crystalline (amorphous) compounds. Ionic bonds are strong and non-directional, thus the melting temperatures of ceramics are higher than those of metals (metallic bonds) and polymers (covalent bonds). The difference between covalent and ionic bonds is illustrated in Figure 6.1. It is important to note that pure

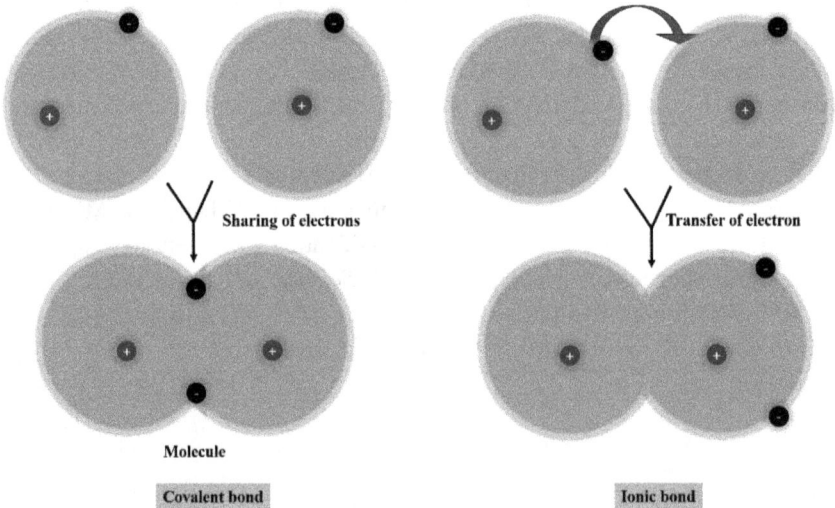

Figure 6.1: Difference between covalent and ionic bonds.

ionic bonds do not exist. All ionic bonds have some degree of covalency. Thus, a bond is deemed as an ionic bond when the ionic character is higher than that of the covalent character. Like all other materials, the properties of ceramics are determined by the kind of atoms present, the bonding between them, and the way the atoms are packed together. Stoichiometrically stable ionic ceramics are regularly created by combining groups of cations and anions to create crystal structures with repeating unit cell shape and size.

Most ceramics currently available consist of two or more elements, known as a compound. Alumina (Al_2O_3), for instance, is a constituent compound of aluminium and oxygen atoms. In general, ceramics have:

- high melting points, which implies they are heat-resistant
- excellent hardness and strength
- significant durability, which implies they last for a long time and have excellent wear resistance properties
- low electrical and thermal conductivity, which implies they are good insulators
- high chemical inertness, which implies they are unreactive with other chemicals

6.2 Ceramic biomaterials

Ceramics form a major subclass of biomaterials, especially in orthopaedics and dental applications (Figure 6.2). Like all other biomaterials, the success rate of bioceramics is determined by two indispensable factors: composition and morphology. They usually have a greater reaction to the surrounding tissues than polymers or metals. Most of the ceramic biomaterials do not discharge their elements into the body but are bioresorbed. Ceramics are typically characterized by excellent biocompatibility, high corrosion resistance, high wear, high strength, extremely high stiffness, and hardness. Further, they are sub-grouped according to their reactivity with surrounding tissues: bioinert ceramics, bioactive ceramics, and bioresorbable ceramics (Figure 6.2 and Table 6.1).

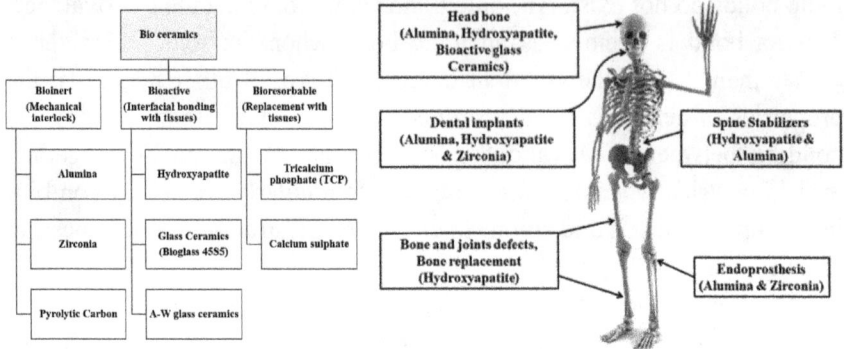

Figure 6.2: Categorization of bioceramics according to their reaction with surrounding tissues and applications in the human body (Farid, 2019; Gul *et al.*, 2020; Naik, 2019).

Table 6.1: Typical bioceramics used in the human body and their applications.

Bioceramics		Tissue reaction	Applications
Alumina		Bioinert	Hip ball and cup, knee joint
Zirconia		Bioinert	Dental crowns and brackets, dental implants
Carbon		Bioinert	Heart valves, spinal inserts
Bioactive glass		Bioactive	Dental implants, bone grafts, bone cements
Calcium phosphates	Hydroxyapatite Tricalcium phosphate Calcium sulphate	Bioresorbable	Repair of periodontal defects, bone defects and regeneration

- **Bioactive ceramics:** Provide a favorable reaction within the biological system at the boundary between the host tissue and the material. This gives rise to direct bonding with the living bone immediately after implantation. This feature of direct attachment to the bone is incredibly helpful for quick recovery and reduces implant failure. This feature is found only in bioceramics among biomaterials. Examples are calcium phosphates, bioactive glasses, and glass-ceramics.
- **Bioinert ceramics:** Do not instigate response or interact with the body's environment, i.e., possess high chemical stability with surrounding tissue after implantation. In other words, adding the bioinert material to the body does not cause the host to respond. Examples are alumina (Al_2O_3), zirconia (Zr_2O_3), and pyrolytic carbon.

- **Bioresorbable ceramics:** Gradually and steadily resorbed in the body after a specified period of interaction with the tissues. They are degraded, solubilized or phagocytosed by the body and substituted by bone over time. An example is tricalcium phosphate $[Ca_3(PO_4)_2]$.

6.3 Bioactive ceramics

6.3.1 *Bioactive glasses*

Bioactive glasses are a subclass of inorganic bioactive ceramics distinguished by their capacity to chemically react with living tissues and create a mechanical and durable bond with them. Hench and his colleagues in 1969 first initiated the concept of bioactive glass as a substitute to nearly or complete inert implant materials. This innovative new class of material has led to major changes in healthcare medicine and modern biomaterial-motivated products. In fact, this laid a foundation for the development of many other well-known materials now, including hydroxyapatite and other calcium phosphates.

The silicate glasses built on $[SiO_4]^{4-}$ tetrahedral units are the most commonly used bioactive glasses. Silica (SiO_2) is the best known glass network-forming oxide and is the key constituent material in glass products, typically containing 50–75% of total configuration. Unlike most ceramics that crystallize upon solidification, SiO_2 naturally transforms from liquid to glassy state upon cooling. Various materials such as sodium oxide (Na_2O), calcium oxide (CaO), Al_2O_3, magnesium oxide (MgO), potassium oxide (K_2O), lead oxide (PbO), and boron oxide (B_2O_3) are added to enhance the material properties (Figure 6.3). The cations of these materials, such as Na^+, K^+, Ca^{2+}, Mg^{2+}, etc., act as network modifiers by forming non-bridging oxygen bonds with silica.

Moreover, the addition of these materials promotes fusion (flux) during heating, increases fluidity in processing molten glass, improves chemical resistance against various acids and basic substances, and improves bone-bonding strength. Over the past few years, several new combinations and other forms of bioglass were developed in order to adapt the corpus response to different clinical uses. The compositions of various bioactive glasses are shown in Table 6.2. When the glass contains more than 60% of SiO_2, bonding to tissues is no longer supported.

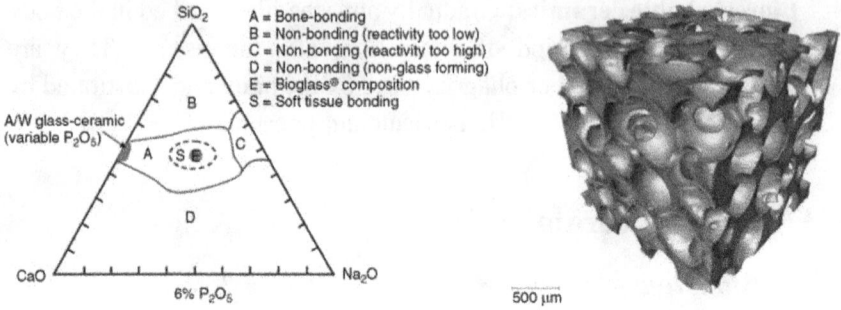

Figure 6.3: (Left) Compositional figure for bone-bonding. The composition achieved in region S is where bioactive glasses bond to both bone and soft tissues. (Right) Typical X-ray microtomography picture of bioactive glass scaffold fabricated by the sol-gel foaming method (Jones, 2008; Mala *et al.*, 2018).

Table 6.2: Compositions of various bioactive glasses.

Name	Composition (mol%)			
	SiO_2	Na_2O	CaO	P_2O_5
45S5 Bioglass®	46.1	24.4	26.9	2.6
58S (Sol-gel derived) Bioglass	60	0	36	4
S53P4 AbminDent1	53	23	20	4

6.3.1.1 *45S5 Bioglass*

Bioactive glasses, especially 45S5 bioglass, represent a group of reactive materials that are solid, non-porous, and hard. Bioglass® represents the title for the native 45S5 composition fabricated by the University of Florida. Thus, it can only be used with regard to this composition and not for other bioactive glasses. It is an Na_2O-CaO-SiO_2-P_2O_5 system (Figure 6.3) distinguished by high amounts of Na_2O and CaO, as well as a comparatively high CaO/P_2O_5 ratio. The two important materials, CaO and P_2O_5, distribute crucial components of the hydroxyapatite (HA), namely Ca^{2+} and PO_4^{3-} ions, while the other oxides, Na_2O and SiO_2, consist of elements abundant in the human body. Precisely, Bioglass® is constituted of 46.1 mol% of SiO_2, 24.4 mol% of Na_2O, 26.9 mol% of CaO, and 2.6 mol% of P_2O_5. It offers remarkable advantages such as high bioactivity index and capability to attach to soft and hard connective tissues. Under physiological conditions, this combination of reactive materials is able to bond to mineralized bone tissue and has presented good results in bone regeneration (Figure 6.3). 45S5 Bioglass®, upon interaction with tissues and body fluids, forms a sensitive, reactive layer with a gel-like texture. This offers a compatible glass-to-tissue interface and forms a biologically active layer of HA. In fact, the first 45S5 Bioglass® was approved in the United States to replace the middle ear's small bones.

6.3.1.2 *The mechanism of HA layer formation on 45S5 Bioglass*

The bioactivity and bone tissue interaction mechanisms of 45S5 Bioglass® were studied extensively. Positive interactions with the bone tissue have been widely credited to the development of a unique hydroxycarbonate apatite (HCA)-like layer on the 45S5 Bioglass® surface. The mechanism consists of several stages. Figure 6.4 outlines a series of interfacial kinetic reactions involving the formation of a bond between the bone and bioactive glass, which are addressed in detail below.

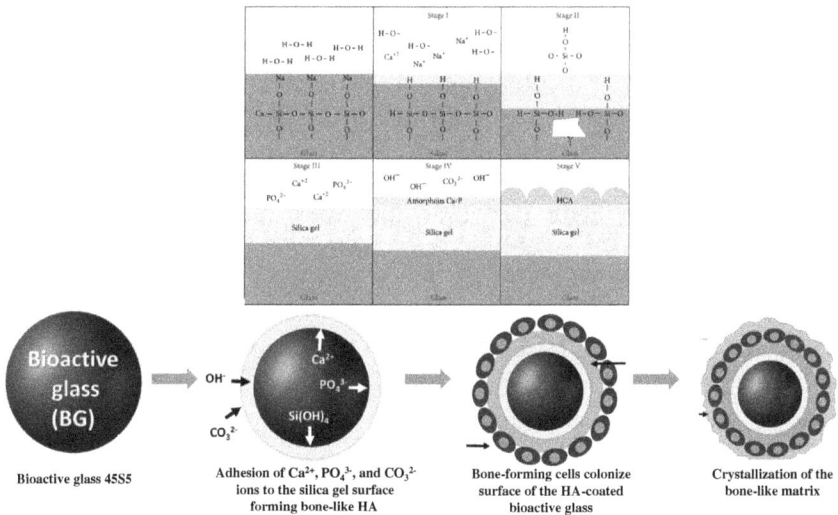

Figure 6.4: (Top) Illustration of hydroxycarbonate apatite (HCA) formation on the surface of bioactive glass upon interaction with body fluids. (Bottom) Mechanism of bioglass bioactivity facilitating the enhanced proliferation of bone cells (Mala *et al.*, 2018; Mondal *et al.*, 2018; Renno *et al.*, 2013).

- **Stage 1:** The silica gel flexible structure allows the ion exchange to begin. Ion exchange occurs among the alkali (Ca^{2+} and Na^+) and hydrogen ions (H^+). The alkali ions are available from glass, and H^+ from the solution. The ion exchange mainly facilitates the hydrolysis of silica groups and formation of silanol groups (Si-OHs).

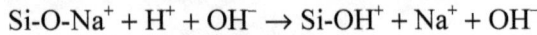

$$Si\text{-}O\text{-}Na^+ + H^+ + OH^- \rightarrow Si\text{-}OH^+ + Na^+ + OH^-$$

- **Stage 2:** The above reaction causes an increase in local pH, which initiates the disintegration of siloxane (Si-O-Si) bonds by interfacial network dissolution. This releases Si ions and forms large Si-OH factions on the surface.

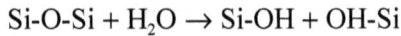

$$Si\text{-}O\text{-}Si + H_2O \rightarrow Si\text{-}OH + OH\text{-}Si$$

- **Stage 3:** Condensation and polymerization of the SiO_2-rich layer take place on the surface when the native pH is lower than 9.5. This process facilitates the development of a thin silica gel layer on the surface.
- **Stage 4:** Development of amorphous calcium phosphate layer materializes due to the migration of Ca^{2+} and PO_3^{4-} ions.
- **Stage 5:** The final stage involves the crystallization of the HCA layer. The carbonate ions (CO_3^{2-}) substitute OH^- ions in the crystal and lead to the establishment of desired HCA.

6.3.2 *Hydroxyapatite*

Understanding of the structural and chemical composition of bones has accumulated over time. Human bone is a natural composite made up of 60–70% acicular hydroxyapatite (HA, $Ca_{10}(PO_4)_6(OH)_2$) and collagen fibers. The structure of HA crystals is shown in Figure 6.5. The human bone also contains a very minimum quantity of other mineral phases, such as dicalcium phosphate ($Ca_2P_2O_7$) and dibasic calcium phosphate (DCP, $CaHPO_4$). However, only HA and DCP are chemically stable at physiological conditions. Due to its close chemical resemblance with the inorganic portion of the bone and teeth, HA hexagonal crystal system with density 3.14–3.16 g/cm^3 is a commonly used synthetic CaP ceramic for bone substitution.

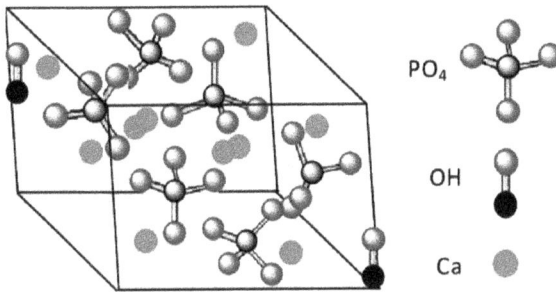

Figure 6.5: The structure of hydroxyapatite crystals (Rujitanapanich *et al.*, 2014).

Table 6.3: Ca/P ratio of various calcium phosphates.

Name	Symbol	Chemical structure	Ca/P ratio	Density (g/cm^3)
Monocalcium phosphate anhydrous	MCPA	$Ca(H_2PO_4)_2$	0.5	2.58
Monocalcium phosphate monohydrate	MCPM	$Ca(H_2PO_4)_2 \cdot H_2O$	0.5	2.23
Dicalcium phosphate (montite)	DCPA	$CaHPO_4$	1.0	2.92
Dicalcium phosphate dihydrate (brushite)	DCPD	$CaHPO_4 \cdot 2 H_2O$	1.0	2.27
Tricalcium phosphate (TCP)	α-TCP	α-$Ca_3(PO_4)_2$	1.5	2.86
	β-TCP	β-$Ca_3(PO_4)_2$	1.5	3.07
Amorphous calcium phosphate	ACP	$Ca_9(HPO_4)(PO_4)_5(OH)$	~1.5	3.01
Calcium hydroxyapatite	HA	$Ca_{10}(PO_4)_6(OH)_2$	1.67	3.16
Fluorapatite	FA	$Ca_{10}(PO_4)_6F_2$	1.67	3.18
Tetracalcium phosphate	TTCP	$Ca_4O(PO_4)_2$	2.0	3.05

HA exists in both monoclinic and hexagonal phases. However, the stable hexagonal structure is preferred in biological applications. The surface of HA acts as a prime nucleating site for bone minerals present in biological fluids to get adsorbed. Among various CaPs (Table 6.3), HA is considered as more stable than any other with minimal solubility in physiological environments such as temperature, pH (4.2–8.0), body fluids, etc. It has a theoretical composition of Ca 39.69 wt%, P 18.46 wt%, OH 3.38%, Ca/P weight ratio of 2.151, and Ca/P molar ratio of 1.667.

Significant efforts are being put into using HA as the standard reference for bone regeneration and mineralization. HA stoichiometry is incredibly important when thermal processing is needed for the material. Slight fluctuations in the Ca/P ratio can contribute to undesirable phase appearances.

- If the Ca/P ratio is below 1.67, β-tricalcium phosphate (β-TCP) and other additional phases, including tetracalcium phosphate (TTCP), may appear within HA.
- If the Ca/P is more than 1.67, calcium oxide (CaO) may be present within the HA phase.

6.3.2.1 *Synthesis of hydroxyapatite*

HA can be obtained naturally and economically from various sources. Natural HA is typically obtained economically from various biological resources including mammalian bone (e.g., bovine), marine or aquatic sources (e.g., fishbone, fish shells, and oyster shells), shells (e.g., eggshell and seashell), plants and algae, and also mineral sources (e.g., limestone). The preparation of HA via biogenic sources is illustrated in Figure 6.6. HA obtained from biological sources is distinct from conventional HA as it is composed of CO_3 groups with small quantities of Mg, Na and traces of other metals. This substance typically has a Ca/P ratio greater than that of the stoichiometric equivalent.

The properties of HA can be modified and controlled, such as particle size, chemical composition, and surface morphology (spherical, rod-shaped, needle-like, etc.). Several chemical processing routes such as solid-state reaction, wet chemical methods, co-precipitation method, sol-gel synthesis, pyrolysis of aerosols, microemulsion, and hydrothermal reactions have been developed to prepare HA. Based on controllability, different methods yield HA crystals in various morphologies, stoichiometries, levels of crystallinity, and sizes such as nanometric, sub-nanometric, and micrometric (Figure 6.7). The processing requirements vary considerably for each of these methods. For instance, the reaction

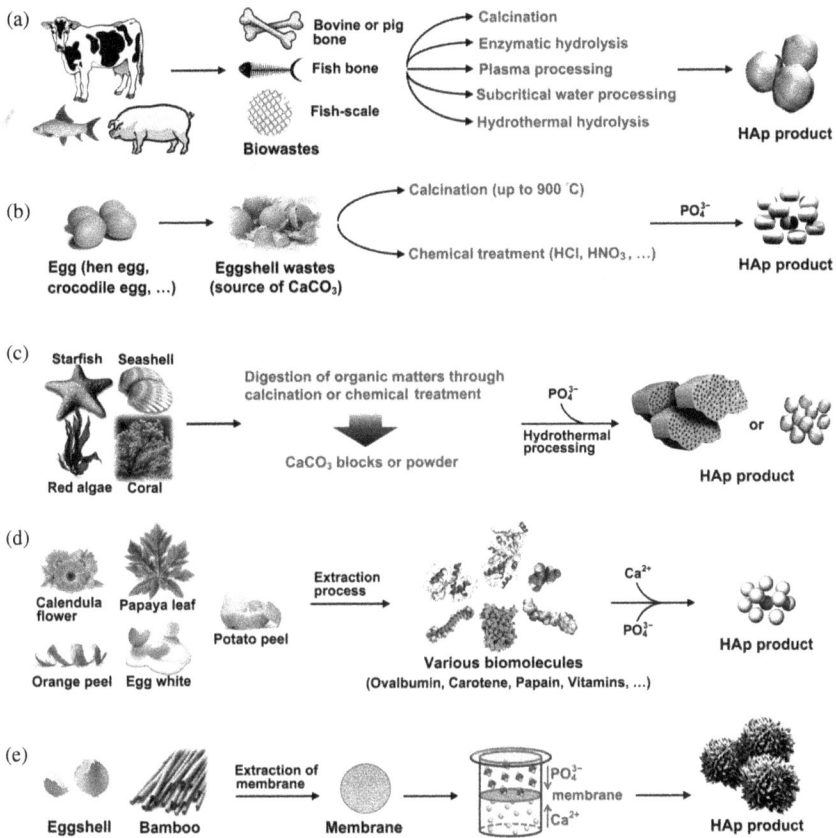

Figure 6.6: Preparation of HA via biogenic sources: (a) extraction of minerals from biowaste; (b) synthesis from eggshells; (c) synthesis from the exoskeleton of marine organisms; (d) synthesis with the aid of naturally derived biomolecules; and (e) synthesis using biomembranes (Sadat-Shojai *et al.*, 2013).

temperature varies from 1000–1250°C for solid-state synthesis methods to less than 350°C for the hydrothermal process and room temperature for aqueous precipitation and emulsion processes.

A. Solid-state reaction

The solid-state reaction involves mix-grinding dry powders by mortar and crusher (Figure 6.8). This process does not involve any solvents and is generally used for mass production. Solid-state reactions typically

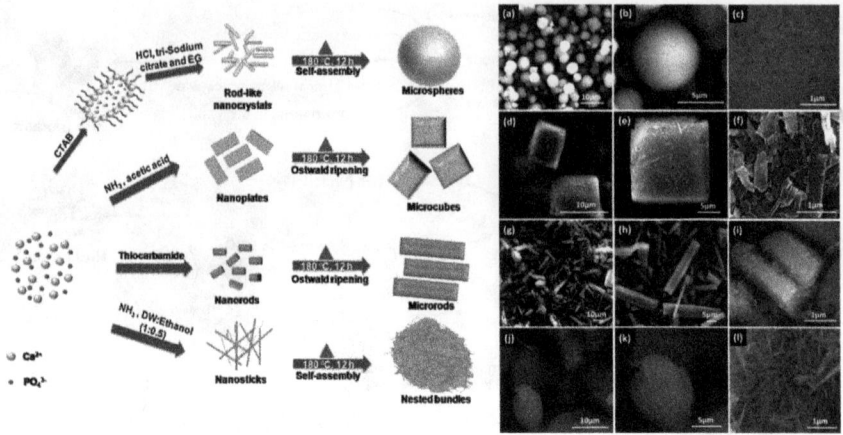

Figure 6.7: Graphic representation of growth processes of HA microstructures and FESEM images with separate magnifications of (a–c) spheres, (d–f) cubes, (g–i) hexagonal rods and (j–l) nested bundles (Mary *et al.*, 2016).

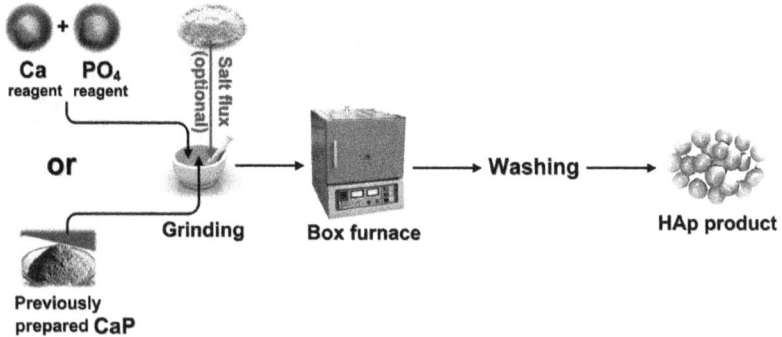

Figure 6.8: Preparation of HA powder through solid-state method (Sadat-Shojai *et al.*, 2013).

give HA that is stoichiometric and well crystallized but requires fairly high temperatures (approximately 1000°C) and long treatment times. The following is an example of a solid-state chemical reaction of preparing HA at room temperature.

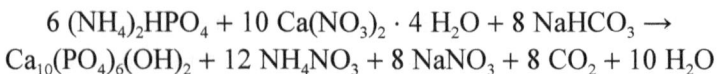

$$6 \ (NH_4)_2HPO_4 + 10 \ Ca(NO_3)_2 \cdot 4 \ H_2O + 8 \ NaHCO_3 \rightarrow$$
$$Ca_{10}(PO_4)_6(OH)_2 + 12 \ NH_4NO_3 + 8 \ NaNO_3 + 8 \ CO_2 + 10 \ H_2O$$

B. Hydrolysis

In contrast to wet-chemical processes, a simple hydrolysis reaction generally replicates better HA crystal composition and morphology. This is primarily due to a limited number of synthesis parameters such as pH, temperature, reaction period, and initial reagents. HA can be produced by the hydrolysis of dicalcium phosphate dihydrate ($CaHPO_4 \cdot 2\ H_2O$), calcium hydrogen phosphate ($CaHPO_4$), alpha-tricalcium phosphate ($\alpha\text{-}Ca_3(PO_4)_2$), beta-tricalcium phosphate ($\beta\text{-}Ca_3(PO_4)_2$), octacalcium phosphate ($Ca_8H_2(PO_4)_6 \cdot 5\ H_2O$), tetracalcium phosphate ($Ca_4(PO_4)_2O$), and their mixtures at low temperatures. These individual phosphates and their mixtures result in needle or blade shape morphology with the size in microns. However, most of the morphologies obtained by the hydrolysis method are highly non-stoichiometric.

For example, the hydrolysis of $CaHPO_4$ is given by

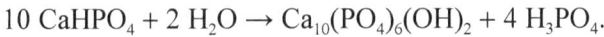

$$10\ CaHPO_4 + 2\ H_2O \rightarrow Ca_{10}(PO_4)_6(OH)_2 + 4\ H_3PO_4.$$

Often, in solution conditions HA precipitation gives a lower Ca/P ratio, that is, less than 1.67, with an excess of water. In the case of tricalcium phosphate, hydrolysis can result in a nonstoichiometric HA, i.e., calcium-deficient hydroxyapatite (CDHA) with a Ca/P ratio extending to 1.5.

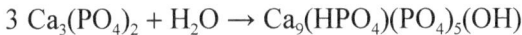

$$3\ Ca_3(PO_4)_2 + H_2O \rightarrow Ca_9(HPO_4)(PO_4)_5(OH)$$

C. Hydrothermal method

Hydrothermal method refers to the use of high temperature (generally <350°C) and high pressure to convert slurries, solutions, or gels into the necessary crystalline phase. The hydrothermal method is commonly used in the synthesis of HA material for its strong reproducibility, lack of defects, and strong control over crystallinity. The hydrothermal approach typically gives high crystallinity HA with a Ca/P ratio close to the stoichiometric value, i.e., 1.67. Many studies have reported that the desired shape and size of HA crystals can be easily regulated by altering the hydrothermal temperature, time, and reaction concentrations. HA is typically synthesized in the $Ca\text{-}PO_4\text{-}H_2O$ hydrothermal system via a chemical reaction between the initial precursors containing Ca^{2+} and PO_4^{3-} ions.

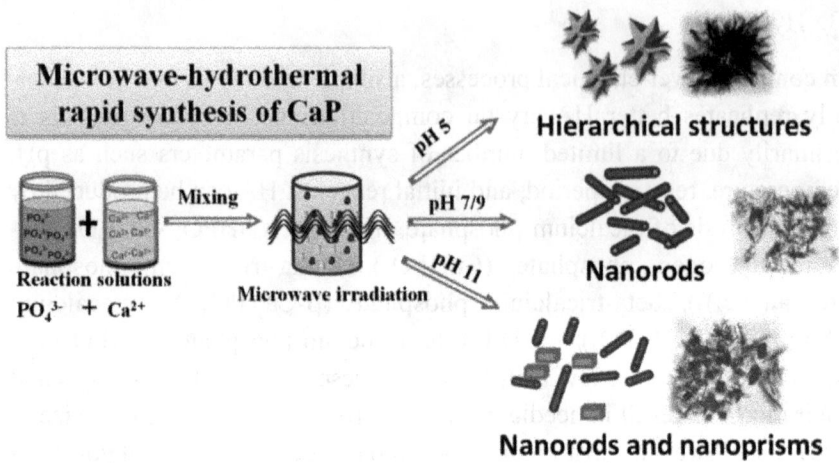

Figure 6.9:   Graphical description to produce CaP nanostructures with the microwave-assisted hydrothermal method under different pH values (Cai *et al.*, 2015).

Graphical representation to produce CaP nanostructures by the hydrothermal method is shown in Figure 6.9.

D. Chemical precipitation method

Chemical precipitation method (Figure 6.10) is a simple, versatile, and economical route for the preparation of HA by mixing molar ratios of calcium salt and phosphate solutions in basic conditions. The formed precipitation is then dried and calcined to obtain ultrafine HA crystals with nanometer size and different shapes (blades, needles, rods, or equiaxed). In precipitation method, the source of calcium for HA synthesis can be obtained from various sources such as corals, animal bones, shells of snails, limestone, etc., with the popular source being eggshell waste. Eggshell waste is a high source of calcium carbonate ($CaCO_3$), which is calcined at 1000°C to convert into calcium oxide (CaO). CaO is then reacted with water (H_2O) to produce the calcium precursor for HA synthesis, i.e., $Ca(OH)_2$.

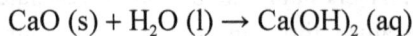

$$CaO \text{ (s)} + H_2O \text{ (l)} \rightarrow Ca(OH)_2 \text{ (aq)}$$

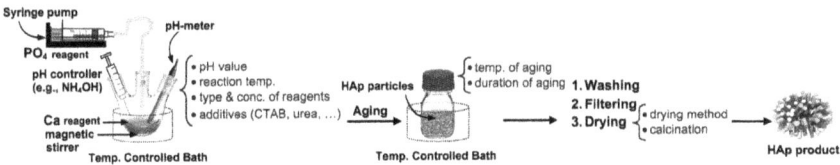

Figure 6.10:   Synthesis of HA nanoparticles through conventional chemical precipitation (Sadat-Shojai *et al.*, 2013).

Option 1: Preparation of HA using $Ca(OH)_2$ and ortho-phosphoric acid (H_3PO_4) as calcium and phosphorus sources, respectively.

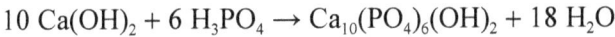

$$10\ Ca(OH)_2 + 6\ H_3PO_4 \rightarrow Ca_{10}(PO_4)_6(OH)_2 + 18\ H_2O$$

Option 2: Preparation of HA utilizing calcium nitrate tetrahydrate, $Ca(NO_3)_2 \cdot 4\ H_2O$, and ammonium phosphate dibasic, $(NH_4)_2HPO_4$, as preliminary materials.

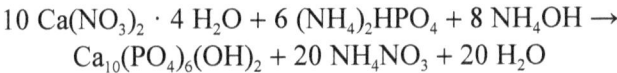

$$10\ Ca(NO_3)_2 \cdot 4\ H_2O + 6\ (NH_4)_2HPO_4 + 8\ NH_4OH \rightarrow$$
$$Ca_{10}(PO_4)_6(OH)_2 + 20\ NH_4NO_3 + 20\ H_2O$$

However, the HA particles synthesized by the chemical precipitation process often have very poor uniformity and may be agglomerated. Due to these issues, CDHA with lattice defects and a Ca/P ratio of less than 1.67 is obtained. Occasionally, high pH value is used to prevent the growth and development of the CDHA phase. Additionally, high calcining temperature is required to obtain crystalline HA. Therefore, the reaction parameters, including pH, temperature, and solution conditions, are controlled extensively to obtain homogenous colloidal HA without the formation of CDHA.

E. Sol-gel

The sol-gel procedure is a wet chemical technique that does not require harsh processing parameters such as high pH or a high sintering temperature (Figure 6.11). This approach provides an atomic mixture of Ca and P that can enhance the homogeneity of chemical substances. Additionally,

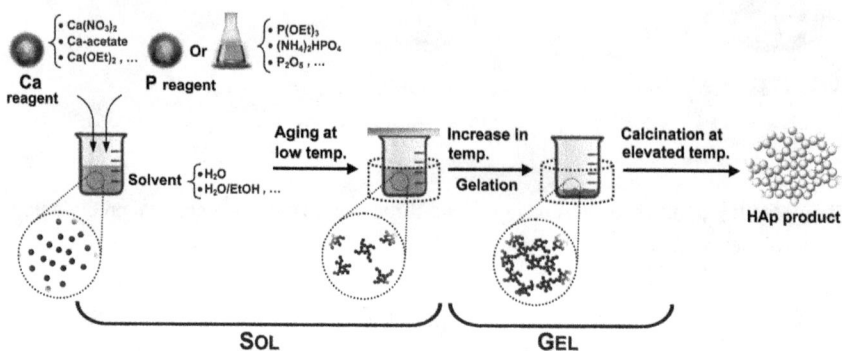

Figure 6.11: Synthesis of HA nanoparticles through the sol-gel process (Sadat-Shojai *et al.*, 2013).

the high chemical reactiveness of the sol-gel powders favors the production of fine particles, homogeneity, reduced processing temperatures, and the possibility of degradation during sintering. For HA synthesis, the sol-gel method involves preparing a solution from alkoxides, inorganic metal salts or other suitable precursors such as nitrates. Moreover, the sol-gel process is easily applicable as a surface coating technique for metallic materials. It allows the deposition of high-quality uniform HA thin films (see Chapter 9). However, studies on sol-gel-derived HA have suggested that HA production is often followed by hydrolysis of the phosphate, forming secondary calcium oxide (CaO). This compound has negative effects on the biocompatibility of HA. Moreover, the HA synthesized by this technique sometimes results in relatively inferior crystallinity and thermal stability.

F. Microemulsion

A microemulsion is a thermodynamically stable and optically transparent dispersion of two immiscible liquids, for instance water and oil, which is regulated by an amphiphilic surface-active agent or surfactant (Figure 6.12). Usually, a high dielectric constant compound (water) is mixed with a low dielectric constant solvent (oil) under stirring conditions. To regulate the interfacial stress, the addition of a surfactant between the two immiscible phases is required. The method could offer precise control over HA size,

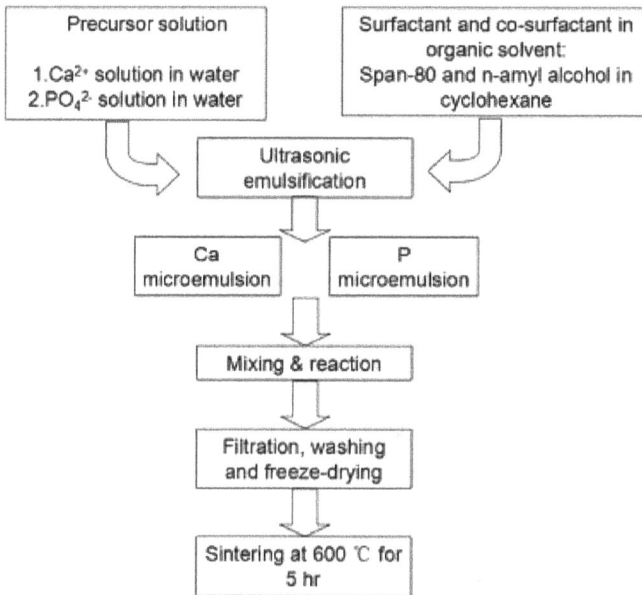

Figure 6.12: Synthesis of HA by microemulsion method (Ma *et al.*, 2016).

size distribution, stability, and shape by manipulating or adjusting the water-to-oil ratio and concentration of surfactants. Microemulsion is one of the few methods that can generate a uniform particle size in the range of nanometers with minimal agglomeration.

6.4 Bioinert ceramics

6.4.1 *Alumina*

Alumina (Al_2O_3) is a well-recognized bioinert, biocompatible, and highly stable oxide ceramic material. Its applications are extensive in the fields of engineering and biomedical science. Depending on heat treatment conditions, Al_2O_3 may be found in many metastable phases such as γ, η, θ, ρ, and χ but transforms into a thermodynamically stable α-Al_2O_3 phase when heated above 1200°C. Al_2O_3 has a rhombohedral structure with a close-packed hexagonal positioning of O^{2-} ions and lattice parameters $a = 4.758$ Å, $c = 12.991$ Å, and $\gamma = 120°$.

Al_2O_3 has been investigated since the late 1960s as implant biomaterial. Today, high purity (>99.5%) polycrystalline α-Al_2O_3 is primarily used as an alternative to metal alloys for structural biomedical applications. The strong chemical bonds between the Al^{3+} and O^{2-} ions are the source of the superior properties of α-alumina. Their extensive use in the biomedical industry is due to decent mechanical properties (high hardness, high wear resistance, and high abrasion resistance) and strong chemical resistance to corrosion. The excellent corrosive properties are due to the development of a thin, compact, and chemically stable oxide layer on the surface. Large quantities of Al_2O_3 are commercially extracted using the Bayer process, a hydrometallurgical extraction and refinement procedure, from mineral ores such as bauxite and cryolite. It can be consolidated briefly into three stages.

- **Stage 1 — Extraction:** crushed bauxite is dissolved in concentrated sodium hydroxide solution at a temperature of 270°C.

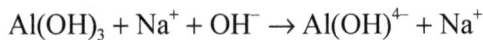

$$Al(OH)_3 + Na^+ + OH^- \rightarrow Al(OH)^{4-} + Na^+$$

- **Stage 2 — Precipitation:** crystalline aluminum trihydroxide ($Al(OH)_3$), also known as gibbsite, is precipitated by cooling the solution. This stage is exactly the reverse of the previous stage.

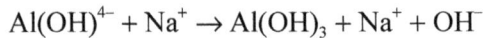

$$Al(OH)^{4-} + Na^+ \rightarrow Al(OH)_3 + Na^+ + OH^-$$

- **Stage 3 — Calcination:** the gibbsite is then converted to Al_2O_3 by calcination.

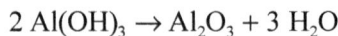

$$2\ Al(OH)_3 \rightarrow Al_2O_3 + 3\ H_2O$$

Since the 1970s, Al_2O_3 has been used in orthopaedic surgery as hip prostheses (acetabula and femoral heads), in dentistry as dental implants, and in surgical devices. Due to excellent wear surface properties and capacity to obtain high surface finish, Al_2O_3 is often employed to manufacture femoral heads for hip prostheses and wear plates for knee replacement implants. Over the last 40 years, Al_2O_3 has been the standard source for total hip replacement (THR) components, both as ceramic heads and in ceramic bearings. THR is a device set formed from a femoral stem component, a femoral head component, and an acetabular cup component.

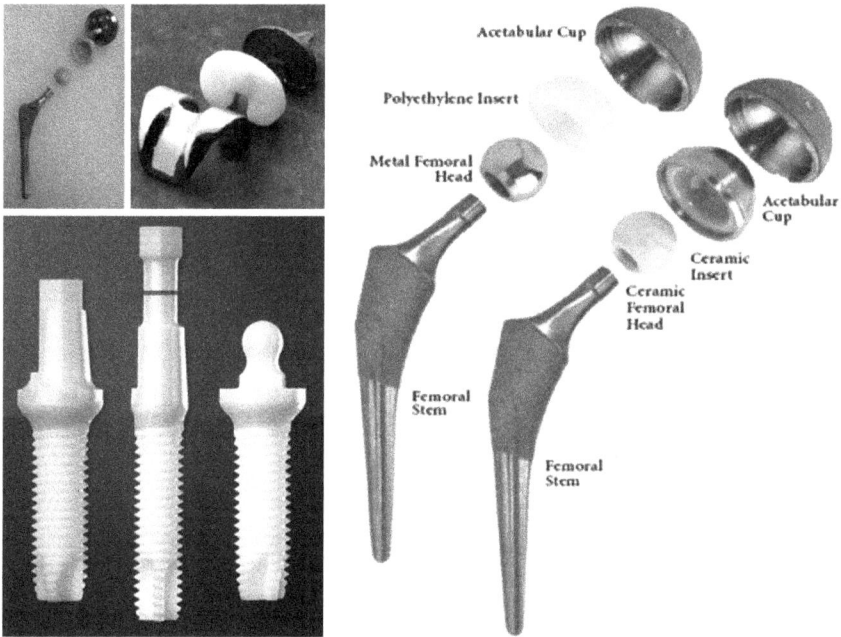

Figure 6.13: Total hip replacement implants (left-top left), total knee replacement implants (left-top right), ceramic dental implants (left-bottom) and total hip replacement component construction (right) (Farid, 2019; Popat *et al.*, 2013; hipandkneesurgery).

The ball and socket part of the implant system (e.g., acetabular cup) has several complications, including high material wear and rapid degradation in a corrosive environment (Figure 6.13). Tribology studies and developments have contributed dramatically to improved wearing surfaces by having diverse potential combinations of the head and cup material, such as "*hard on soft*" and "*hard on hard*" bearings.

a) Hard on Soft

- Metal or Ceramic with traditional polyethylene liner
- Metal or Ceramic with UHMWPE

Hard on soft bearings involving polyethylene is discussed in detail in the polymeric biomaterials chapter. Traditional polyethylene cups with metals are affected by early failures due to poor fracture resistance and early wear debris. However, when coated with Al_2O_3, the wearing rates are nearly 20 times lower on UHMWPE than metal, contributing to a decrease in debris formation.

b) Hard on Hard

- Metal on Metal Devices
- Ceramic on Ceramic Devices

In addition to the core application, alumina is also utilized as a coating material for femoral stems and porous alumina spacers. In particular, ceramic on ceramic devices, i.e., Al_2O_3-Al_2O_3 ceramic bearings in THR, have shown to have even more superior properties than Al_2O_3-UHMWPE or metal-UHMWPE, ensuing in improved wear resistance properties and avoiding toxic reaction in the body. The exceptional frictional and wear properties of Al_2O_3 ceramics are expected due to the very low surface roughness and high surface strength.

Specifically, dense Al_2O_3 (specific gravity of 3.97) has been employed widely in dental applications, explicitly for the substitution of teeth. In most cases, dental implants use single-crystal Al_2O_3 with a superior bending strength (13000 kg/cm^2) in contrast to lower bending strength polycrystalline Al_2O_3 (3500 kg/cm^2). It is because polycrystalline Al_2O_3 is prone to fracturing while implanting the material in the dental root.

6.4.2 *Zirconia*

Zirconia (ZrO_2) has become a popular substitute to Al_2O_3 owing to significantly superior fracture toughness and strength, and remarkably low wear properties. Over time, it has become one of the most extensively used inert bioceramics in the biomedical industry. ZrO_2 has a polymorphic structure (Figure 6.14) with three different crystal forms: monoclinic (below 1170°C), tetragonal (1170–2370°C), and cubic (above 2690°C).

monoclinic (1170°C)↔tetragonal (2370°C)↔cubic (2690°C)↔liquid

From Table 6.4, it can be observed that when compared to Al_2O_3, ZrO_2 has superior mechanical properties in terms of fracture toughness, tensile

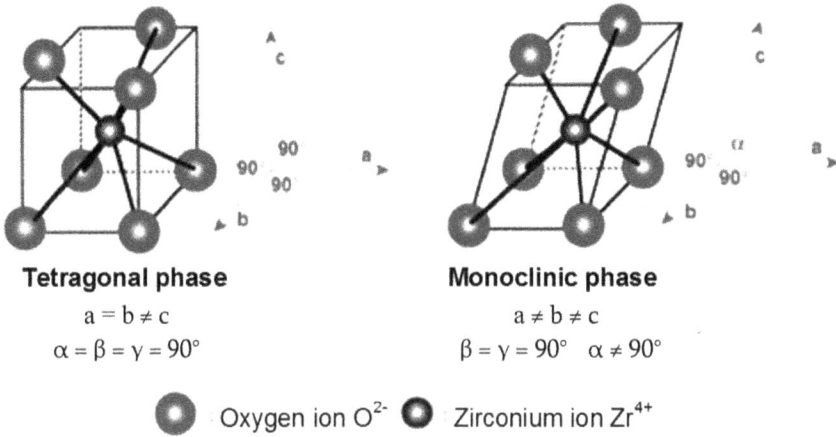

Tetragonal phase

$a = b \neq c$

$\alpha = \beta = \gamma = 90°$

Monoclinic phase

$a \neq b \neq c$

$\beta = \gamma = 90°$ $\alpha \neq 90°$

Oxygen ion O^{2-} Zirconium ion Zr^{4+}

Figure 6.14:   Tetragonal and monoclinic zirconia structures (Reclaru *et al.*, 2020).

Table 6.4:   Mechanical properties of bioceramics.

Ceramics	Density (g/cm^3)	Young's modulus (GPa)	Fracture toughness (MPa m$^{1/2}$)	Compressive strength (MPa)	Tensile strength (MPa)
Alumina	>3.97	440–500	4–5.4	4500	282–551
Zirconia	5.74–6.08	210–240	6.4–10.9	1990	810–1490
Silicon nitride	3.3	303	3.3–5.4	3720	720–1110
Hydroxyapatite (3% porosity)	–	7–13	3.05–3.15	350–450	38–48

strength, and relatively lower Young's modulus. Above all, ZrO_2 demonstrates a unique transformation toughening mechanism that resists cracking propagation. At low temperatures, the stable phase of pure ZrO_2 is monoclinic, but the tetragonal phase is often obtained before the formation of the monoclinic phase. Due to the detrimental extreme monoclinic-tetragonal phase transition, pure ZrO_2 is not used for biomedical applications. The phase transition induces shape and volume changes and may result in structural deterioration and cracking. This instability of phases in ZrO_2 is mainly caused by either mechanical or chemical energy, or by aging. However, the incorporation of stabilizers such as magnesia

(MgO), yttria (Y_2O_3), calcia (CaO) or other rare-earth metal oxides limits the phase transformation and facilitates transformation toughening. Therefore, partially stabilized zirconia (PSZ), a blend of cubic and tetragonal and/or monoclinic phases, yttria-stabilized zirconia (Y_2O_3-ZrO_2) and tetragonal zirconia polycrystals (TZP) are extensively exploited for biomedical applications. Y_2O_3 is included in ZrO_2 to stabilize the tetragonal or cubic phase and to prevent conversion back to the monoclinic phase. Table 6.5 presents different types of ZrO_2 ceramic systems and their applications in the biomedical industry.

Additionally, ZrO_2 has a high affinity for bone tissues and does not result in any potential oncogenic effect. Due to the unique transformation-toughening mechanisms functioning in their microstructures, these ceramics have found applications in total hip prostheses and dentistry, such as implant and tooth-reinforced restorations. In fact, ZrO_2 is holistic, which implies it is the only viable choice for absolute metal-free dentistry. In aesthetical terms, titanium dental implant creates a dark line around the gum, whereas ZrO_2 has a high degree of translucency, and no unattractive coloration occurs.

Table 6.5: Different types of ZrO_2 ceramic systems and their biomedical applications.

ZrO_2 system	Abbreviation	Description	Biomedical applications
Fully stabilized zirconia	FSZ	100% cubic; ZrO_2 combined with about 10 mol% of CaO, MgO or Y_2O_3 to retain cubic structure at room temperature	Oxygen sensors and solid oxide fuel cells (SOFC)
Partially stabilized zirconia	PSZ	Cubic ZrO_2 matrix with a dispersion of tetragonal precipitates	Dental applications
Tetragonal zirconia polycrystals	TZP	ZrO_2 stabilized with 3 mol% of Y_2O_3	Dental crowns
Yttrium cation-doped tetragonal zirconia polycrystals	Y-TZP	Y_2O_3 is substituted in the range of 2–3 mol% Y_2O_3–ZrO_2 (2–3Y-TZP)	Dental frameworks
Zirconia-toughened alumina	ZTA	Al_2O_3-x ZrO_2 (x = 1.5–20 vol%); ZrO_2 particles are placed among alumina particles	Hip implants

6.5 Bioresorbable ceramics

6.5.1 *Calcium phosphate ceramics*

For hard tissue engineering, especially bone fracture healing, bone repair, and bone augmentation, it involves a diligent structural stabilization strategy. In addition to well-known casting and forged metals, bone-implant interfaces can also be treated using stable consolidated ceramics.

Calcium phosphates (CaP) are of particular importance to the human body as they are the most important inorganic constituent of bones and teeth (Table 6.6). Because of chemical and structural similarity with biological apatite, CaP ceramics have strong potential for application as biomaterials. Comparatively, these materials can be synthesized economically and have exceptional biological properties, such as biocompatibility, osteoconductivity, and bioresorbability, thus allowing high bone integration with living tissues. However, owing to their weak mechanical properties (very brittle and low fatigue resistance), CaPs are mostly limited to fillers for treatments such as skull-maxillofacial and bone defect reconstructions. Several different types of CaP exist with different Ca/P ratios (Table 6.3). These different CaPs can be formulated by combining Ca and P solutions under acidic or basic conditions. Because of their high solubility, complexes with a Ca/P ratio less than 1 are not considered as appropriate materials for biological implantation. Many CaP ceramics exhibit distinct differences in their chemical and structural compositions. However, only certain ceramics have an identical composition with the original bone mineral. The most commonly used bioresorbable

Table 6.6: Comparative composition of inorganic minerals in adult humans with respect to HA (Al-Sanabani *et al.*, 2013; Dorozhkin, 2015; Shanmugam *et al.*, 2018).

Composition (wt%)	Enamel	Dentine	Bone	HA
Calcium	36.5	35.1	34.8	39.6
Phosphorous	17.1	16.9	15.2	18.5
Ca/P ratio	1.63	1.61	1.71	1.67
Total inorganic	97	70	65	100
Total organic	1.5	20	25	—
Water	1.5	10	10	—

bioceramics based on CaP in medical applications are β-tricalcium phosphates.

6.5.1.1 *Tricalcium phosphate*

Tricalcium phosphate (TCP; $Ca_3(PO_4)_2$), with a Ca/P ratio of 1.5, is one of the widely studied CaP ceramics along with HA. TCP has two polymorphs, namely α-TCP and β-TCP. Even though they have identical chemical compositions, they are distinguishable by the crystal structure, solubility, physical, and chemical properties. Both polymorphs of TCP can be synthesized only at high temperatures. Therefore, under normal conditions, it is difficult to precipitate TCP from low-temperature aqueous solutions.

- α-TCP has a monoclinic crystal structure and is synthesized at 1125°C or higher.
- β-TCP has a rhombohedral crystal structure and is synthesized at 900–1100°C.

β-TCP is the most broadly used phase in bone tissue engineering applications due to low-temperature synthesis (relative to α-TCP), balanced stable structure, and a superior biodegradation rate. Due to these properties, β-TCP is extensively studied for bone regeneration and commonly employed in bone cements and substitution. When compared to HA, β-TCP has low stability but has a rapid degradation rate and better solubility. β-TCP can be synthesized directly above 800°C by thermal decomposition of CDHA or by solid-state interaction of acidic calcium orthophosphates. In an ideal scenario, natural tissue is slowly resorbed and replaced by an implanted biodegradable material over a period.

Nevertheless, a major challenge in these circumstances is balancing the resorption rate of the implant material with that of the bone tissue's predicted regeneration. The biodegradable implant may not fulfil its purpose if the resorption rate is too high. TCP with Ca/P ratio of 1.5 is more quickly resorbed than HA with Ca/P ratio of 1.67. Due to this, biphasic calcium phosphate materials with a combination of HA and β-TCP were developed in order to potentially exploit the exceptional characteristics of more soluble TCP and more stable HA. These tailored chemical properties varying the ratio of HA/β-TCP have several applications in bone grafts, bone substitute materials, and dental materials.

α-TCP is a high-temperature phase, formed by the transformation of β-TCP at temperatures above ~1125°C. Chemically pure α-TCP is of little significance for biomedical applications due to a faster resorption rate than the bone.

6.6 Multiple choice questions

1. Ceramic head is favoured over metal head against the UHMWPE acetabular cup because of
   (a) longer lifetimes and lower wear rates
   (b) high melting temperatures
   (c) brittleness
   (d) none of the above

2. Which type of atomic bonding characterizes the ceramics?
   (a) covalent bonding
   (b) ionic bonding and metallic bonding
   (c) covalent and ionic bonding
   (d) metallic bonding

3. Which of the following is TRUE regarding characteristic properties of ceramic materials?
   (a) high-temperature stability; high mechanical strength; low elongation; low hardness
   (b) high-temperature stability; high mechanical strength; low elongation; high hardness
   (c) low-temperature stability; high mechanical strength; high elongation; low hardness
   (d) low-temperature stability; low mechanical strength; high elongation; high hardness

4. Which of the following is NOT true of crystalline solids?
   (a) they have long-range and short-range order
   (b) they contain a repeating pattern of atoms or ions or molecules
   (c) they contain a random arrangement of constituents
   (d) they have well-defined melting points

5. Which type of material, with example, upon placement in the human body starts to dissolve slowly and is replaced by advancing tissue?
   (a) bioinert; alumina
   (b) bioactive; hydroxyapatite
   (c) bioresorbable; tricalcium phosphate
   (d) bioinert; tricalcium phosphate

6. Which type of material, with example, has minimal interaction with surrounding tissue?
   (a) bioinert; alumina
   (b) all biomaterials
   (c) bioresorbable; tricalcium phosphate
   (d) bioinert; tricalcium phosphate

7. Which of the following classes of bioinert materials is used as coating component on metallic biomaterials to enhance biological properties?
   (a) bioceramics
   (b) biopolymers
   (c) titanium
   (d) particulate suspension

8. During sintering, densification is not due to
   (a) atomic diffusion
   (b) surface diffusion
   (c) bulk diffusion
   (d) grain growth

9. Which of the following is TRUE about biodegradation of bioceramic bone fillers?
   (a) biodegradation of the component should match the healing rate of the bone
   (b) the component can degrade faster irrespective of healing
   (c) no relation between biodegradation and bone healing
   (d) faster biodegradation of components will help bone to heal faster

10. Which of the following is/are NOT true about bioglass?
    I. carbonate-substituted hydroxyapatite enhances bioactivity and biocompatibility
    II. thin oxide layer of TiO_2 is formed on the substrate
    III. the rate of ion release from the bioglass surface is determined by the Ca:P ratio
    IV. bioglass composition and microstructure do not have any role in determining bioactivity
    (a) only I and III
    (b) only III
    (c) only II and IV
    (d) only I, II and IV

11. Which of the following is/are TRUE regarding HCA of bioglass?
    I. HCA enhances bioactivity and biocompatibility
    II. HCA crystals provide a base for adsorption of components of ECM
    III. HCA crystals improve the melting temperature of bioglass
    IV. HCA crystals facilitate chemical bonding with neighbouring bone
    (a) only I and II
    (b) all of the above
    (c) only I, III and IV
    (d) only I, II, and IV

12. Which of the following is/are NOT true about hydroxyapatite?
    I. used in bone tissue engineering owing to its chemical similarity to the mineral of bone
    II. cannot be used in bone repair due to low melting point
    III. also used as a coating material on metallic implants to improve bioactive properties
    IV. does not have any effect on improving osseointegration
    (a) only III and IV
    (b) only I, II and IV
    (c) only I and II
    (d) only II and IV

13. An example of amorphous material is
    (a) glass
    (b) zinc
    (c) carbon
    (d) iron

14. Select the TRUE statement(s) about hydroxyapatite phase.
    (a) it has low solubility under physiological conditions (pH 7.4)
    (b) it has high solubility under physiological conditions (pH 7.4)
    (c) it has higher dissolution in acidic conditions (pH 6.5)
    (d) it has lower dissolution in acidic conditions (pH 6.5)

15. Select the TRUE statement(s) about effect of the crystallinity of hydroxyapatite.
    (a) has an influence on solubility
    (b) does not have an influence on solubility
    (c) affects protein adsorption
    (d) does not have an effect on protein adsorption

References & Further Reading

Al-Sanabani, J. S., Madfa, A. A., & Al-Sanabani, F. A. (2013). Application of calcium phosphate materials in dentistry. *International Journal of Biomaterials, 2013*, 876132. doi:10.1155/2013/876132.

Cai, Z.-Y., Peng, F., Zi, Y.-P., Chen, F., *et al.* (2015). Microwave-assisted hydrothermal rapid synthesis of calcium phosphates: Structural control and application in protein adsorption. *Nanomaterials, 5*(3), 1284–1296. doi:10.3390/nano5031284.

Dorozhkin, S. V. (2015). Calcium orthophosphate bioceramics. *Ceramics International, 41*(10, Part B), 13913–13966. doi:10.1016/j.ceramint.2015.08.004.

Farid, S. B. H. (2019). Chapter 2 — Structure, microstructure, and properties of bioceramics. In S. B. H. Farid (Ed.), *Bioceramics: For Materials Science and Engineering* (pp. 39–76): Woodhead Publishing.

Gul, H., Khan, M., & Khan, A. S. (2020). Chapter 3 — Bioceramics: Types and clinical applications. In A. S. Khan & A. A. Chaudhry (Eds.), *Handbook of Ionic Substituted Hydroxyapatites* (pp. 53–83): Woodhead Publishing.

Jones, J. R. (2008). Chapter 12 — Bioactive glass. In T. Kokubo (Ed.), *Bioceramics and their Clinical Applications* (pp. 266–283): Woodhead Publishing.

Ma, X., Chen, Y., Qian, J., Yuan, Y., *et al.* (2016). Controllable synthesis of spherical hydroxyapatite nanoparticles using inverse microemulsion method. *Materials Chemistry and Physics, 183*, 220–229. doi:10.1016/j.matchemphys.2016.08.021.

Mala, R., & Ruby Celsia, A. S. (2018). Chapter 8 — Bioceramics in orthopaedics: A review. In S. Thomas, P. Balakrishnan, & M. S. Sreekala (Eds.), *Fundamental Biomaterials: Ceramics* (pp. 195–221): Woodhead Publishing.

Mary, I. R., Sonia, S., Viji, S., Mangalaraj, D., *et al.* (2016). Novel multiform morphologies of hydroxyapatite: Synthesis and growth mechanism. *Applied Surface Science, 361*, 25–32. doi:10.1016/j.apsusc.2015.11.123.

Mondal, S., Hoang, G., Manivasagan, P., Moorthy, M. S., *et al.* (2018). Nano-hydroxyapatite bioactive glass composite scaffold with enhanced mechanical and biological performance for tissue engineering application. *Ceramics International, 44*(13), 15735–15746. doi:10.1016/j.ceramint.2018.05.248.

Naik, K. S. (2019). Chapter 25 — Advanced bioceramics. In S. N. Meena & M. M. Naik (Eds.), *Advances in Biological Science Research* (pp. 411–417): Academic Press.

Popat, K. C., & Desai, T. A. (2013). Chapter B — Alumina. In B. D. Ratner, A. S. Hoffman, F. J. Schoen, & J. E. Lemons (Eds.), *Biomaterials Science (Third Edition)* (pp. 162–166): Academic Press.

Reclaru, L., Ardelean, L. C., Miu, C. A., & Grecu, A. F. (2020). Are zirconia bioceramics and ceramics intended to come in contact with skin inert? *materials, 13*(7), 1697. doi:10.3390/ma13071697.

Renno, A. C. M., Bossini, P. S., Crovace, M. C., Rodrigues, A. C. M., *et al.* (2013). Characterization and *in vivo* biological performance of biosilicate. *BioMed Research International, 2013*, 141427. doi:10.1155/2013/141427.

Rujitanapanich, S., Kumpapan, P., & Wanjanoi, P. (2014). Synthesis of hydroxyapatite from oyster shell via precipitation. *Energy Procedia, 56*, 112–117. doi:10.1016/j.egypro.2014.07.138.

Sadat-Shojai, M., Khorasani, M.-T., Dinpanah-Khoshdargi, E., & Jamshidi, A. (2013). Synthesis methods for nanosized hydroxyapatite with diverse structures. *Acta Biomaterialia, 9*(8), 7591–7621. doi:10.1016/j.actbio.2013.04.012.

Shanmugam, K., & Sahadevan, R. (2018). Chapter 1 — Bioceramics — An introductory overview. In S. Thomas, P. Balakrishnan, & M. S. Sreekala (Eds.), *Fundamental Biomaterials: Ceramics* (pp. 1–46): Woodhead Publishing.

Chapter 7
Metallic biomaterials

7.1 Introduction

Human beings are able to perform daily activities because of the flexibility of joints. However, the movement of joints or bones can be severely impaired by accidents and diseases such as osteoarthritis (inflammation in joints) and osteoporosis (brittleness in bones) associated with general aging. These traumas, diseases or geometrical abnormalities cause pain and discomfort for performing daily activities. Via internal or external fixations, bone fractures or inflammations may be stabilized, mechanical integrity can be restored to an acceptable level, and the quality of life can be improved. Metallic implants that are commonly used for biomedical applications are shown in Figure 7.1. These implants aid in the replacement of diseased/damaged tissues, and also assist in healing, improving function, correcting functional abnormalities and cosmetic problems, and facilitating diagnosis and medical treatments.

Metallic implant production has been largely inspired by demands for bone repair, typically long bones with internal fractures. They are predominantly used in load-bearing parts, to assist the body weight on bones and joints and facilitate the rebuilding of tissues. The various kinds of conventional metallic implant procedures are shown in Table 7.1. Metallic materials usually have high elastic modulus, and sufficient yield points to bear heavy loads without any substantial elastic and permanent deformation. Unlike ceramics, metals have ductile properties, which implies that surpassing the yield point generates a plastic deformation instead of sudden brittle fracture. Metals also benefit from adequate plasticity and thus have high fatigue endurance limits. These properties have

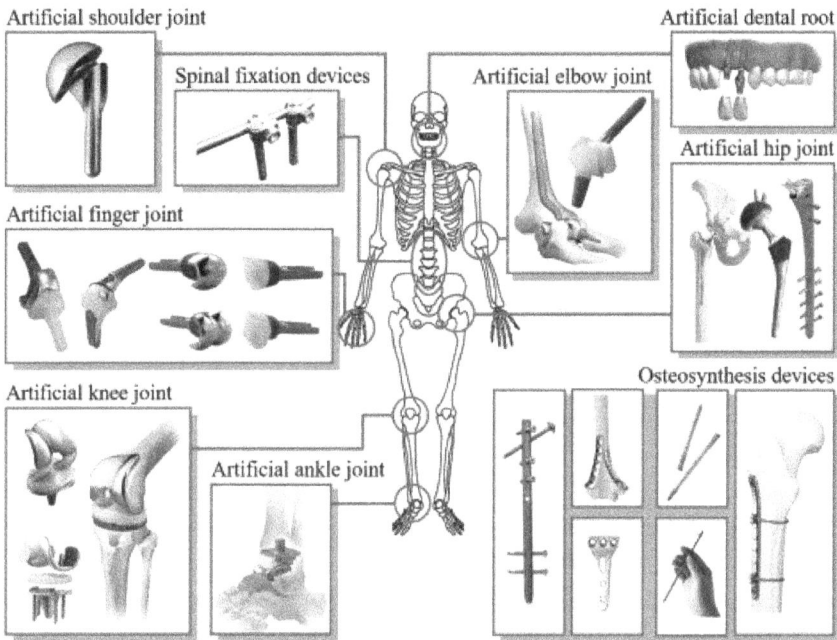

Figure 7.1: Various metallic implants used in orthopaedic surgery and dentistry (Nakano, 2019).

Table 7.1: Various kinds of conventional metallic implant procedures. The corresponding images are presented in Figure 7.2.

Procedure	Summary
Fixation of a bone	Also termed as osteosynthesis, this is a surgical procedure for restoration or stabilization of bones by joining the ends of fractured/broken parts with screws, plates, nails, and pins. It is a widely acknowledged practice to achieve bone healing.
Total joint replacement	Total joint replacement is a surgical procedure that replaces damaged or diseased parts of a joint with a metal device known as prosthesis. It aids in the eradication of discomfort and rebuilding of normal function without any limitations. Hips and knees are replaced most often. Apart from metals, polymers, ceramics, or a combination of these materials, they can also be used to enhance the implant's longevity.

(Continued)

Table 7.1: (*Continued*)

Procedure	Summary
Vascular and functional devices	Stents; pacemakers or cochlear implants
Modular tumor implants	Modular tumor prosthesis is used for segmental bone and joint replacement. It is frequently applied for femur and tibia.
Spine implants	Spinal implants are devices used primarily for rectifying abnormalities like scoliosis and kyphosis and to treat degenerative diseases like spondylolisthesis. These devices are also used to stabilize and strengthen the spine and facilitate the fusion of two vertebrae.

facilitated metallic materials to become the most desirable biomaterial for load-bearing applications, thereby permitting corrective measures prior to the serious loss of mechanical integrity.

In accordance with the fundamental definition, materials that are bonded via metallic bonds are primarily labelled as metals. Metallic materials are inorganic substances, which include alloys and pure elements, ferrous and non-ferrous metals. While about 80% of the elements in the periodic table are metals, very few are being used in clinical applications because of their inadequate biocompatibility caused by corrosion and wear. Nevertheless, metallic biomaterials (metals and alloys) are amongst the extensively used materials for hard tissue engineering applications. It is due to their outstanding mechanical (high fatigue strength, high mechanical loading, high tensile strength, and fracture resistance), physical, and chemical (corrosion resistance) properties. For load-bearing applications, these properties make metallic materials superior to polymers and ceramics. They are most often used to reconstruct failed hard tissues such as orthopaedic implants (hip and knee prostheses), fracture fixations (wires, pins, screws, and plates), maxillofacial reconstructions, dental implants, and cardiovascular interventions (Figure 7.2 and Table 7.2). The following properties are usually expected in metals designed for biological applications:

- excellent mechanical properties (i.e., fracture toughness, fatigue strength, ductility, and yield strength)

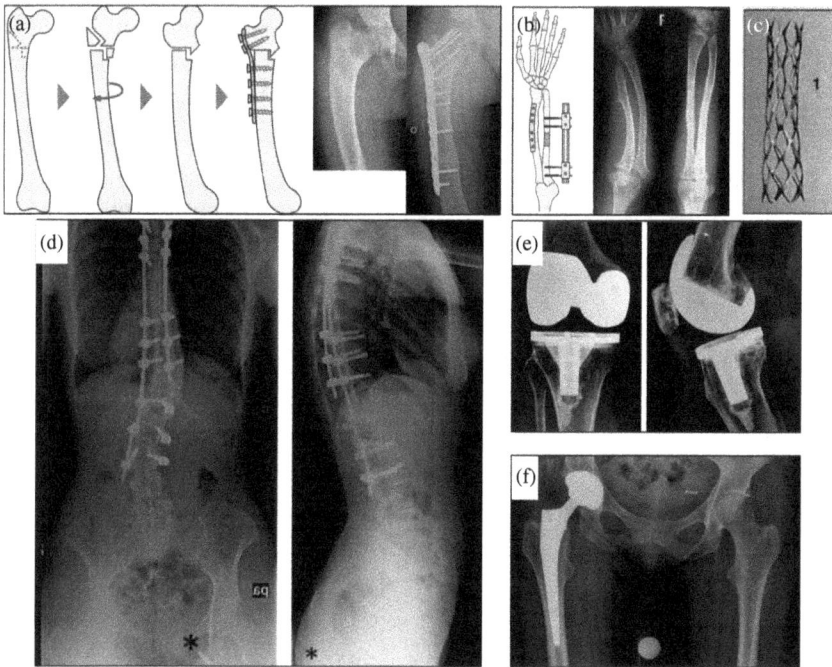

Figure 7.2: (a) Bone internal fixation with corresponding X-ray image; (b) hand internal and external fixation with corresponding X-ray image; (c) stent; X-ray images of (d) spine fixation; (e) total knee replacement; and (f) total hip replacement (Dailey *et al.*, 2015; Geavlete *et al.*, 2016; Loughenbury *et al.*, 2018; Matsubara *et al.*, 2019; Mullaji *et al.*, 2015).

Table 7.2: Applications of metallic biomaterials.

System	Application	Metallic biomaterials
Skeletal system	Joint replacements (hip and knee prostheses)	Titanium, stainless steel, Co-Cr alloys
	Fracture fixation (wires, pins, screws, and plates)	Almost all bio-metals
	Dental implants	Titanium
Cardiovascular system	Heart valve	Dacron, carbon, metal
	Pacemaker	Titanium in combination with polyurethane
	Implantable defibrillator	Titanium in combination with polyurethane
	Stent	Stainless steel and degradable Mg alloys
Organs	Heart assist device	Titanium and stainless steel in combination with polyurethane

- high biocompatibility (i.e., negligible long-term toxicity to the host locally or at systemic level)
- high corrosion and wear resistance (i.e., excellent long-term stability and no circulation of any toxic metal ions or wear fragments into the biological medium)
- appropriate osseointegration (i.e., able to integrate positively with adjacent bones, if needed)

To attain these properties, often pure metals are used. However, alloys (metals that contain two or more elements) can enhance material properties, including biocompatibility, strength, and resistance to wear and corrosion. They are produced by merging two or more metallic materials using various processing methods, such as casting or forging. The various metallic implant materials commonly considered and used in the biomedical field are tabulated in Table 7.3 with their individual mechanical properties.

Key metallic biomaterials

- Stainless steel (SS316 and SS316L, L denotes low carbon content)
- Titanium and its alloys (α, $\alpha + \beta$, and β)
- Cobalt-chromium and cobalt-chromium-molybdenum alloys
- Magnesium alloys
- Tantalum alloys

Table 7.3: Comparison of mechanical properties of metallic biomaterials.

Material	Young's modulus (GPa)	Yield strength (MPa)	Tensile strength (MPa)	Fatigue limit (MPa)
Stainless steel	189	220–1212	585–1350	242–821
Co-Cr alloys	211–250	441–1605	654–1895	207–948
Titanium	112	484	758	302
Ti-6Al-4V	112	894–1031	963–1102	619
Magnesium	41–45	—	—	—
Cortical bone	15–35	32–69	72–152	—

The earliest metallic components to be used successfully in orthopaedic applications were stainless steel and Co-Cr alloys, whereas Ti and its alloys were established later in the late 1940s. It is noteworthy to mention that most materials, except Mg and Ta alloys, were originally designed and developed for specific commercial reasons and only later introduced for biomedical applications owing to their favourable biological properties. Also, all these metals and their alloys can be manufactured effortlessly with conventional (turning, milling, drilling, grinding, forging, pressing, etc.) and unconventional (sintering, laser cutting, net-shape technology) methods.

7.2 Wolff's Law: Stress shielding

Before understanding the various kinds of metallic biomaterials employed in the human body, it is important to realize the importance of the bone-implant mechanical interface. A bone is in a constant state of flux that remodels its micro- and macro-structure accordingly in response to the loads applied throughout its life. This is achieved by means of a subtle balance between the osteogenic (bone-forming) and osteoclastic (bone-removing) processes. By altering the balance between osteogenesis and osteoclasis, bones can adapt to a new mechanical environment. For example, as presented in Figure 7.3, in its natural condition a femur bears all

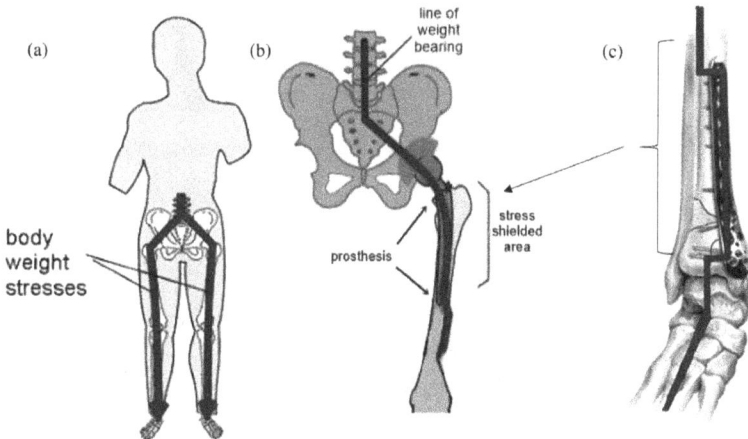

Figure 7.3: (a) Loads from the body weight on the lower limb skeleton; (b) stress shielding in hip prosthesis (Copyright © HB Valdemar Surin, 2005); (c) stress shielding in locking compression plate fixing fractures in distal tibia (Salahshoor *et al.*, 2011). The blue lines represent the transmission paths of the loads (Arifin *et al.*, 2014).

external (hip joint and muscle) loads by itself. An internal fixation surgical procedure is performed due to disease or accident, and the femur is supplied with an intramedullary stem. Now the femur shares the load-carrying capacity with the implant. Where one structure, the bone, had carried all the load at the beginning (before surgery), now the load is being shared by the stem and the bone (after surgery). As a result, the bone is now subjected to reduced stresses, and is stress shielded. The stiffness mismatch between the implant and the bone can persist in causing the implant to receive most of the stress and leads to a phenomenon known as stress shielding.

In simple terms, stress shielding is a biomechanical phenomenon where there is a decrease in bone density, bone strength, or rigidity around the implant due to the withdrawal of typical stress from the bone by an external implant. This situation commonly happens when the implant material has a higher elastic modulus than the associated bone. Elastic modulus and ultimate tensile strength of bone in comparison with common metallic implant materials are presented in Figure 7.4. Wolff's Law

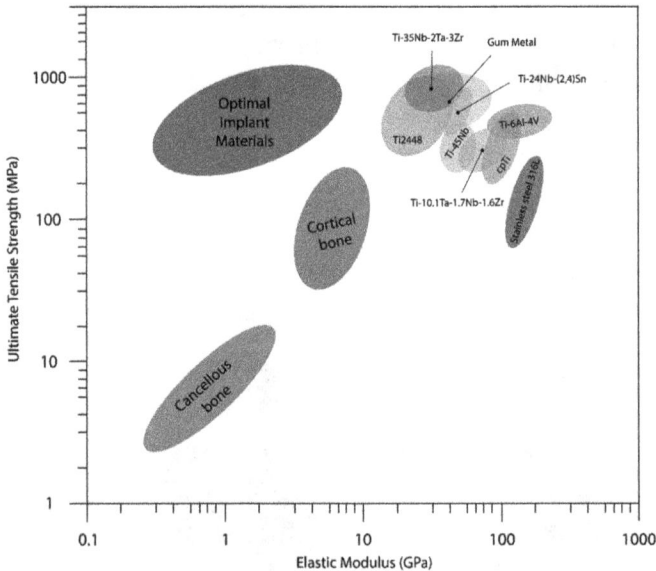

Figure 7.4: Elastic modulus and ultimate tensile strength of bone in comparison with common metallic implant materials (Li *et al.*, 2020).

dictates that the density of bone is reliant on the stress condition. The significant decrease of stress compared with the natural situation causes the bone to adapt to the changing mechanical environment by decreasing its mass, either by converting itself to become more porous (internal remodeling) or by becoming depleted (external remodeling). This phenomenon of resorption causes or contributes to the failure of the fixation and loosening of implants.

7.3 Stainless steel

Stainless steel (SS), a special type of steel alloy, belongs to iron-based alloys, and has the longest record of practical usage in the biomedical industry. Since the 1800s, steel alloys made from iron and carbon were used as surgical instruments. Depending on the individual quantities of nickel (Ni) and chromium (Cr) and their crystal phases, there are several alloys which are part of the SS group, including martensitic (Fe–Cr system), ferritic (Fe–Cr system), austenitic (Fe–Cr–Ni system), duplex and precipitation-hardening SS. These different types of SS have different properties, and microstructures can be precisely produced by adjusting the steel chemistry.

- **Austenitic SS:** face-centered cubic and non-magnetic
- **Martensitic SS:** magnetic
- **Ferrite SS:** body-centered cubic and magnetic
- **Duplex SS:** mixed microstructure comprising ferrite and austenite phases

However, only austenitic SS (AISI 316L, ASTM F-55, and F-138) with low carbon content (Table 7.4) is commonly used for biomedical applications. SS contains at least 10.5% Cr and varying alloying elements such as Ni, molybdenum (Mo), copper (Cu), manganese (Mn), silicon (Si), nitrogen (N), etc. Typical chemical compositions of medical-grade SS are presented in Table 7.4. The Cr present in SS has a high affinity for oxygen, allowing the development of an inert Cr-rich oxide film with approximately 3 nm thickness. This thin oxide layer is responsible for endorsing self-healing by accelerating passivation. Mo

Table 7.4:   Comparison of different properties of stainless steel.

Alloy	Fe	Cr	Ni	Mo	Mn	Si	S	C	P
						Composition			
SS302	Balance	17.0–19.0	8.0–10.0	—	≤2.00	0.75–1.00	≤0.030	≤0.15	≤0.045
SS316	Balance	16.0–18.0	10.0–14.0	2.0–3.0	≤2.00	≤0.75	≤0.030	≤0.08	≤0.045
SS316L	Balance	16.0–18.0	10.0–14.0	2.0–3.0	≤2.00	≤0.75	≤0.030	≤0.03	≤0.045

promotes passive film stability and enhances resistance against pitting corrosion in chloride solutions while Mg and Si improve machinability. Mn strengths the required austenitic phase, improves the solubility of N, and reduces the magnetic susceptibility. The presence of N stabilizes the austenitic phase of Fe at room temperature, whereas Ni is responsible for increasing strength and hardness without losing ductility and toughness. SS alloys can be casted (hot liquid metal poured into a mold), forged (forming and shaping metals) or strengthened by cold-working.

Since 1926, due to its superior resistance to various corrosive agents, ductility, cost, high hardness values, and relative ease of fabrication, SS has been primarily used in orthopaedic implants such as joint replacements and plates screws, pins, rods, coronary stents, and surgical instruments. SS shows a mild to high elastic modulus and tensile strength among the metals used in orthopaedics. Furthermore, it has strong ductility, which makes it easy to be machined into desired shapes.

Important terms and definitions

Crevice corrosion: This refers to corrosion that occurs in a confined area, to which the underlying fluid has restricted access.

Pitting corrosion: This refers to a form of extremely concentrated corrosion that leads to the formation of small holes in metals.

Deacetylation: This is the reverse reaction of acetylation, where an acetyl group is disconnected from a molecule.

Osteoconductive: This refers to the property of a material that allows for possible integration of the new bone with the host bone.

7.3.1 *SS 316L*

The design of type 316L SS is mainly established via modifying type 302 SS by adding an additional element of Mo (2.0–3.0%) to improve corrosive resistance, increasing Ni composition from 8.0–10.0% to 10.0–14.0%, and decreasing C composition to less than or equal to 0.030%. Medical-grade SS 316L ('L' implies low carbon content where C $\leq$ 0.030%) is currently the most commonly used SS type (Table 7.4) for load-bearing applications. SS 316L has sufficient biocompatibility and density to withstand loads which makes it an acceptable surgical-implant material. This class of SS is non-magnetic and has a greater resistance to corrosion than any other steel alloy. The most common locations for SS 316L are concentrated on fracture fixation plates, femoral intramedullary stabilization rods, screws, and other cohesive fixtures tied to predominantly orthopedic structures.

Even though Ni is responsible for increasing the strength and hardness and maintaining the austenite microstructure's stability, it is highly associated with metal allergy. When alloyed beyond biological limits and even slightly less than it, Ni shows cytotoxic behaviour, haemolytic behaviour in fine particulate form (destruction of red blood cells), genotoxicity (damaging the genetic information), carcinogenicity (inducement of tumors), and potential mutagenicity. As a result, nickel-free austenitic stainless steels with high N content are being researched over the past few decades. Commercially available CarTech® BioDur® 108 is such alloy, which contains less than 0.05% Ni content. Overall, irrespective of their excellent properties for orthopaedic applications, SS implants also experience significant drawbacks such as:

- the difference in Young's modulus between the implant and bone (190 GPa vs. 15–35 GPa for cortical bone, and 1–3 GPa for cancellous bone), which may trigger stress shielding,
- the high specific weight of metals,
- relative lower strength,
- relatively poor wear resistance, and
- the inability to absorb X-rays.

Also, clinical applications have shown that SS-passivated surfaces release an appreciably large concentration of metallic ions into the biological medium which may negatively influence surrounding tissues in the long term.

Key points

Stainless steels

- 316L alloy, i.e., Mo-containing and low-carbon content SS are used for implant applications. The important alloy additions are:
  - Ni stabilizes the austenitic microstructure of steel but is susceptible to allergic reactions.
  - Cr generates thin passivating oxide layer.
  - Mo has a positive effect on pitting and crevice corrosion resistance.
- Very high Young's modulus — can cause stress shielding.

7.4 Cobalt-chromium alloys

Since the 1900s, Co-based alloys, the second-generation implant metals, have demonstrated outstanding wear resistance and surface hardness that supplemented SS in hard tissue engineering. These alloys are widely studied and developed for artificial knee and hip joints, such as femoral component in total knee replacement and femoral head in total hip replacement (Figure 7.5).

Back in the 1930s, alloys based on Co were first established for dental applications. The Co-Cr-Mo critical alloy (Vitallium) was employed

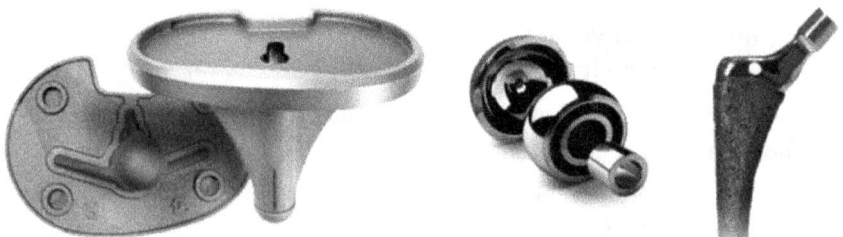

Figure 7.5: Components of artificial hips and knees manufactured from the Co–Cr superalloy (Image courtesy Zimmer Biomet).

initially as a cast dental alloy and eventually tailored to fit for orthopaedic treatments in the 1940s. The improved wear resistance (higher than SS and even Ti-based alloys) has made it possible to use Co-based implants for artificial hip joints where wear can result from direct close contact between the bone plate and the femoral head. These alloys demonstrate exceptionally high resistance to corrosion even in Cl environments owing to the instinctive development of a passive layer of chromium oxide (Cr_2O_3) in the human body. When compared with SS, Co-based alloys exhibit a superior balance between mechanical properties and biocompatibility. Co-Cr alloys which are commonly used for hip and knee replacements can be predominantly categorized into two groups: (i) Co-Cr-Mo alloys; and (ii) Co-Ni-Cr-Mo alloys.

Co-Cr alloys with Mo

- ASTM F75: Co-28Cr-6Mo, a casting alloy, has been broadly employed in the manufacture of femoral stems.
- ASTM F799: Co-28Cr-6Mo, a thermodynamically processed alloy, has a similar chemical configuration to F75 but is hot-forged after casting to increase mechanical properties.

Co-Cr alloys with Ni

- ASTM F90: Co-20Cr-15W-10Ni, a wrought alloy, possesses high strength and corrosion resistance making it suitable for surgical implant and stent applications.
- ASTM F562: Co-35Ni-20Cr-10Mo, a wrought alloy, is used in cardiac pacing and neurostimulation lead conductor applications.

Cast F75 Co-Cr alloy has been primarily used in the stem, ball, and cup of artificial hip joints and also in the sliding components of artificial knee joints. To improve wear resistance surface properties, Co-Cr components are usually coated with UHMWPE polymer. F90 and F562 systems containing Ni as alloying part demonstrate outstanding hot/cold workability, good ductility, and formability. These features make the F90 and F562 alloys suitable for fabricating coronary stents, intracranial aneurysm clips, and orthodontic dental arch wires. The complete applications of various Co-Cr alloys are tabulated in Table 7.5.

Table 7.5: Applications of Co-Cr alloys.

ASTM Standard	Alloys (mass%)	Application
F75	Co-28Cr-6Mo	Stem, ball, and cup of artificial joints
F799	Co-28Cr-6Mo	Joint replacements (hip, knee, shoulder)
F90	Co-20Cr-15W-10Ni	Fixation wires, vascular stents, heart
F1091		valves
F562	Co-35Ni-20Cr-10Mo	Lead conductor wires, orthopaedic
F688		cables, catheters, cardiovascular
F961		stents
F1058	40Co-20Cr-16Fe-15Ni-7Mo	Arch wires, surgical clips, lead conductor wires, stents

Key points

Co-Cr alloys
- Wear resistance is higher than SS and even Ti-based alloys
- Extensively used to manufacture heads of artificial hip joints and sliding parts of artificial knee joints
- Toxicity issues with Cr and Ni

7.5 Titanium and its alloys

Compared with SS and Co-Cr alloys, the next-generation element titanium (Ti) and its alloys are comparatively new materials. Since its inception and for a variety of factors, Ti and its alloys are progressively being used as viable alternatives to SS and Co-Cr alloys for biomedical applications. Owing to the exceptional combination of properties and remarkable biocompatibility with bones, commercially pure titanium (Cp-Ti; ASTM F67), Ti-6Al-4V (ASTM 136), Ti-Nb, Ti-Ta-Nb/Zr/Sn, Ti-Zr, and Ni-Ta are some of the Ti-based alloys employed for use in hard tissue engineering. More importantly, Ti alloys are characterized by low density (4.5 g/cm^3, which is around 62 % of iron's density and nearly half of cobalt's density), good mechanical strength, and excellent corrosion resistance to body fluids.

Furthermore, the low elastic modulus of Ti (two times lower in comparison to SS and Co–Cr) tends to minimize stress shielding around implants. Apart from exceptional mechanical properties, Ti was found to be the only metallic biomaterial to be osseointegrated directly with bone. It is possibly due to the slow growth of hydrated natural titanium oxide (TiO_2) with a layer thickness of 5–20 nm on the surface of the Ti implant. It is important to note that at temperatures above 530°C the surface oxide depletes its structural continuity, radically decreasing the corrosion resistance of the material.

Ti is an allotropic element, meaning it exists in different crystallographic forms. There are two crystalline phases of Ti: a low-temperature alpha (α) phase that has a hexagonal close-packed (HCP) crystal structure, and a high-temperature beta (β) phase that has a body-centered cubic (BCC) crystal structure (Figure 7.6). This allotropic transformation from HCP to BCC crystal structure occurs at 882°C. This temperature is also known as beta transus temperature, where the β phase remains stable beyond this point up to the melting point, i.e., 1668°C.

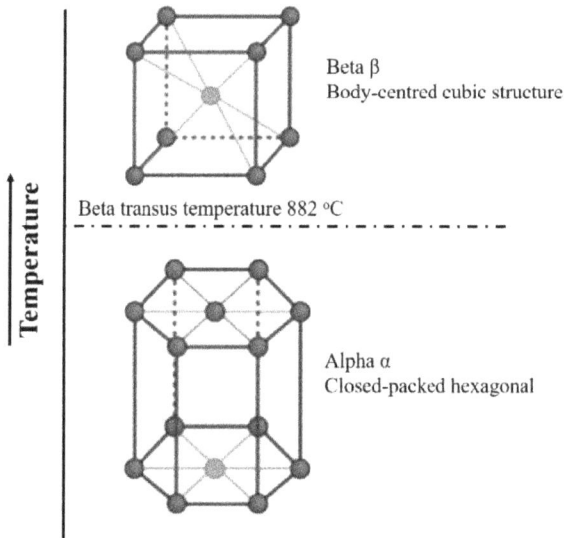

Figure 7.6: Crystal structures of titanium.

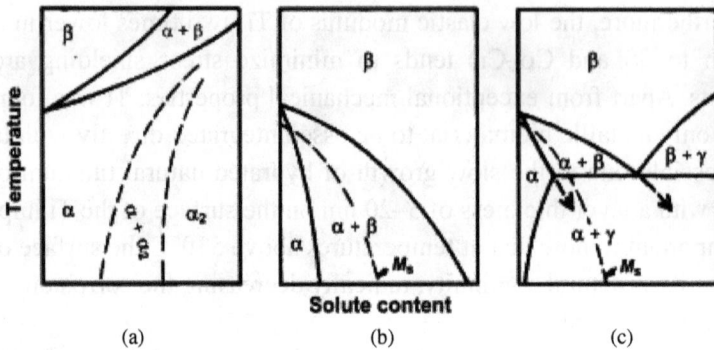

Figure 7.7:   Basic phase diagrams for Ti alloys (Polmear *et al.*, 2017).

The basic crystal structures of Ti are the basis for the classification of the three widely-recognized types as described below (Figure 7.7).

- **α type:** also known as Cp-Ti. Based on the oxygen content, Cp-Ti can be classified into four grades (grade 1 to grade 4). All four grades have an HCP crystal structure and are stable up to a temperature of 882°C.

- **$\alpha + \beta$ type:** the most common biomedical alloy under this category is Ti-6Al-4V with 6 wt.% of Al and 4 wt.% of V and an elastic modulus of 110–120 GPa.

- **β type:** these are low-modulus titanium alloys with β stabilizers consisting of V, Ta, Mo, Nb, W, Cr, Fe, Co, Ni, Cu, and Mn. These alloys are researched and developed to address the stress shielding effect.

Alloying Ti metal with other elements allows for the selective stabilization of either the HCP or BCC crystal structure at lower temperatures, facilitating the development of stable α-type Ti, $\alpha + \beta$-type Ti or β-type Ti alloys (Figure 7.7). Some of the frequent alloying elements used for stabilization of the α phase include Al, Sn, and O. In contrast, those employed to stabilize the β phase include Nb, Mo, Ta, Cr, Fe W, Cr, Si, Co, Mn, H, and V. $\alpha + \beta$ alloys are formed by metallurgically balancing amounts of both α and β stabilizers. The α stabilizers raise the α-to-β transition temperature beyond 882°C, while the β stabilizers lower the transition temperature. Al is the most commonly used alloy element to stabilize and enhance the α phase, increasing thermal stability and reducing alloy density (Figure 7.7).

7.5.1 α type

α-type Ti contains primarily α-phase at temperatures beyond 540°C. α-type Ti is essentially unalloyed material, i.e., pure Ti ($\geq$99%), which consists of various grades often classified into grades 1 to 4. These grades differ primarily in the amount of oxygen content, iron content, and interstitial elements such as C, N, and H. The O content in α-phase defines the grade, which increases significantly from $\leq$0.18% in grade 1 to $\leq$0.50% in grade 4 (Table 7.6). In fact, the small amounts of increase in O content have a substantial positive effect on yield strength (170 MPa to 480 MPa), UTS (240 MPa to 550 MPa), while the elongation at break drops from 24% to 15%. α-type Ti alloys also contain neutral alloying elements such as Sn (Table 7.6). These are weldable and non-heat-treatable.

7.5.2 $\alpha + \beta$

Two-phase $\alpha + \beta$ metastable Ti alloys comprise one or more of the α and β stabilizer elements. As mentioned earlier, $\alpha + \beta$ alloys generally blend the metallurgically equilibrated quantities of both α and β stabilizers. They are usually employed in applications where ideal concentrated properties are needed.

Table 7.6: Classification of Cp-Ti and Ti-6Al-4V alloys and their typical mechanical properties (Niinomi, 1998). YS: Yield strength; UTS: Ultimate tensile strength.

	Composition (wt%)								Mechanical Properties		
	O	Fe	H	N	C	Ti	Al	V	YS (MPa)	UTS (MPa)	Modulus (GPa)
Grade 1	$\leq$0.18	$\leq$0.2	$\leq$0.015	$\leq$0.03	$\leq$0.1	$\geq$99.5	—	—	170	240	102.7
Grade 2	$\leq$0.25	$\leq$0.3	$\leq$0.015	$\leq$0.03	$\leq$0.1	$\geq$99.2	—	—	275	344	102.7
Grade 3	$\leq$0.35	$\leq$0.3	$\leq$0.015	$\leq$0.05	$\leq$0.1	$\geq$99.1	—	—	377	440	103.4
Grade 4	$\leq$0.5	$\leq$0.3	$\leq$0.015	$\leq$0.05	$\leq$0.1	$\geq$99	—	—	480	550	104.1
Ti-6Al-4V	0.20	0.30	0.015	0.05	0.08	Balance	5.50–6.75	3.50–4.50	825–869	895–930	110–114
Ti-6Al-4V (ELI)	0.13	0.10	0.012	0.05	0.08	Balance	5.50–6.50	3.50–4.50	795–875	860–965	101–110

Table 7.7:   Melting points and densities used for alloying titanium.

Element	Melting point (°C)	Density (g/cm³)	Effect on phase stability
Ti	1668	4.506	—
V	1910	6.11	β-stabilizer
Ta	3017	16.69	β-stabilizer
Nb	2477	8.57	β-stabilizer
Al	660.32	2.70	α-stabilizer
Zr	1855	6.52	Neutral
Mo	2623	10.28	β-stabilizer
Fe	1538	7.874	β-stabilizer
Ni	1455	8.908	β-stabilizer
Co	1495	8.90	β-stabilizer
Mn	1246	7.21	β-stabilizer
W	3422	19.3	β-stabilizer
Cr	1907	7.19	β-stabilizer

The most common $\alpha + \beta$ alloy of Ti is Ti-6Al-4V (grade 5), a composition of 6% α stabilizer element Al and 4% β stabilizer element V (Table 7.7). It was originally developed for aerospace applications but is now comprehensively used as an orthopaedic implant due to its improved mechanical properties when compared to pure Ti. For biomedical applications, Ti-6Al-4V with ELI grade (grade 23), i.e., extra-low interstitial content of O, C, N, and H, is used. The reduced levels of O (lowered to 0.13%), Fe (lowered to 0.25%), and Ni (lowered to 0.03%) are demonstrated to have better biological properties and improved fracture toughness when contrasted with Ti-6Al-4V (Table 7.6). However, the gradual leaching of Al and V ions has stirred alarm about the long-term use of Ti-6Al-4V as an implant material. Normally, Al in human body accelerates acute metabolic bone disorders including osteomalacia and neurodegenerative diseases such as Alzheimer's, while V ions are vulnerable to causing cytotoxic conditions.

7.5.3 *Low-modulus β alloys*

Although Ti has a low elastic modulus in contrast with other metallic biomaterials, it is still 4–6 times higher than that of cortical bone. The elastic modulus mismatch between bone and implant still exists. Third generation β-type Ti alloys with non-toxic and non-allergenic components have been comprehensively researched and developed to match the elastic modulus between the biomaterial and adjoining bone and to remove the toxic effect of V and Al in Ti-6Al-4V alloy. These have excellent mechanical properties and high workability.

The overall composition in β alloys has more β stabilizers and less α stabilizers than $\alpha + \beta$ alloys. Ti-6Al-7Nb, Ti-5Al-2.5Fe, Ti-35Nb-5Ta-7Zr, and Ti-15Zr-4Nb-4Ta are some of the alloys developed recently. In particular, the alloy developed with Nb, Ta, and Zr as alloying elements has an elastic modulus of 48–55 GPa, which is about half of the traditional Ti-6Al-4V alloy (Figure 7.8). Nevertheless, most β Ti alloys produced are denser than the other types of Ti alloys due to the addition of higher-density alloying elements (such as Mo, Ta, Nb, Zr). Melting points and densities used for alloying Ti are presented in Table 7.7.

Ti and its alloys are most affected by their extremely low wear resistance. This adverse feature makes the material inappropriate for load-bearing articulating surfaces. Surface modification is usually performed to provide a better wear resistance property. Various surface modification techniques performed on metallic implants are discussed in detail in Chapter 9.

Overall, the biocompatibility of metals and alloys, the material's resistance to corrosion, and the impact that corrosion has on the tissue are the main

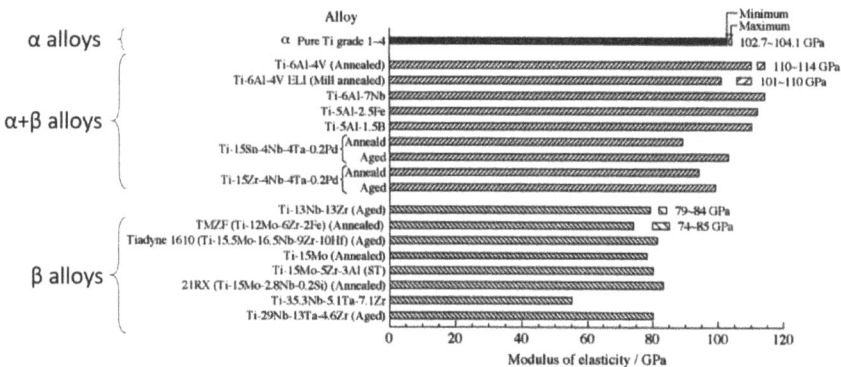

Figure 7.8:   Comparison of modulus of elasticity among α, $\alpha + \beta$, and β alloys (Niinomi, 1998).

aspects that determine the material's longevity *in vivo*. The corrosion resistance of the 316L stainless steel, Co-Cr, and Ti-based implant alloys usually depends on their passivation through a thin oxide surface layer. SS is one of those least resistant to corrosion, and never appears to be completely integrated with bone or soft tissue, so it is typically only used for temporary implants. On the other hand, Ti and Co-Cr alloys are the least corroded alloys in the body; however, over a long period of time, the metal ions gradually migrate through the oxide layer and accumulate in the tissue.

Key points

α **alloys**
- corrosion resistance, better biocompatibility
- weldability
- poor forgeability, low strength

α + *β* **alloys**
- mechanical properties can be improved by heat treatment
- leaching of Al and V ions; harmful over a long period of implantation

α **alloys**
- high hardenability and low elastic modulus
- reduce stress shielding effect
- have high density due to high-density alloy additions

7.6 Other metallic biomaterials

7.6.1 *Magnesium alloys*

As stated previously, most of the orthopaedic implants have been employed as wires, screws, pins, plates, spinal fixing, and others. The well-established orthopaedic implants discussed in previous sections tend to be severely restricted by their ion leaching, corrosion, and inadequate wear resistance. Once exposed to physiological environments, the degradation products released from these alloys possess huge human body risk. As mentioned in earlier chapters, polymers such as polyethylene, PMMA, PLGA, PLLA, collagen, and chitosan have been employed to address these issues by using them as bone cements or scaffolds. Nevertheless, due to inadequate mechanical properties, polymers are not suited well for load-bearing implant applications.

In view of this, considerable attention has been given to the development of biodegradable implants for orthopaedic and cardiovascular applications. More importantly, many modern methods were used to develop biodegradable metals instead of biodegradable polymers. Biodegradable metals are one of the desirable alternatives for the regeneration of tissues made from temporary metals for fixing of fractures. But as mentioned in section 7.2, matching the elastic modulus of the implant material to that of the neighbouring bone is one of the most critical challenges while designing a material for orthopaedic implants. As discussed, inadequate matching of the elastic modulus results in stress shielding, bone resorption, and the ultimate collapse of the implant.

Following major advances in biomaterials over the past few years, developing long-lasting metallic implants with a matching elastic modulus have become a major research area. Zn, Fe, and magnesium (Mg) are some of the best-explored biodegradable metals, used widely for cardiovascular and orthopaedic temporary implant applications.

Mg, the fourth most abundant element present in the human body, possesses properties that are very close to those of bone, and consequently can help reduce the risk of stress shielding. Mg-based biodegradable alloys hold high specific strength and also relatively lower density (1.75 g/cm^3) and elastic modulus (40 GPa), which are relatively close to that of human bones (density 1.8 g/cm^3; elastic modulus 2–20 GPa) and much lower than other well-established implant materials.

Mg-based materials are being used in manufacturing as temporary supportive structures due to their distinctive characteristic to biodegrade *in vivo* by means of surface pitting corrosion. Mg-based cardiovascular stents and fracture fixation devices such as rods, plates, and screws possess superior biocompatibility, provide superior mechanical strength needed, and slowly degrade, thus providing room for bone tissue regeneration.

Nonetheless, Mg is extremely dynamic of all engineering materials, and has a high driving force for corrosion, especially in environments full of biological fluids (Figure 7.9b). Mg-based biodegradable implants are highly corrosive due to high ionization tendency and do not form stable, protective oxide films like Ti at neutral pH. The corrosion in Mg and its alloys occurs through an electrochemical process, given as:

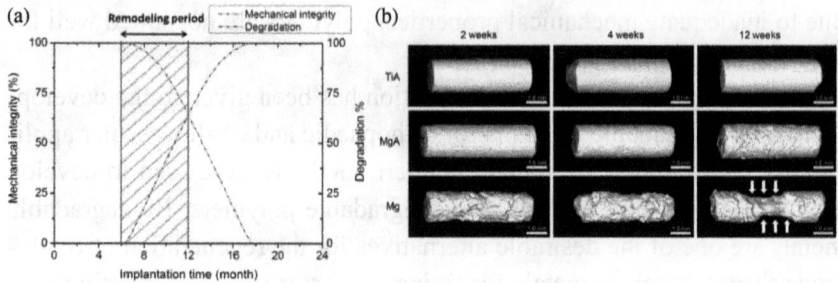

Figure 7.9:   (a) Schematic trend of mechanical integrity and degradation rate of an ideal Mg or Mg alloy; (b) micro-computed tomography data images showing degradation behaviour of Mg and Mg alloy compared with Ti alloy (Kawamura *et al.*, 2020; Mostaed *et al.*, 2019).

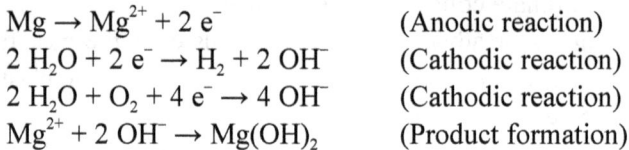

$$Mg \rightarrow Mg^{2+} + 2\ e^- \qquad \text{(Anodic reaction)}$$
$$2\ H_2O + 2\ e^- \rightarrow H_2 + 2\ OH^- \qquad \text{(Cathodic reaction)}$$
$$2\ H_2O + O_2 + 4\ e^- \rightarrow 4\ OH^- \qquad \text{(Cathodic reaction)}$$
$$Mg^{2+} + 2\ OH^- \rightarrow Mg(OH)_2 \qquad \text{(Product formation)}$$

The formed $Mg(OH)_2$ serves as a protective layer and increases its resistance against corrosion. However, the thin protective layer of $Mg(OH)_2$ breaks down under physiological conditions because of the presence of high concentrations of Cl^- ions. This reaction contributes to pitting corrosion. Corrosion mechanism of Mg in the presence of Cl^- ions is given by:

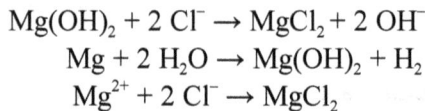

$$Mg(OH)_2 + 2\ Cl^- \rightarrow MgCl_2 + 2\ OH^-$$
$$Mg + 2\ H_2O \rightarrow Mg(OH)_2 + H_2$$
$$Mg^{2+} + 2\ Cl^- \rightarrow MgCl_2$$

Nevertheless, the degradation kinetics of Mg can be controlled via alloying such that a balance between tissue regeneration and degradation can be achieved (Figure 7.9a). Mg corrosion products are largely non-toxic and are excreted via urine with no identified destruction to the liver or kidneys. However, the rapid corrosion rate causes large amounts of Mg^{2+} ions to be released, which results in the premature loss of implant mechanical strength. In addition, hydrogen gas release from Mg-based alloys is also rapid and can lead to the formation of gas pockets around the implant.

7.6.2 *Tantalum*

Tantalum (Ta), a refractory metal, is also regarded as one of the key ortho-pedic metals due to its relatively low cytotoxicity, high resistance to cor-rosion, and excellent biocompatibility. Ta is a biologically inert material, but several studies showed that the Ta_2O_5 protective layer has the capabil-ity to augment bone in-growth under the biological environment by the development of calcium phosphate (CaP) layers. CaP boosts hard and soft tissue adhesion and increases implant longevity. Due to this unique prop-erty, Ta is used as a separate bulk material or coating material on Ti and SS bioimplants, loaning them better osseointegration properties.

Porous Ta (Figure 7.10) is chemically and electrically neutral and is beneficial for bone-tissue in-growth and enhancing implant stability through biological fixation. Foam structures are also being used as bone augmentation templates. When the Ta metal is made porous, its Young's modulus reduces drastically from ~185 GPa to ~3 GPa, a value close to that of subchondral bone. For orthopaedic applications, Ta with pore sizes in the range of 400–600 μm results in 75–85% porosity, facilitating con-siderable tissue infiltration and strong cell attachment. Its high volumetric porosity is much better when contrasted to other porous materials used in orthopaedic applications such as sintered beads and fiber metals.

Ta is primarily used to manufacture acetabular components in total hip arthroplasty, whereas porous Ta implant is used for treating the early stages

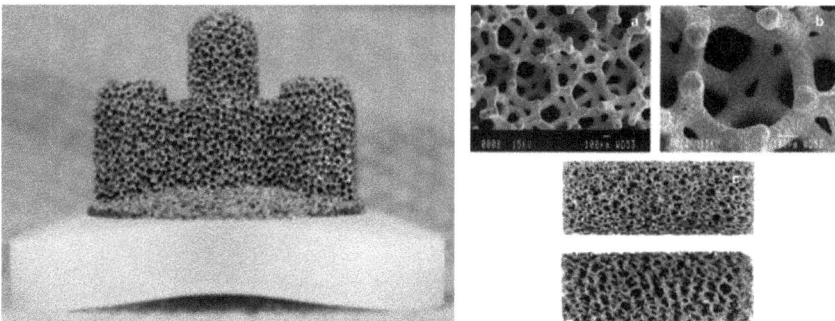

Figure 7.10: (Left) Ta-based porous implant utilized for total shoulder arthroplasty; (Right) SEM image of porous Ta showing the cellular structure formed by the tantalum struts (George *et al.*, 2018; Wilson, 2018; Bobyn *et al.*, 1999).

of osteonecrosis disease. However, the use of Ta in the orthopedic industry is very much restricted due to its extremely high melting temperature (3017°C), higher elastic modulus of bulk Ta (185 GPa), high density (16.6 g/cm³), high affinity towards oxygen, high manufacturing costs and processing routes, together with short-term clinical results.

7.6.3 *Nitinol*

Nitinol, the acronym for Nickel Titanium Naval Ordinance Laboratory, is an Ni-Ti alloy with a near-equiatomic composition, i.e., 49–51% of Ni and Ti each. Since its discovery in 1960, this alloy has become a revolutionary innovation in the field of dental orthodontics wires, endovascular devices (catheters, stents, vena cava filters), and superelastic needles (Figure 7.11). Nitinol alloys are known to have thermal memory and belong to the class of shape memory alloys (SMAs) with superelastic and pseudo-elasticity properties. They act in response to stress or heating by undergoing a transition in their metallic crystal structure (Figure 7.11). SMAs deform at a low temperature but can recover to its previous permanent shape when heated to above the transformation temperature. The two distinct temperature-dependent crystal structures are recognized as martensite (low-temperature phase) and austenite (high-temperature phase). In simple terms, when martensite NiTi is heated it transforms into austenite, and returns back to martensite when cooled. Changes in the ratio of Ni to Ti result in substantial fluctuations in the metal alloy's transition temperature.

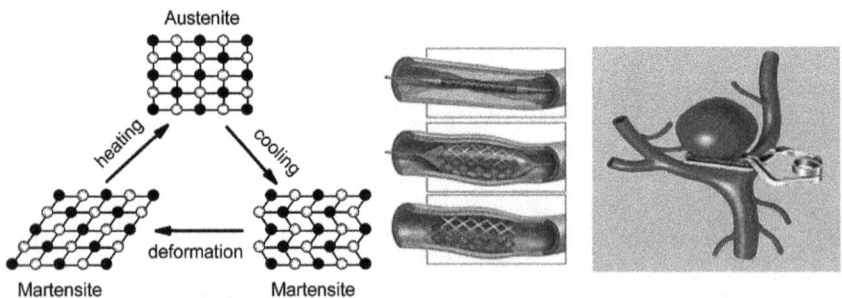

Figure 7.11: (Left) Reshaping of Ni-Ti alloy and procedure of shape memory effect; (Right) vascular stent and aneurysm clip made from Ni-Ti alloy (Wilson, 2018).

Owing to the superior Ti composition, nitinol alloy demonstrates excellent corrosion resistance and superior biocompatibility *in vivo*. Nevertheless, while superelasticity and shape memory effect of nitinol alloys are highly beneficial, the risk of Ni metallic allergy is still high.

7.7 Other biomedical applications

7.7.1 *Heart pacemakers*

The heart pacemaker or cardiac pacemaker is an artificial biomedical implantable electronic device that regulates inappropriate cardiac rhythms through a rhythmic electric stimulus when the natural regulating mechanisms break down. A pacemaker (Figure 7.12) is usually implanted just under the skin, either over or under the pectoral muscle (below the collarbone). The main parts of an artificial pacemaker are pulse generator (consists of a metallic casing, battery, circuit, and connector block), pacing leads and electrodes. The various components of the pacemaker, including the casing, microelectronics, and the leads, are all made with biocompatible materials. The biomaterial aspect of the pacemaker is critical not only to overcome the challenges presented by any device/body physiological interaction but also in constructing the appropriate electrical supply and insulation. Typically, the pulse generator case is fabricated from Ti or its alloys, and electrodes are made from titanium nitride, platinum-iridium alloys, or activated carbon.

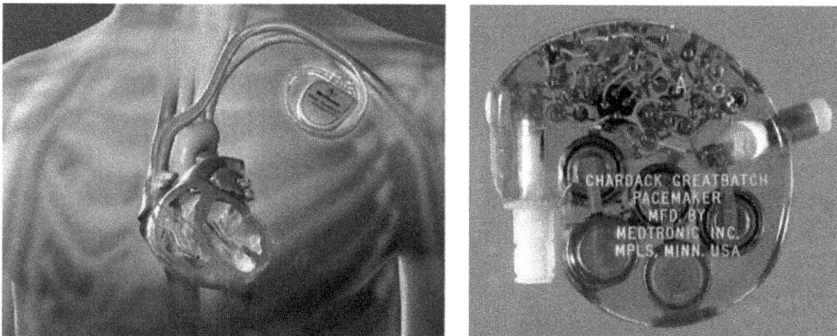

Figure 7.12: (Left) A cardiac resynchronization therapy pacing and defibrillation system; (Right) the Chardack–Greatbatch pacemaker (Mattson *et al.*, 2019).

7.7.2 *Deep brain stimulator*

Deep brain stimulation (DBS) is a highly effective therapy to implant a device that transmits electrical signals to brain regions intended for the movement of the body. It is sometimes referred to as a "*brain pacemaker*". DBS was developed to relieve symptoms of tremor, rigidity, and bradykinesia in patients with neuropsychiatric disorders, especially those suffering from Parkinson's disease. The DBS system comprises three modules: the implanted pulse generator (IPG), the lead, and an extension. The IPG is a battery-powered neurostimulator enclosed in a Ti metal housing. During DBS surgery, a wire, known as lead, is injected into a specific area of the brain. The lead with four electrodes produces electric current to exact brain sites in control of body movement.

7.8 Multiple choice questions

1. Select the statement(s) which is/are TRUE about metallic implants.
    I. metallic implants do not encounter any issue with wear
    II. metallic implants comprise two or more metals
    III. a thin stable oxide layer is formed on top of biometals which further resists corrosion
    IV. metallic implants are used as bone fillers
      (a) only I
      (b) only II and IV
      (c) only II and III
      (d) all of the above

2. Stress shielding usually occurs in
      (a) polymeric biomaterials
      (b) bioceramics
      (c) metallic implant materials
      (d) any biomaterial

3. High elastic modulus in materials arises from
      (a) high strength of metallic bonds
      (b) hydrogen bonds
      (c) covalent bonds
      (d) none of the above

4. Which of the following is/are NOT true about stress shielding?
   - I.   it usually occurs due to modulus mismatch between bone and implanted material
   - II. it is associated with polymeric scaffold materials
   - III. the lower modulus provides for the possibility of less stress shielding effects
   - IV. it leads to implant stabilization
     - (a) only I
     - (b) only II and IV
     - (c) only II, III and IV
     - (d) only IV

5. Which of the following is/are TRUE?
   - I.   Ti-6Al-4V alloy has less stress shielding effect than α alloy
   - II. β alloys for orthopaedics are developed to increase the melting temperature
   - III. β alloys have lower stress shielding effect than α and $\alpha + \beta$ alloys
     - (a) only I
     - (b) only III
     - (c) only II and III
     - (d) all of the above

6. Which is a *unique* characteristic of Ti implants which is NOT present in other metallic implant materials?
   - (a) osseointegration
   - (b) formation of a native oxide layer
   - (c) used for permanent implants as internal and external fixation devices
   - (d) biocompatibility

7. Implants for hard tissue engineering are most often made of
   - (a) titanium
   - (b) hydroxyapatite
   - (c) calcium carbonate
   - (d) alumina and zirconia

8. Select the TRUE statement(s) about magnesium alloys for bone tissue engineering.
   (a) have lower Young's modulus compared to other Ti SS316 alloys
   (b) have unique osseointegration properties
   (c) reduce the stress shielding-related problems of orthopaedic/cardiovascular implants
   (d) all of the above

9. Select the TRUE issue(s) about magnesium alloys when utilized for bone tissue engineering.
   (a) fast corrosion rate in physiological environment
   (b) evolution of H_2 gas in physiological environment
   (c) low Young's modulus
   (d) all of the above

10. Which of the following is TRUE regarding the formation of $Mg(OH)_2$ on Mg alloys?
    (a) enhances the osteointegration bone-bonding like TiO_2 layer
    (b) accelerates corrosion because of reaction with Cl^- in physiological conditions
    (c) improves bone-tissue integration
    (d) all of the above

11. Which type of stainless steel is commonly used in orthopaedic implants?
    (a) austenitic stainless steel
    (b) ferritic stainless steel
    (c) martensitic stainless steel
    (d) duplex stainless steel

12. In stainless steel, this element is added for improving corrosion resistance; and the presence of hydrogen in steel causes this effect.
    (a) tungsten; increases corrosion resistance
    (b) magnesium; improves cell adhesion
    (c) carbon; decreases cell adhesion
    (d) chromium; embrittlement

13. The capability of an orthodontic wire to spring back to its original shape is assessed by
    (a) Young's modulus
    (b) stiffness
    (c) resilience
    (d) elasticity and plasticity

References & Further Reading

Arifin, A., Sulong, A. B., Muhamad, N., Syarif, J., *et al.* (2014). Material processing of hydroxyapatite and titanium alloy (HA/Ti) composite as implant materials using powder metallurgy: A review. *Materials & Design, 55,* 165–175. doi:10.1016/j.matdes.2013.09.045.

Bobyn, J. D., Toh, K. K., Hacking, S. A., Tanzer, M., & Krygier, J. J. (1999). Tissue response to porous tantalum acetabular cups: a canine model. *Journal of Arthroplasty, 14*(3), 347–354. doi:10.1016/s0883-5403(99)90062-1.

Dailey, S. K., Crawford, A. H., & Asghar, F. S. (2015). Implant Failure Following Posterior Spinal Fusion–Caudal Migration of a Fractured Rod: Case Report. *Spine Deformity, 3*(4), 380–385. doi:10.1016/j.jspd.2015.02.001.

Geavlete, P., Niță, G., Mulțescu, R., Moldoveanu, C., *et al.* (2016). Chapter 11 — Prostatic Stents. In P. A. Geavlete (Ed.), *Endoscopic Diagnosis and Treatment in Prostate Pathology* (pp. 161–170): Academic Press.

George, N., & Nair, A. B. (2018). Chapter 11 — Porous tantalum: A new biomaterial in orthopedic surgery. In P. Balakrishnan, S. M. S., & S. Thomas (Eds.), *Fundamental Biomaterials: Metals* (pp. 243–268): Woodhead Publishing.

Kawamura, N., Nakao, Y., Ishikawa, R., Tsuchida, D., *et al.* (2020). Degradation and Biocompatibility of AZ31 Magnesium Alloy Implants In Vitro and In Vivo: A Micro-Computed Tomography Study in Rats. *Materials, 13*(2), 473. doi:10.3390/ma13020473.

Li, J., Jansen, J. A., Walboomers, X. F., & van den Beucken, J. J. J. P. (2020). Mechanical aspects of dental implants and osseointegration: A narrative review. *Journal of the Mechanical Behavior of Biomedical Materials, 103,* 103574. doi:10.1016/j.jmbbm.2019.103574.

Loughenbury, F., McWilliams, A., Smith, M., Pandit, H., *et al.* (2018). Leg length inequality after primary total hip arthroplasty. *Orthopaedics and Trauma, 32*(1), 27–33. doi:10.1016/j.mporth.2017.11.006.

Matsubara, H., & Tsuchiya, H. (2019). Treatment of bone tumor using external fixator. *Journal of Orthopaedic Science, 24*(1), 1–8. doi:10.1016/j. jos.2018.06.022.

Mattson, A. R., Eggen, M. D., & Iaizzo, P. A. (2019). Chapter 6 — The Cardiac Pacemaker: A Crossroads of Engineering and Medicine. In P. A. Iaizzo (Ed.), *Engineering in Medicine* (pp. 153–178): Academic Press.

Mostaed, E., Sikora-Jasinska, M., & Vedani, M. (2019). Zinc-Based Degradable Implants. In R. Narayan (Ed.), *Encyclopedia of Biomedical Engineering* (pp. 478–487): Elsevier.

Mullaji, A., & Shetty, G. (2015). Cemented total knee arthroplasty remains the "gold standard". *Seminars in Arthroplasty, 26*(2), 62–64. doi:10.1053/j. sart.2015.08.006.

Nakano, T. (2019). 3 — Physical and mechanical properties of metallic biomaterials. In M. Niinomi (Ed.), *Metals for Biomedical Devices (Second Edition)* (pp. 97–129): Woodhead Publishing.

Niinomi, M. (1998). Mechanical properties of biomedical titanium alloys. *Materials Science and Engineering: A, 243*(1), 231–236. doi:10.1016/ S0921-5093(97)00806-X.

Polmear, I., StJohn, D., Nie, J.-F., & Qian, M. (2017). Chapter 7 — Titanium Alloys. In I. Polmear, D. StJohn, J.-F. Nie, & M. Qian (Eds.), *Light Alloys (Fifth Edition)* (pp. 369–460): Butterworth-Heinemann.

Salahshoor, M., & Guo, Y. (2012). Biodegradable Orthopedic Magnesium-Calcium (MgCa) Alloys, Processing, and Corrosion Performance. *Materials (Basel), 5*, 135–155. doi:10.3390/ma5010135.

Surin, H. B. V. (2005). Stress shielding effect of the shaft component. Retrieved from http://www.bananarepublican.info/Stress_shielding.htm.

Wilson, J. (2018). Chapter 1 — Metallic biomaterials: State of the art and new challenges. In P. Balakrishnan, S. M. S., & S. Thomas (Eds.), *Fundamental Biomaterials: Metals* (pp. 1–33): Woodhead Publishing.

Chapter 8
Medical devices: Standards, regulations and sterilization

8.1 Medical devices

The term "*medical devices*" refers to any device, apparatus, machine, or appliance intended to diagnose, prevent, investigate, evaluate, or treat medical conditions. Medical devices come in many forms, purposes, and degrees of complexity. They cover a vast range from extremely advanced computerized medical equipment or programmable pacemakers to simple surgical gloves, bandages, and band-aids. Besides, medical devices also encompass *in vitro* diagnostic (IVD) units such as test kits (pregnancy, COVID-19) and blood glucose meters. Some examples of medical devices are shown in Figure 8.1. In the healthcare sector, innovative and advanced

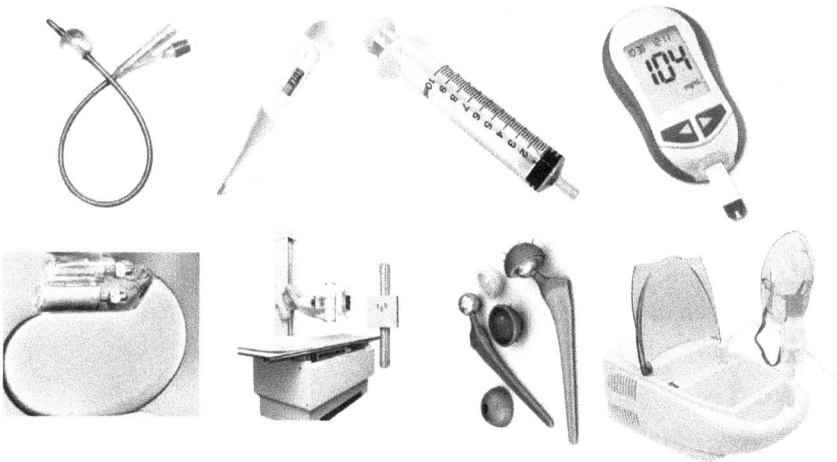

Figure 8.1: Examples of medical devices.

biomedical technologies are increasingly being promoted to improve medicine's reputation, healthcare, and the human condition itself. These drastically changing advancements create substantial debates, challenges and disputes for law, regulation, and governance.

8.2 Standards versus regulations

Before going into detail about various standards and regulations for medical device manufacturing, it is crucial to understand the critical differences between the terms *"regulations"* and *"standards"*. The differences between laws, standards, and regulations are often confused by the complex terminologies and varying definitions. Hence, it is crucial to understand the definitions and how they relate to each other.

8.2.1 *Standards*

Standards are documented agreements containing technical specifications or other precise norms/conditions that must continuously be used to guarantee that devices, materials, equipment, processes, and facilities are suited for the objective they are intended for. Standards across industries are essential to safeguard quality reliability while harmonizing requirements, both nationally and globally. Medical devices are subject to strict operational laws and procedural regulations. Various regulatory bodies and standards associations are working together to set mutually agreed guidelines for medical equipment. The two associations that usually issue international standards are the International Organization for Standardization (ISO) and the International Electrotechnical Commission (IEC). Their typical tasks include defining performance indicators, characterizing and evaluating methodologies, production methods, quality requirements, scientific guidelines, and regulatory criteria. A region or country has an organization of standards that may adopt and modify international standards or restrict them in some cases.

8.2.2 *Regulations*

Regulations refer to constitutional laws laid down by government authorities, which dictate what can be done and how it should or should not be executed. They surface as a crucial pillar of the technology plan, and function to ensure uniform application of the law. This is primarily aimed at guaranteeing product safety and fundamentally safeguarding public health. Oversight of healthcare technology over the past few decades has become more critical and debatable. In the case of biomaterials, the regulations can include how a specific biomaterial should be fabricated, measured, and tested for a specific application. Owing to the existing significant unfavorable effects of short- and long-term devices, strict regulations ensure that inventors need to apply for medical device approval before they can be used. In general, legislative institutions pass laws, government organizations develop regulations to implement these laws, and product development organizations adopt accredited standards.

Key points

Objectives of standards and regulations

- Provide equal opportunities for international trade and entry to open markets
- Improve human wellbeing and safeguard health promotion
- Provide powerful government-industry connections and global synchronization in agreements

---

8.3 Classification of medical devices

A medical device classification for regulatory objectives is associated with the device's related risks such as severity, contact length, the infected body system, and systemic and non-systemic impacts. The range of evaluation of medical equipment is dependent on the level of risk involved. Usually, low-risk devices like medical gloves and tongue depressors are pre-evaluated by manufacturers. In contrast, essential scientific evidence such as efficiency and safety complications data are needed in high-risk devices. For these kinds of devices, the procedure consists of broad pre- and post-market investigations. Obtaining basic knowledge of regulatory product categorization of each country/region will be invaluable and help in designing the new products to meet standards. The classification of medical devices by risk level and regulatory checks in various countries are presented in Figure 8.2.

Country/organization	Classification			
US	Class I	Class II		Class III
EU	Class I	Class IIa	Class IIb	Class III
China	Class I	Class II		Class III
Japan	Class I	Class II	Class III	Class IV
Australia	Class I	Class IIa	Class IIb	Class III
Singapore	Class A	Class B	Class C	Class D
Risk	Low risk	Low-moderate risk	Moderate-high risk	High risk

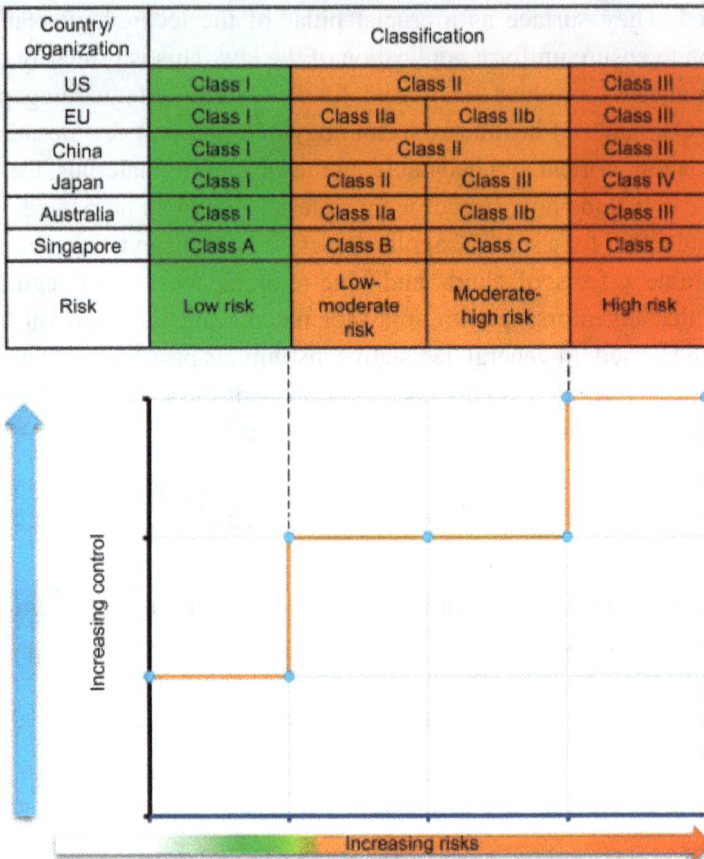

Figure 8.2:   The classification of medical devices by risk level and regulatory checks in various countries (Gudeppu *et al.*, 2020; Ramakrishna *et al.*, 2015; Shan *et al.*, 2020).

8.3.1 *Classification by country*

8.3.1.1 *Classification in the United States*

In the United States (U.S.), all marketed medical devices are regulated by the Food and Drug Administration (FDA). The Center for Devices and Radiological Health, a division of FDA, is solely accountable for guaranteeing the safety and effectiveness of medical equipment, pre-market approvals, and providing information to help the industries to comply with FDA regulations. The medical devices are classified using a predicate-based system either as Class I, II, or III. The categorization is primarily based on the device's threat, invasiveness, and effect on the patient's complete health condition.

- **Class I:** low to moderate-risk medical devices; general controls
- **Class II:** moderate to high-risk medical devices; general and special controls and require pre-market notification 510(k)
- **Class III:** high-risk medical devices; general controls and pre-market approval (PMA)

Class I medical devices possess the lowest level of risk with uncomplicated or unsophisticated designs that can be found in every household. Class I devices have minimum contact with patients' bodies and have very minimal influence on a patient's overall health. Examples of this device class include adhesive bandages, tongue depressors, wheelchairs, scalpels, etc. Class II devices are moderate risk since they are expected to come into continuous contact with a patient. They are much more complex in design when compared to Class I. If failed, this device class has a small chance of immediate risk of severe harm or death. General controls for the regulation of Class II devices are deemed insufficient, which calls for special controls. Many Class I and some Class II devices are exempted from pre-market notification 510(k). Class III medical devices are the most innovative and cutting-edge medical devices with the highest risk level, meaning failure of device can possibly lead to death or cause significant medical difficulties. All Class III devices are expected to go through a PMA procedure. Examples include life-saving devices such as pacemakers, coronary stents, and implants. Classification with examples is shown in Figure 8.3.

8.3.1.2 *Classification in the European Union*

After the U.S., Europe occupies the second-largest market for medical device technology. The regulations for a medical device in the European Union (E.U.) are formulated by the European Commission as Medical Device Directives (MDD). Unlike in the U.S., there is no centralized approach at the E.U. The European Medicines Agency operates as a decentralized scientific agency responsible for medical devices for human

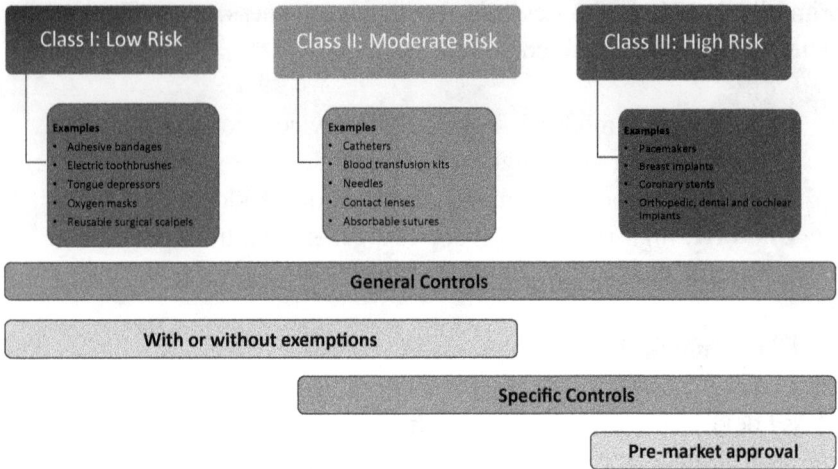

Figure 8.3:   Classification of Class I, Class II, and Class III medical devices in the U.S. with examples.

or animal use. A list of current E.U. medical device regulations and directives are mentioned below.

- Council Directive 90/385/EEC: Active Implantable Medical Devices Directive (AIMDD)
- Council Directive 93/42/EEC: Medical Devices Directive (MDD)
- Directive 93/68/EEC: CE marking
- Directive 98/79/EC: *in vitro* Diagnostic Medical Devices Directive (IVDD)
- Directive 2000/70/EC: Amending Council Directive 93/42/EEC
- Directive 2001/104/EC: Amending Council Directive 93/42/EEC concerning medical devices
- Regulation (E.U.) 2017/745: Medical Device Regulation (MDR). It repels the council directive of 90/385/EEC and 93/42/EEC.
- Regulation (E.U.) 2017/746: *in vitro* Diagnostic Medical Device Regulation (IVDR). It repels the directive of 98/79/EC.

For general medical devices, manufacturers need to comply with the MDD Council Directive 93/42/EEC and MDR No. 2017/745. The AIMDD Council Directive 90/385/EEC is for higher risk devices, whereas IVDD 98/79/EC applies to IVDs (E.U. 2017/746). More details and instructions about the European classification system are found in MEDDEV 2.4/1, and the division regulations are found in Annex IX of Directive 93/42/EEC. The MDD's and MDR's objective is to bring attention to the patient and medical device consumer safety. The new unique device identification (UDI) and a European database (EUDAMED) are currently being developed by the E.U. to facilitate easier traceability and significantly improve the efficacy of post-market safety-related activities.

Medical device corporations who wish to sell or advertise their products in Europe must obtain a Conformité Européenne (C.E.) marking certification by demonstrating their fulfilment with the appropriate European regulations. The C.E. marking offers the extra benefit of free movement of the medical device in all 30 member countries of the European Free Trade Area. The MDD and the MDR group medical devices are divided into four basic categories (Figure 8.4) with 18 rules for classification:

- **Non-invasive devices (Rules 1–4):** Any instrument or device that does not infiltrate the body via an orifice or the surface of the body

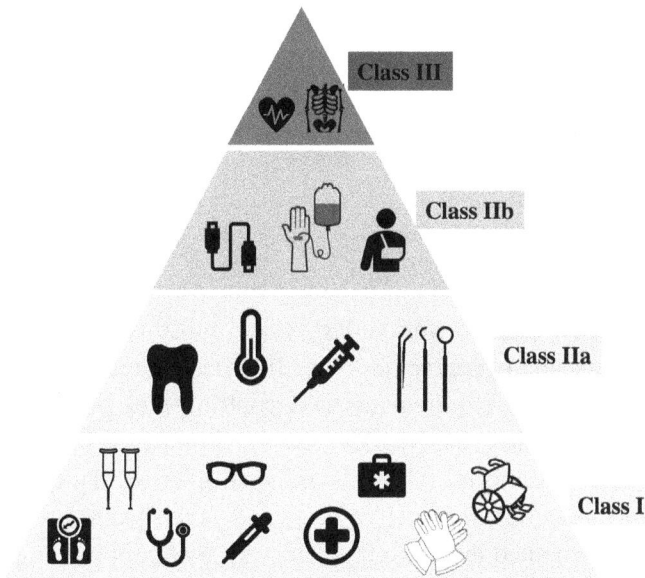

Figure 8.4: Medical device classification in Europe.

- **Invasive medical devices (Rules 5–8):** Any instrument or device that penetrates into the body in whole or in part, through an orifice or the body's surface
- **Active medical devices (Rules 9–12):** An instrument or device which relies on energy
- **Special Rules (Rules 13–18):** Includes contraceptives, disinfectants, drug-device combinations, diagnostic medical devices, etc.

Recently, four new rules (rules 19–22) are included in the MDR.

According to the European framework MDD 93/42/EEC, general medical devices are further segmented into four sections, similar to the product classification system in the U.S. A comparison of device approval processes in the U.S. and E.U. is presented in Figure 8.5. Active implantable medical devices are not classified, and IVDs are grouped separately as Class A, B, C, and D.

- **Class I:** lowest-risk medical devices that are non-sterile or do not have a quantifying task or function. Examples include glasses, stethoscopes, etc.
- **Class IIa:** medium-risk medical devices which are sterile and/or have a quantifying function. A conformity assessment is required.
- **Class IIb:** medium-to-high risk medical devices. A conformity assessment is required.
- **Class III:** highest-risk medical devices. A conformity assessment is required.

8.3.1.3 *Classification in Singapore*

Singapore has among the world's largest and most advanced health systems despite its small geographical size. In order to meet adequate safety, quality, and efficacy requirements and contribute to the expansion of national drug policies, the Medical Device Branch of the Singapore's Health Sciences Authority (HSA) is assigned with regulating drugs and advanced therapeutics, medical devices, and other health products. The HSA has implemented the latest regulatory system built on the principles supported and recommended by the Global Harmonization Task Force

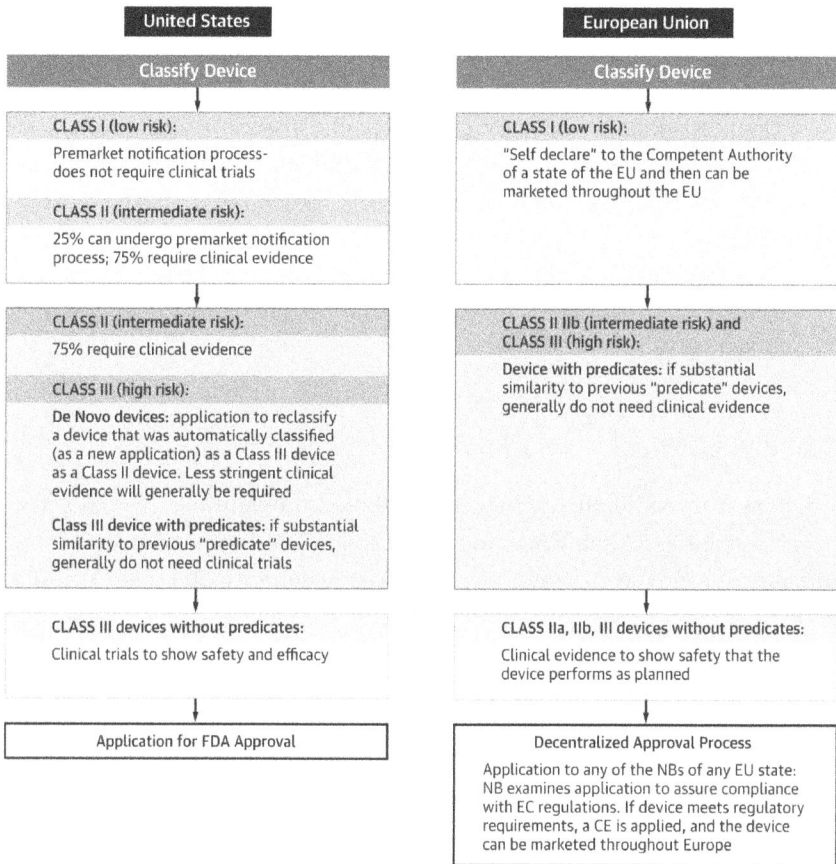

Figure 8.5: Comparison of device approval processes in the US and EU (Ogrodnik, 2020; Van Norman, 2016).

with revisions to match the Singapore context. A database containing a registry of all medical devices commonly used in hospitals, clinics or healthcare departments is the Singapore Medical Devices Register. Based on the extent of medical device interaction with the body and level of invasiveness, they are categorized into four classes:

- **Class A:** Low specific risk and low public health risk. They do not require pre-market registration but must be listed with the HSA. Examples include wheelchairs and tongue depressors.

184 An Introduction to Biomaterials Science and Engineering

- **Class B:** Low to moderate risk or low public health risk. If no safety concerns are registered in any of the reference countries for three years, devices are eligible for Immediate Class B Registration. Examples include hypodermic needles and suction equipment.
- **Class C:** Moderate to high risk or moderate public health risk. Examples include ventilators and hip, knee, and shoulder joint replacements.
- **Class D:** High individual risk and high public health risk. Examples include HIV blood diagnostics, heart valves, and implantable defibrillators.

8.3.1.4 *Classification in China*

In China, the National Medical Products Administration (NMPA), formerly dubbed as China Food and Drug Administration, is the governing organization for food, drugs, biological products, cosmetics, and medical devices. Medical devices in China, including manufacturing, marketing, and sale, are subject to a mandatory filing/registration administrated and controlled by the NMPA. Similar to the U.S. FDA, the NMPA categorizes medical devices according to their potential risk into three classes (I to III). The class is defined by the "product panel", which links specific devices with standard uses and product codes. Class I equipment has the lowest risk and can be adequately supervised via frequent administration. In contrast, Class III equipment are complicated implants or life supportive devices that are linked with high risks. A clinical assessment is compulsory for trade-in class II and III medical devices. China is adamant about national standards. Thankfully, these are often indistinguishable from, or at least comparable to, international standards. Their abbreviations usually differentiate national and industry standards.

- GB: Binding/mandatory national standard
- GB/T: Non-binding/recommended national standard
- YY: Binding/mandatory industry standard for medicine
- YY/T: Non-binding/recommended industry standard for medicine
- JJG: Metrology measurement standard

8.3.1.5 *Classification in India*

Over the years, the regulatory framework for Indian health equipment has grown from the absence of regulation, to inadequate regulation, to consistent regulation. The Indian medical device market value was evaluated at US\$4.5 billion in 2012, and its market now positions itself in the top 20 in the world and the top 5 amongst Asian countries. The industry is highly competitive and has about 750–800 domestic medical device manufacturers in the country. In India, all medical devices, instruments, diagnostic devices, life support and monitoring equipment and cosmetics are controlled by the Drug Controller General of India within the Central Drugs Standard Control Organization (CDSCO), a part of the Ministry of Health and Family Welfare. Together with CDSCO, the Bureau of Indian Standards standardizes a few other low technology devices. According to Medical Devices (Amendment) Rules 2020, effective from 1st April 2020 all medical devices in India are labeled as *"drugs"* and regulated under the Drugs and Cosmetics Act of 1940. Like Singapore, medical devices in India other than *in vitro* diagnostic medical devices are categorized as Class A (low risk) to Class D (high risk). To obtain registration in India, all the importers and manufacturers need to be compliant with ISO-13485 (Medical Devices-Quality Management Systems-Requirements for Regulatory Purposes). Some of the important classifications of medical devices in India are:

- CT scan, MRI, PET equipment and X-ray machine: Class C
- Defibrillators: Class C
- Dialysis Machine: Class C
- Bone marrow cell separator: Class B
- Digital thermometer: Class B
- Blood pressure monitoring devices: Class B
- Implantable infusion pumps with catheters: Class D

However, Indian medical device companies are predominantly involved in low technology. In contrast, more than 70% of high-end devices such as imaging equipment, heart pacemakers, orthopaedic implants, respiration devices, and dental equipment are traded in from countries such as the U.S., Japan, U.K., and Germany.

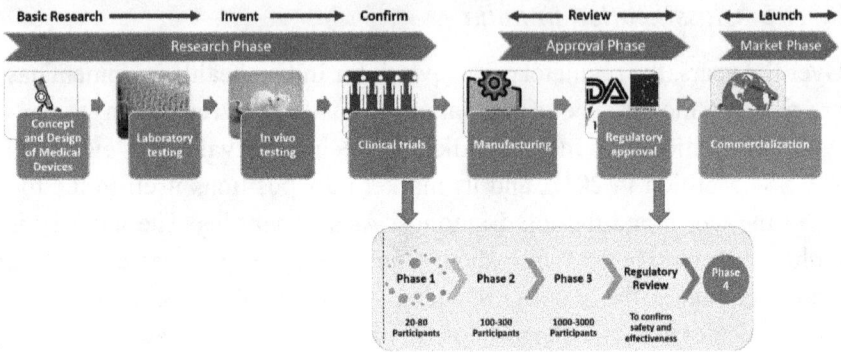

Figure 8.6: Medical device life cycle from concept phase to market phase.

8.3.2 *Life cycle*

Regardless of their purpose, all these devices will go through the same five general stages: basic research, design, validation *in vitro* and *in vivo*, review and launch, and post-market review. The product life cycle of medical devices is associated with regulatory frameworks in the U.S., the E.U., and other industry leaders who follow their policies. The medical device life cycle from concept phase to market phase is shown in Figure 8.6.

8.4 Sterilization

Over the past few decades, the medical device market has changed considerably. Many new biological devices are being added to the market every year with more advanced technologies and more novel combinations of various biological materials. These medical devices are one way by which healthcare-associated infections can be transmitted. Over the duration of the manufacturing process, all viable microbial life forms, including fungi, bacteria, viruses, and spore types, accumulate and live on the surface of the product. If not disinfected, these microbial contaminations could result in disease transmission. In the medical sector, the risk of disease transmission due to bacterial contamination is a subject of rising concern. In view of this, irrespective of the size and complexity, development of sterile medical devices has been a central objective of all manufacturers. Two main terms are associated with sterilization: bioburden and sterility assurance level (SAL).

Bioburden is generally described as the number of viable bacteria living on a surface or within a liquid that has not been sterilized. In simple terms, it implies the overall state of cleanliness of the device at the molecular level before it is sterilized. Over several years, bioburden testing or microbial limit testing has been employed in the pharmaceutical and medical device manufacturing industries to determine amounts of microbial adhesion on raw materials, fluids, media, device components, and finished goods. The bioburden level is often a contributing factor when determining the sterilization dose for any given product/device. For example, higher bioburden levels may require a higher dose of sterilization when compared to the dose selected for a device with lower bioburden levels. Factors affecting bioburden are shown in Figure 8.7. Sterilization can be defined as any method that efficiently eradicates or kills all viable forms of microorganisms from equipment, food, medicines, or biological culture media to attain an acceptable

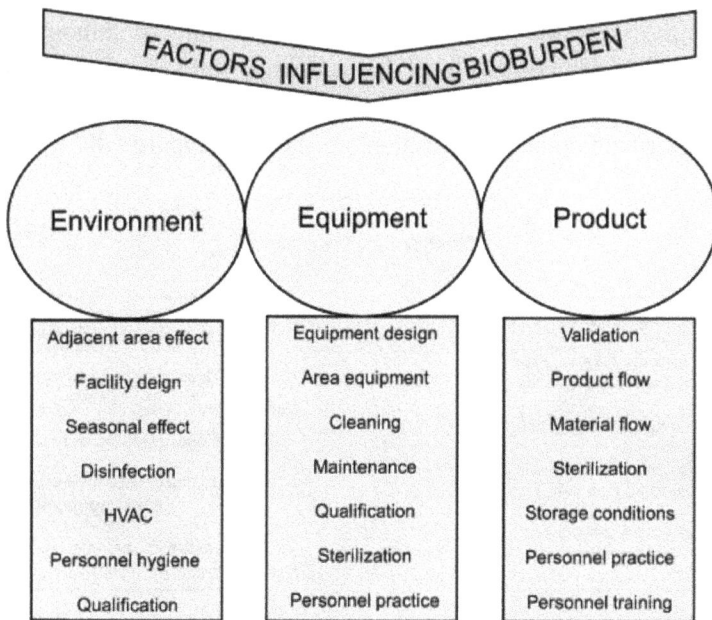

Figure 8.7: Factors affecting bioburden (Branaghan *et al.*, 2020; Moondra *et al.*, 2018).

SAL. Ideally, this implies that there are no viable microorganisms at all on the surface and the bulk. Since the accomplishment of absolute sterility cannot be verified, a medicinal preparation's sterility can only be described in terms of probability. Currently, an SAL of 10^{-6} (SAL6) is deemed as the standard for medical devices, i.e., a probability of 1 in 1,000,000 that the device is non-sterile (Sadeque *et al.*, 2020; Sandle, 2016).

While sterilization can be employed in various industry sectors, medical and surgical fields are some of the fields where sterilization is a must. The sterilization of implant materials is a prerequisite event before implantation to reduce the possibility of instituting unwanted microorganisms or pathogens by these materials and prevent disease transmission. The field of medical sterilization has become progressively challenging due to the need to avoid exposure of patients to infections caused by organisms on instruments and devices used during their treatment. Failure to sterilize medical instruments leads to significant hospital costs associated with patient nosocomial infections and mortality/morbidity issues.

Sterilization should not be confused with the terms disinfection or sanitization. Sterilization eliminates all microorganisms present. Disinfection and sanitization, on the opposite, minimize the quantity of pathogenic species on medical devices to a level that is not harmful to health so that they cannot reach vulnerable sites to cause infection. The significant differences between sterilization and disinfection are shown in Figure 8.8.

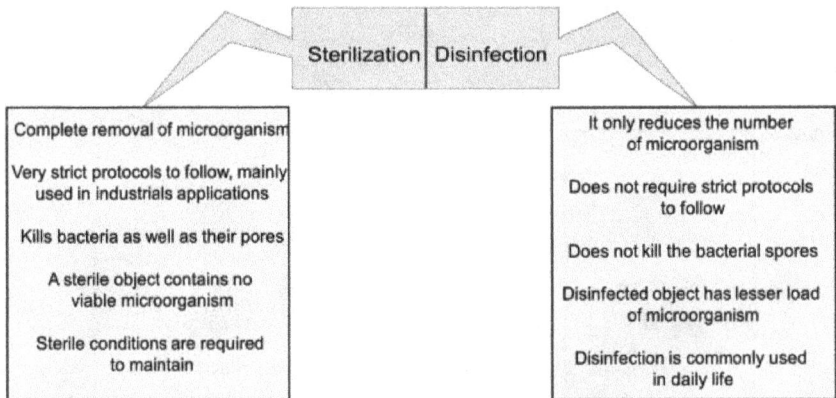

Figure 8.8:   Difference between sterilization and disinfection (Lerouge, 2019; Moondra *et al.*, 2018).

8.5 Sterilization methods

Sterilization methods (Figure 8.9) operate chemically or physically on microorganisms. Typically, each procedure results in a modification in the structure or function of the organic macromolecules in the microorganism, resulting in death or the inability to reproduce. Medical instruments are sterilized in various ways, such as:

- Moist heat (steam) sterilization or autoclaving
- Dry heat sterilization
- Ethylene oxide sterilization
- Gamma radiation sterilization
- Electron beam sterilization
- Ultraviolet radiation
- Chemical treatment
- Low-temperature gas plasma treatment
- Gaseous chlorine dioxide treatment

While several procedures are available, it is widely accepted that no single process will sterilize all medical devices without negative effects.

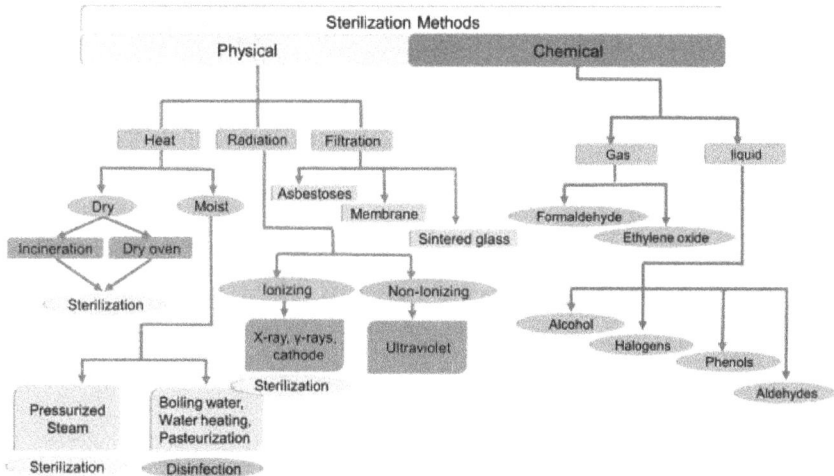

Figure 8.9: Various methods of sterilization (Harrington *et al.*, 2020; Moondra *et al.*, 2018; Sadeque *et al.*, 2020).

A list of all sterilization methods and their common biomaterial applications are displayed at the end of this chapter in Table 8.4. The required sterilization dose largely depends on the quantity of bioburden (living microorganisms) present on the device prior to irradiation. All procedures have their intrinsic advantages and disadvantages. Many negative effects are due to incompatibilities between the products used in medical devices, sterilization process parameters, and the release of harmful gases or radiation. In addition, specific procedures often involve environmental problems for the manufacturing personnel and negative reactions in patients.

8.5.1 *Autoclaving*

Of all the methods available for sterilization, steam sterilization or autoclaving is extensively used and is a highly dependable sterilization method (Figure 8.10a and b). This is a reasonably simple process and is

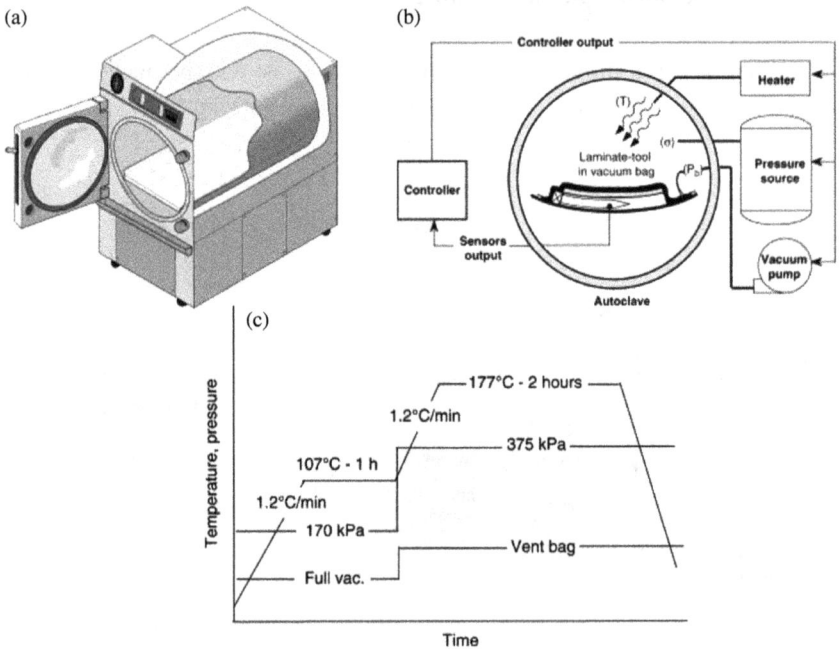

Figure 8.10:   (a) Schematic of cylindrical research autoclave; (b) Typical autoclave processing system; (c) Typical autoclave process cycle (Hubert *et al.*, 2012).

accomplished by subjecting the material system to saturated water vapor within a sealed chamber under high pressure (121 kPa) and high temperature (121°C) for a certain amount of time. The chamber is then allowed to cool slowly or by passive heat dissipation (Figure 8.10c). The process kills attached microorganisms by damaging critical metabolizing and structural elements for their replication. At this high moist heat temperature, autoclaving is able to deactivate all microbes, fungi, the most resilient bacterial spores, mold (e.g., *Pyronema domesticatum*), and prions.

Autoclaving is an efficient, effective, fast, and relatively simple procedure that does not result in toxic residues. This sterilization technique is generally used for culture media, glassware, flammable and heat-sensitive items, liquids and dense loads, heat-resistant surgical instruments, and intravenous fluid sterilization. Medical devices made from metallic alloys are well-suited for autoclaving. For biomedical polymers, the high temperature (121°C), humidity, and pressure used in the process will cause many of them to hydrolyze, soften, or degrade. Based on the way the air is removed from the chamber, autoclave sterilization is classified into three types:

- **Type N:** Air removal is by passive displacement with steam; recommended only for non-wrapped solid instruments and non-porous materials
- **Type B:** Air removal is by vacuum deaeration; recommended for all kinds of materials containing packaged, hollow, and porous structures
- **Type S:** Air removal and applications in this type are not defined by any standards; the manufacturer usually specifies the application and performance capabilities

8.5.2 *Dry heat sterilization*

Dry heat sterilization is an alternative to steam sterilization whereby objects are exposed to dry heat in an oven for a prolonged period (e.g., 180°C for 1–2 h). Primary differences between autoclaving and dry heat sterilization are tabulated in Table 8.1. Dry heat destroys microorganisms and bacterial spores by causing a coagulation of proteins. Sterilizing by dry heat is achieved by conduction and usually requires higher

Table 8.1: Advantages and disadvantages of autoclaving and dry heat sterilization.

	Pros	Cons
Autoclaving	Increased productivity with lower energy expenditure	Incompatible for sterilization of powders and oils
	Requires significantly less time and reduced heat	Moisture retention
Dry heat	Non-corrosive for metallic materials as no moisture is used	Instruments need to be dry when loaded to avoid reaction with water molecules
	Involves no toxic agents, so no harmful substances need to be discarded	Due to high temperatures, only metallic objects are preferred
		Time-consuming as it takes more time to achieve sterilization
		Issue with overexposure

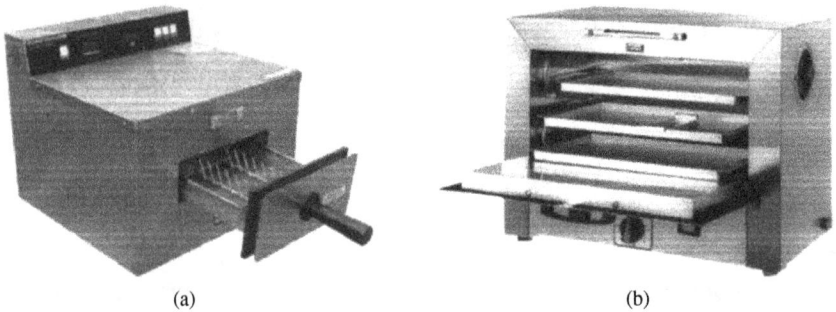

Figure 8.11: The two commercial dry-heat sterilizers: (a) Cox fastest dry-heat sterilizer (6 min unwrapped at 190 °C; 12 min wrapped) and (b) Wayne S1000 dry-heat sterilizer (standard 160–180°C oven for instruments) (Rogers, 2013; Sadeque *et al.*, 2020).

temperatures than steam sterilization (autoclaving, 121°C). In this process, the heat is initially absorbed by the object's exterior surface, then flows through to the object's core, layer by layer. In due course, the entire item/body achieves the temperature required for sterilization to occur. The most common time-temperature settings for dry heat sterilization are 180°C for 30–60 min, 160°C for 60–120 min, 150°C for 150–240 min, and 120°C for 240–360 min. These may be set differently or extended subject to the volume of the product and particular application. The two commercial dry-heat sterilizers are presented in Figure 8.11. In most cases, dry heat furnaces are employed to disinfect objects that may be harmed by or are impermeable to moist heat (e.g., powders, petroleum products). Except for silicon prostheses, dry heat sterilization is not frequently utilized in the medical device industry and is usually not recommended in healthcare environments. Advantages include low operation cost (dry heat cabinet), non-toxicity, and non-corrosivity for metals. However, this process is time-consuming and has a very slow heat penetration rate. Sometimes it is difficult to monitor the cycle consistently and it varies for different substances. Dry heat sterilization is generally used for metallic instruments, oils, and glassware. There are several different categories of dry heat sterilization, such as:

- **Static-air type:** The hot air oven has heating coils on the bottom of the device, which works on the principle of gravity convection. This type of device usually needs lengthier times to achieve the desired temperature, and the temperature may not be uniform throughout the oven.
- **Forced-air type:** This type has a motorized blower to disseminate the heat more efficiently throughout the oven at a certain velocity.

8.5.3 *Ethylene oxide*

Ethylene oxide (EO or EtO) sterilization is a low-temperature gaseous process widely applied to sterilize a variety of medical devices and healthcare products that cannot withstand the high temperatures of autoclaving and dry heat sterilization. At concentrations below 500 ppm, EtO is colourless and odourless, and at concentrations above 500 ppm, EtO is sweet and has an ether-like smell. Due to toxicity, flammability, carcinogenic and explosive nature of EtO gas, it is rarely used in its pure form and is often mixed with other inert gases such as N_2 or CO_2. The efficiency, effectiveness, and reliability of EtO gas as a surface sterilant is undeniable. EtO sterilization can effectively infiltrate through solid matrices, reach inner surfaces of most medical devices, and invalidate various infectious agents such as bacteria, microorganisms, yeasts, molds, and viruses. The EtO killing mechanism is alkylation (transfer of an alkyl group from one molecule to another) of side chains of enzymes, deoxyribonucleic acid (DNA) and ribonucleic acid (RNA). The alkylation disrupts the regular cellular metabolism and reproductive processes, making the affected microbes non-viable. A typical EtO sterilization cycle is usually more than 14 hours and has at least three stages:

- **Preconditioning:** EtO is only productive in a humid environment. Therefore, to achieve intended sterility and preserve product stability, the moisture state of a device/material must be controlled during EtO sterilization. Preconditioning provides ideal temperature and humidity conditions to infectious agents so that the endospores will come out of hibernation and become exposed. Typical settings for this preconditioning stage are a temperature of 40–60°C and a relative humidity of 50–65%.
- **Sterilization/Conditioning:** This involves exposure of the device to the sterilizing agent in a vacuum chamber at the specified temperature. The chamber is maintained at a predefined pressure.
- **Aeration (Degassing):** Aeration is the most crucial and lengthiest part of the EtO sterilization cycle. In this step, the leftover EtO gas is removed and absorbed gas is permitted to evaporate again from the sterilized objects by flowing HEPA (high-efficiency particulate air) filtered air at a temperature of 30–50°C. This step helps in removing any remaining EtO particles and meeting the residual limit guidelines outlined in the EN ISO 10993-7.

The lethality of EtO sterilization depends on EtO concentration, exposure time, temperature, and humidity. Its lower temperature process (typically between 37°C and 63°C) makes it compatible with a broad range of materials utilized in the manufacture of medical devices such as polymers (plastic or resin), metals, and glass. The total duration of the EtO sterilizing cycle can vary depending on the product, but average cycles are between 36 and 48 hours. A hypothetical and typical 100% EtO process cycle is shown in Figure 8.12.

Although EtO has proven its effectiveness at much lower temperatures, there is concern that certain humid environments may initiate or accelerate the chain degradation for certain absorbable polymers and have an adverse effect on the material's mechanical properties. Another limitation is that EtO is considered to be highly explosive and carcinogenic, which presents many health issues for operators. Additionally, the

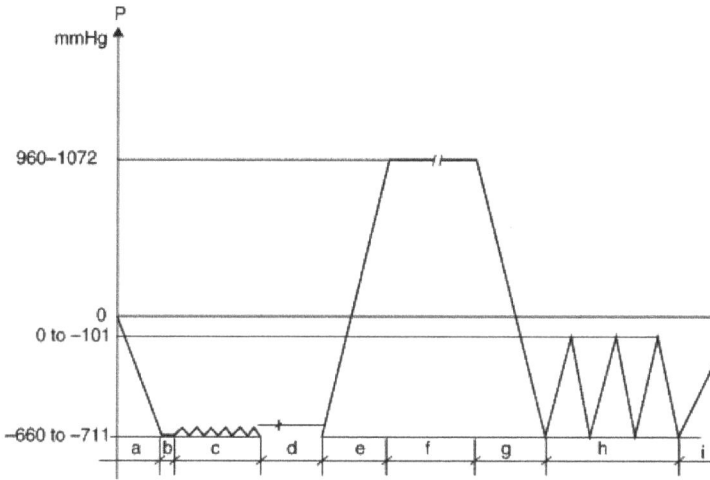

Figure 8.12: A pre-humidification EtO sterilization cycle. Steps: (a) initial evacuation, (b) leak check, (c) pre-humidifying, (d) humidity dwell, (e) ethylene oxide gas mixture injection, (f) ethylene oxide exposure, (g) post-evacuation, (h) 3 air washes, (i) final air inbleed to atmospheric pressure (Rogers, 2013).

Table 8.2: Advantages and disadvantages of EtO sterilization.

Advantages	Disadvantages
Propagation in all places and highly efficient	Leftover EtO residues
Sterilization at very low temperatures	Safety concerns: EtO is carcinogenic, toxic and flammable
Ideal for thermo-sensitive materials	Needs distinctive room requirements, safety kit, and individual ventilation system
Effective and compatible with most materials	

EtO gas can interact with the disinfected polymer, and incomplete removal of EtO leaves behind the residual gas. Ethylene chlorohydrin and ethylene glycol, by-products of this reaction, are of major concern in the healthcare industry. It should also be noted that EtO is essentially a surface sterilizing agent, and its efficacy and diffusion into the bulk of a device is very much limited. The efficiency of the EtO sterilization cycle hinges on the relative humidity and temperature in the cycle, so monitoring and validating these parameters through the process is necessary. The typical advantages and disadvantages of EtO sterilization are presented briefly in Table 8.2.

8.5.4 *Radiation sterilization*

Radiation sterilization mainly relies on ionizing radiation, i.e., changing of atoms into charged ions. It primarily uses gamma rays from a cobalt-60 (^{60}Co) isotope and machine-generated electron radiation to neutralize microorganisms such as bacteria, fungi, viruses, and spores. A comparison of sources for radiation sterilization is shown in Figure 8.13. Due to numerous advantages over chemical-based or heat sterilization techniques, this approach is exceptionally attractive in sterilizing medical devices, especially pharmaceuticals. Radiation can be fatal to biological macromolecules by stimulating genetic damage and chemical changes. During sterilization treatment, the sample of interest is bombarded with high energy gamma radiation or high energy electron beam. This leads to the creation of extremely unstable free radicals, molecular ions, and secondary electrons. The radiation by-products then interact with neighbouring molecules to rupture. The unwanted microorganism DNA is highly vulnerable to the destructive effects of ionizing radiation, which can break, depolymerize, mutate and modify the nucleic acid structure.

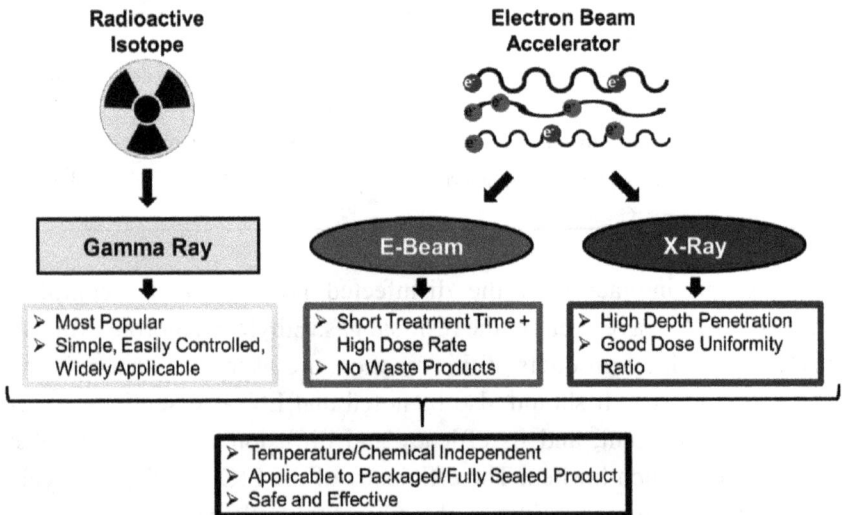

Figure 8.13: Comparison of sources for radiation sterilization (Image courtesy E. Goronzy).

8.5.4.1 *Gamma radiation*

Gamma (γ) irradiation is pure energy (about 1.2 MeV) generated by the spontaneous decay of radioisotopes. It is generated by self-disintegration (decaying) of the radioisotope $^{60}Co_{27}$ to stable non-reactive $^{60}Ni_{28}$ by emitting one negative β particle. Among thousands of γ emitters, only ^{60}Co (rarely ^{137}Cs) is suitable for the emittance of fairly high energy γ rays and reasonably long half-life of 5.27 years. ^{60}Co is prepared via neutron capture, as shown in the following equation:

$$^{59}Co_{27} + {}^{1}n_0 \rightarrow {}^{60}Co_{27}$$

γ sterilization is conducted at room temperature which makes it an appropriate sterilization method for temperature-sensitive materials. The high γ-ray penetrability allows for large sterilization loads and durability, even for intricate structures and tightly packed devices. γ rays either destroy the DNA helix directly or produce free radicals to disrupt chemical bonds within the DNA structure of microorganisms. The amount of energy transmitted and absorbed by a device is expressed in units of absorbed dose called kilo-Gray (kGy). The most regularly authenticated dose used to sterilize medical devices is 25 kGy (2.5 Mrad). Depending on the device, FDA further mandates that the maximum dose should not exceed 50 kGy. Due to its very high penetrating power, γ irradiation is a common procedure in sterilization of disposable medical equipment (syringes, needles) and connective tissue allografts such as skin, cartilage, bone, tendons, heart valves, and corneas.

γ radiation can easily be applied to many materials, including all extremely stable metallic alloys. It has been a common sterilization method for UHMWPE used in total joint replacement. However, in some cases, polymer irradiation may lead to cross-linking or breaking of the molecular chains (degradation) and, most likely, modifying mechanical properties. High levels of γ irradiation, i.e., 30–40 kGy (3.0–4.0 Mrad), have been shown to exhibit detrimental effects on tissue mechanics. Soft tissue allografts are reported to work well when treated at <20 kGy (2.0 Mrad). However, most bioresorbable polymers such as polyvinyl chloride are also too delicate to radiation to be sterilized by this procedure.

For operators' protection, γ radiation demands bulky shielding; it also needs a strong facility to store the radioisotope as it continually emits γ rays irrespective of the procedure (half-life is 5.27 years). Due to safety issues, γ-ray sterilization cannot be conducted in regular healthcare facilities and are instead performed in a few industrial centers.

8.5.4.2 *Electron beam irradiation*

Electron beam (e-beam) radiation energy (between 4 and 6 MeV) is higher than that of γ rays. Sterilization can thus be accomplished alternatively using a high beam of electrons. These scattered electrons destroy nucleic acids, proteins, and enzymes vital for microorganism growth and proliferation. When compared to γ radiation, e-beam is capable of producing the same dose in less time (seconds when compared to hours) but has a disadvantage of low penetration depth. The advantages and disadvantages of radiation sterilization are presented in Table 8.3.

8.5.4.3 *Ultraviolet radiation*

Ultraviolet (UV) radiation, also known as UV disinfection or UV germicidal irradiation, provides a quick, effective inactivation of

Table 8.3:   Advantages and disadvantages of radiation sterilization.

Advantages	Disadvantages
High penetration depth	High cost with specialized facilities is needed. γ radiation needs a nuclear reactor, whereas electrons are generated using e-beam accelerators.
Radiation can be processed in their fully sealed, final packaging.	In some polymeric materials, radiation energy leads to breakage of bonds and chemical cross-linking.
No heat dependence and compatible with temperature-sensitive materials.	In the case of γ radiation, careful disposal of radioactive material is a must.
No residue is left behind on the sterilized product.	
Flexibility of materials	

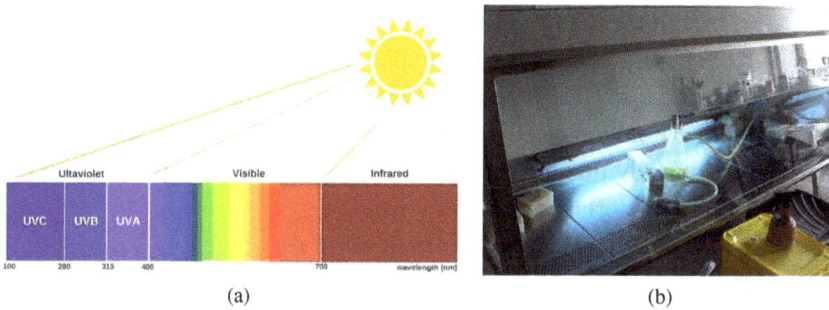

Figure 8.14: (a) Examples of non-ionizing radiation include infrared and UV radiation; (b) UV light employed in research laboratories to irradiate and sterilize laminar flow cabinets between or before experiments (Boundless, 2019; Obodovskiy, 2019).

microorganisms through a physical process. A characteristic germicidal wavelength between 240 and 280 nm can decrease reproduction capability of both vegetative and spore forms of microorganisms by breaking down specific chemical bonds and cluttering the structures of DNA, RNA, and proteins. UV light has three wavelength categories: UV-A, UV-B, and UV-C (Figure 8.14a). Only the high-energy and shorter wavelength UV-C light is used to neutralize microorganisms. Its maximum efficacy relies on the total energy applied, duration of exposure, and distance from the source of light. For instance, a UV lamp placed close to a bacteria-grown petri dish (e.g., *E. coli*) can achieve full sterilization in 1–2 min. On the other hand, it may take 5–10 min to sterilize surgical instruments and about 30 min for a complete biosafety cabinet. UV radiation is particularly useful in hospitals to destroy the spore-forming gram-positive bacteria *Clostridium difficile*, a major source of hospital-acquired infections. The image of UV light-employed laminar flow cabinet typically used in research laboratories to irradiate and sterilize between or before experiments is shown in Figure 8.14b.

8.5.5 *Non-traditional sterilization methods*

8.5.5.1 *Chemical treatments*

Although EtO is the most commonly used chemical for sterilization of devices, other chemicals such as ozone (O_3) gas, hydrogen peroxide

(H_2O_2), nitrogen dioxide (NO_2), glutaraldehyde ($C_5H_8O_2$) and formalde-hyde (CH_2O) solutions, phthalaldehyde, and peracetic acid are used as alternatives to oxidize most organic matter. Alcohol-based solutions, such as ethanol, are not suggested for the sterilization of medical and surgical materials, primarily due to their inefficiency on bacterial spores and fail-ure to infiltrate materials rich in proteins.

O_3, a pale-blue gas and an allotropic form of oxygen, is a robust oxi-dative gas that chemically alters and inactivates chemical impurities and pathogens. It may be considered as one of the most effective natural ger-micides that have the potential to disinfect and sterilize devices with no leftover residues as it decomposes to natural oxygen (O_2). Despite O_3's oxidative efficiency, its use as a sterilizing agent continues to be a concern due to its highly toxic nature and stabilization problems.

Vaporized H_2O_2 (VHP) sterilization is a low-temperature sterilization process that inactivates microorganisms by converting into extremely reactive hydroxyl radicals (OH oxidation) which target membrane lipids, DNA, and other important elements of cells. It can be rapidly decomposed to environmentally safe by-products (water and oxygen) by enzymes known as peroxidases. H_2O_2 sterilization has a quick cycle time (30–45 min) and has relatively good material compatibility. It is commonly used to sterilize reusable metals, non-metallic devices, and heat-sensitive devices employed in healthcare facilities. However, when compared to EtO, VHP has lower penetration capabilities.

Glutaraldehyde is a saturated dialdehyde, which has been generally accepted as an extraordinary-level disinfectant and chemical sterilizer for medical devices such as endoscopes, probes, spirometry tubing, dialyzers, transducers, anaesthesia, and respiratory therapy equipment. As men-tioned earlier, chemical sterilization is employed for devices that are sus-ceptible to the high heat used in steam sterilization, and for devices that can be affected by irradiation. One of the major contrasts between thermal (autoclaving and dry heat) and liquid chemical procedures for sterilization of devices is the ease of penetration into microorganisms by the sterilant. Heat can efficiently infiltrate membranes to destroy bacterial cells, whereas liquids cannot infiltrate these barriers satisfactorily. The major drawbacks of chemical sterilization are post-processing and leftover solvents. Ozone and H_2O_2 sterilization treatments are still under evaluation by the FDA.

8.5.5.2 *Gaseous chlorine dioxide treatment*

Due to its simplicity and low cost, chlorine dioxide (ClO_2) oxidative gas is also used in sterilization methods at temperatures ranging from 25–30°C. It is normally employed for decontaminating surfaces of medical devices. Its deep penetration ability into the slime layers of bacteria has also resulted in its adoption for deactivating most water-borne pathogens such as *Cryptosporidium parvum* oocysts in the drinking water industry. Its sterilization mechanism is by disrupting protein synthesis. In its pure form, ClO_2 is a hazardous gas, but it rapidly breaks down in the air to chlorine (Cl_2) gas and O_2. Cl_2 gas has some harmful effects, such as altering target quality. Hence, although this technology was first introduced in the late 1980s, it has not yet been cleared by the FDA, raising concerns about its efficacy and safety.

Table 8.4:   Sterilization methods and their common biomaterial uses.

Sterilization method		Common biomaterial uses
Steam		Dental, sterile processing, culture media, glassware, flammable and heat-sensitive items, liquids, and dense loads
Dry heat		Metallic instruments, oils, glassware, and ceramics
Ethylene oxide		Most medical devices and endoscopes
Gamma radiation		Biopolymers such as UHMWPE, bone, and musculoskeletal tissue grafts
Electron beam sterilization		Heat-sensitive biomedical devices
Plasma		Endoscopes, soft contact lenses, surgical items, and dental products
Chemical treatment	Ozone	Silicone-based hydrogels and laboratory devices such as pipettes, pipette tips, gloves, and plates
	Glutaraldehyde	Endoscopes, probes, spirometry tubing, dialyzers, transducers, anaesthesia, and respiratory therapy equipment
	Vaporized H_2O_2	Reusable metals, non-metallic devices, and heat-sensitive devices

8.6 Multiple choice questions

1. Sterilization is a process
   (a) by which the microbial burden on objects is reduced or completely removed
   (b) by which the microbial burden on objects is increased
   (c) used to improve surface properties of the object
   (d) used to change the surface topography of the object

2. The absence of all forms of microbial life, including spores, is known as
   (a) cleaning
   (b) sanitization
   (c) disinfection
   (d) sterilization

3. The temperature-pressure combination for typical autoclaving is
   (a) 99°C and 9 psi
   (b) 121°C and 15 psi
   (c) 114°C and 10 psi
   (d) 141°C and 13 psi

4. Which of the following is an accepted sterilant?
   (a) chlorhexidine
   (b) chloroform
   (c) ethylene oxide
   (d) benzene

5. Which of the following is NOT a sterilization method?
   (a) aqueous glutaraldehyde for 10 hours
   (b) dry heating at 180°C for 1–2 hours
   (c) water boiling of medical device at 100°C for 20–25 minutes
   (d) using electrons for sterilization

6. Which of the following is TRUE regarding heat conduction in dry air?
   (a) slower than in steam
   (b) quicker than in steam
   (c) similar to steam
   (d) none of these

7. Which order of reaction describes the destruction of microorganisms by moist heat?
   (a) first-order
   (b) zero-order
   (c) fourth-order
   (d) fifth-order

8. Cell-sensitive media comprising bacterial spores and heat-sensitive materials are usually sterilized by
   (a) autoclaving
   (b) dry heat
   (c) UV radiation
   (d) chemical treatments

9. Which of the following about EtO sterilization is NOT true?
   (a) kills all bacterial spores
   (b) kills all microorganisms
   (c) performed at temperatures identical to autoclaving
   (d) long cycles

10. The long exposure of batch sterilization may cause the following consequence:
    (a) purification of media may happen
    (b) revival of media may happen
    (c) product degradation
    (d) quality of the device may improve

References & Further Reading

Boundless. (2019). Microbiology (Boundless). In *The LibreTexts libraries* (Vol. CC BY-SA 4.0). Department of Education Open Textbook Pilot Project: Powered by MindTouch®.

Branaghan, R. J., Hildebrand, E. A., & Foster, L. B. (2020). Chapter 1 — Designing for medical device safety. In A. Sethumadhavan & F. Sasangohar (Eds.), *Design for Health* (pp. 3–29): Academic Press.

Gudeppu, M., Sawant, S., Chockalingam, C. G., & Timiri Shanmugam, P. S. (2020). Chapter 8 — Medical device regulations. In P. S. Timiri Shanmugam, L. Chokkalingam, & P. Bakthavachalam (Eds.), *Trends in Development of Medical Devices* (pp. 135–152): Academic Press.

Harrington, R. E., Guda, T., Lambert, B., & Martin, J. (2020). Chapter 3.1.4 — Sterilization and Disinfection of Biomaterials for Medical Devices. In W. R. Wagner, S. E. Sakiyama-Elbert, G. Zhang, & M. J. Yaszemski (Eds.), *Biomaterials Science (Fourth Edition)* (pp. 1431–1446): Academic Press.

Hubert, P., Fernlund, G., & Poursartip, A. (2012). Chapter 13 — Autoclave processing for composites. In S. G. Advani & K.-T. Hsiao (Eds.), *Manufacturing Techniques for Polymer Matrix Composites (PMCs)* (pp. 414–434): Woodhead Publishing.

Keene, A. T. (2020). Chapter 16 — Biological evaluation and regulation of medical devices in the European Union. In J. P. Boutrand (Ed.), *Biocompatibility and Performance of Medical Devices (Second Edition)* (pp. 413–440): Woodhead Publishing.

Lerouge, S. (2019). Chapter 16 — Sterilization and cleaning of metallic biomaterials. In M. Niinomi (Ed.), *Metals for Biomedical Devices (Second Edition)* (pp. 405–428): Woodhead Publishing.

Moondra, S., Raval, N., Kuche, K., Maheshwari, R., *et al.* (2018). Chapter 14 — Sterilization of Pharmaceuticals: Technology, Equipment, and Validation. In R. K. Tekade (Ed.), *Dosage Form Design Parameters* (pp. 467–519): Academic Press.

Obodovskiy, I. (2019). Chapter 30 — Radiation Sterilization. In I. Obodovskiy (Ed.), *Radiation* (pp. 373–378): Elsevier.

Ogrodnik, P. (2020). Chapter 2 — Classifying medical devices. In P. Ogrodnik (Ed.), *Medical Device Design (Second Edition)* (pp. 17–49): Academic Press.

Ramakrishna, S., Tian, L., Wang, C., Liao, S., *et al.* (2015). Chapter 2 — General regulations of medical devices. In S. Ramakrishna, L. Tian, C. Wang, S. Liao, & W. E. Teo (Eds.), *Medical Devices* (pp. 21–47): Woodhead Publishing.

Rogers, W. J. (2013). Chapter 4 — The effects of sterilization on medical materials and welded devices. In Y. Zhou & M. D. Breyen (Eds.), *Joining and Assembly of Medical Materials and Devices* (pp. 79–130): Woodhead Publishing.

Sadeque, M., & Balachandran, S. K. (2020). Chapter 10 — Overview of medical device processing. In P. S. Timiri Shanmugam, L. Chokkalingam, & P. Bakthavachalam (Eds.), *Trends in Development of Medical Devices* (pp. 177–188): Academic Press.

Sandle, T. (2013). Chapter 8 — Gaseous sterilization. In T. Sandle (Ed.), *Sterility, Sterilization and Sterility Assurance for Pharmaceuticals* (pp. 111–128): Woodhead Publishing.

Sandle, T. (2016). Chapter 12 — Sterilization and sterility assurance. In T. Sandle (Ed.), *Pharmaceutical Microbiology* (pp. 147–160). Oxford: Woodhead Publishing.

Shan, C., & Liu, M. (2020). Chapter 18 — Medical device regulations in China. In J. P. Boutrand (Ed.), *Biocompatibility and Performance of Medical Devices (Second Edition)* (pp. 475–488): Woodhead Publishing.

Van Norman, G. A. (2016). Drugs and Devices: Comparison of European and U.S. Approval Processes. *JACC: Basic to Translational Science, 1*(5), 399–412. doi:10.1016/j.jacbts.2016.06.003.

Chapter 9
Surface engineering

9.1 Introduction

Since we have studied about cells and their functions in Chapter 1, can we now tell on which surfaces cells attach more: hydrophobic or hydrophilic? If it is hydrophilic, how can we turn a hydrophobic surface hydrophilic? What happens when foreign material is implanted in the body? Is it possible to selectively modify a surface to enhance performance of the biomaterials?

Metallic, polymeric, and ceramic materials used in medical implants obviously meet certain functional property specifications. Still, at various implanted sites, the biological media (extracellular fluid or blood) or the specific biological material (soft or hard tissue) may be different. Although bulk properties such as material design and mechanical modulus may primarily determine its qualification or fitness for a given implant application, the material surface and its chemical properties often have the most significant impact on how the implant interacts with the surrounding biological environment. In nearly all cases, the significant interactions for surgically implanted biomaterials (polymer, ceramic or metal) occur at microscopic, macroscopic, and systemic levels. The interface between these biomaterials and tissues/body fluids, and the reactions at cellular or protein level, are in some way directly or indirectly linked with the surface properties of the biomaterials.

Surface engineering is the method of modifying or coating a material's surface to achieve desired purposes. In tissue engineering and several other biomedical disciplines, surface engineering of the biomaterial surface plays a crucial role in enhancing cell adhesion, proliferation, viability, and improved ECM-secretion functions. In brief, the overall objectives of biomaterial surface engineering are:

- Decontaminate the material surface
- Lower/remove protein adsorption
- Decrease/eliminate undesired cell adhesion
- Decrease/eliminate bacterial adhesion
- Reduce thrombogenicity
- Encourage desired cellular attachment/adhesion
- Modify transport characteristics
- Enhance lubricity, i.e., reduction in friction and/or wear (metallic materials)
- Improve hardness values (metallic materials)
- Augment corrosion/degradation resistance

9.2 Biomaterial-tissue interaction

To understand the importance of surface engineering, it is first essential to understand the interactions that are happening at the interface between implant material and tissue. When a biomaterial is implanted in the individual and comes into contact with biological fluids, the host and the biomaterial engage in a series of interactions/reactions. This body fluid is a corrosive aqueous medium composed of different forms of ions and molecules (proteins, polysaccharides, and enzymes) and distinct cell types that help the tissue to grow and remodel. The early complex events happening on the biomaterial surface can significantly impact its implantation efficacy and effectiveness.

Within nanoseconds (10^{-9} seconds), molecular-level reactions occur where water molecules first touch its surface. The interaction and binding of water on the surface are determined by the surface properties, which affect the proteins and other molecular forms that later appear. Within seconds of implantation, a protein layer is adsorbed. Over a long duration, depending on the biomaterial surface, several macro reactions such as implant collapse and/or new tissue creation may occur. After water adsorption and protein adsorption, the system's surface is still exposed to a sequence of biological occurrences as the exposure time extends from

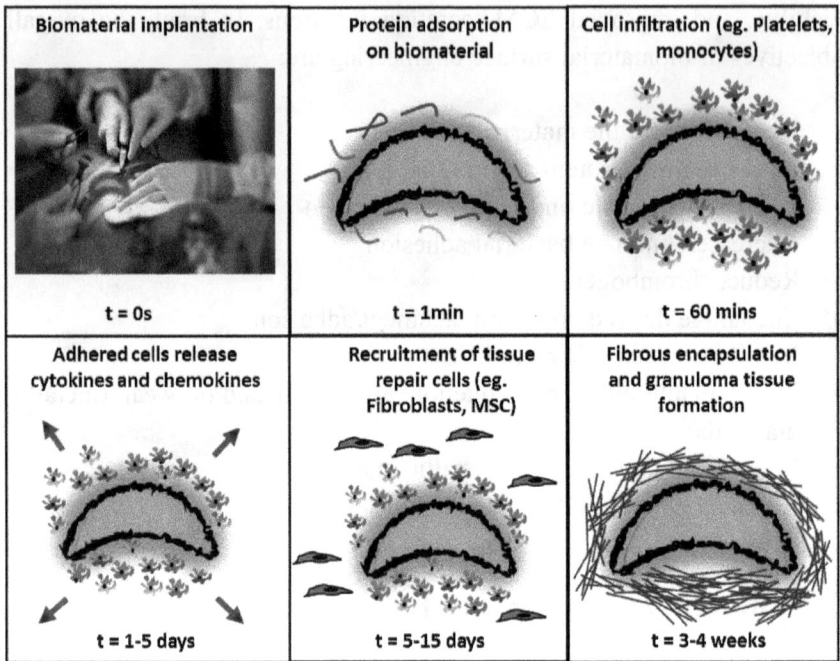

Biomaterial implantation	Protein adsorption on biomaterial	Cell infiltration (eg. Platelets, monocytes)
t = 0s	t = 1min	t = 60 mins
Adhered cells release cytokines and chemokines	Recruitment of tissue repair cells (eg. Fibroblasts, MSC)	Fibrous encapsulation and granuloma tissue formation
t = 1-5 days	t = 5-15 days	t = 3-4 weeks

Figure 9.1:   Instinctive immune reaction following implantation of biomaterial (Sridharan *et al.*, 2015).

minutes to hours, days, and years. These include temporary matrix development, cell adhesion, cell proliferation, and new tissue development on and across the biomaterial being implanted. Figure 9.1 shows a natural instinctive immune reaction following the implantation of biomaterial. If the biomaterial is blood-contacting, as most of the implants are, the first adsorbed protein layer dictates how cells react to the inherent biomaterial, resulting in either successful tissue incorporation or rejection as a foreign body. The protein layer commences a series of cascade trials and regulates the healing actions, including (i) inflammation, (ii) formation of granulation tissue, (iii) foreign body reaction, and (iv) scar growth.

9.3 Wound healing phases

Wound healing is an extremely complex and closely organized mechanism for restoring the tissue's integrity after injury, infection or physical

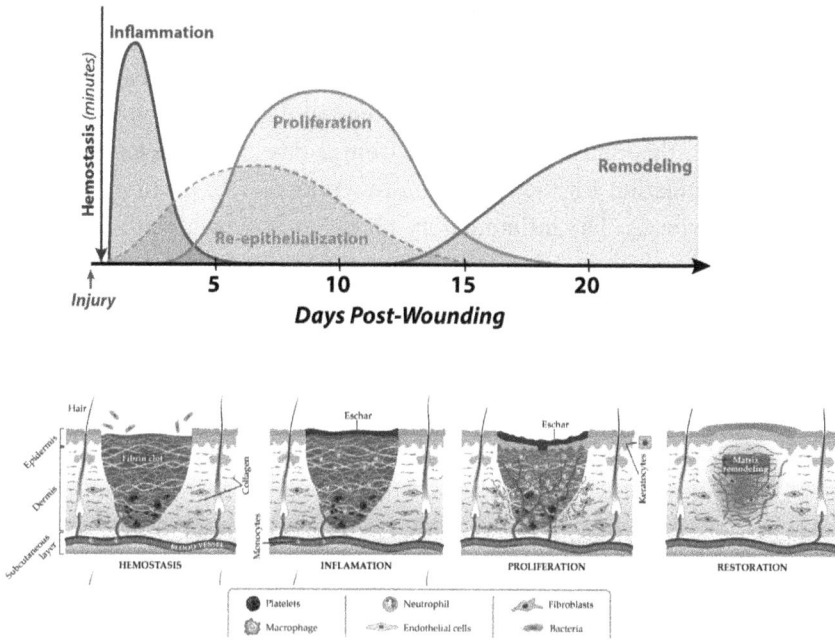

Figure 9.2: (Top) Timeline of a typical human cutaneous wound healing process; (Bottom) schematic representation of the healing phases (des Jardins-Park *et al.*, 2019; Rezvani Ghomi *et al.*, 2019; Walker *et al.*, 2015; Negut *et al.*, 2018).

trauma. As presented in Figure 9.2, this phase can essentially be broken down into three separate phases:

(i) **Coagulation and inflammation phase:** the injury, wound, or tissue damage is temporarily closed by hemostasis, and recruitment of inflammatory cells is instigated.
(ii) **Tissue proliferation/repair:** pro-inflammatory indicators decline slowly, and local growth factors instigate cell proliferation.
(iii) **Tissue remodeling:** wound reorganization restructures the tissue.

9.3.1 *Inflammatory phase*

Inflammation is the body's natural immediate defensive reaction that begins at the time of injury, surgery or infection. Depending on the nature of the wound, this phase usually lasts from 2 days to 3 weeks. It establishes the foundation for the remaining two phases, i.e., proliferative and remodelling phases. The inflammatory phase is associated with hemostasis (prevent and stop bleeding), chemotaxis (cell movement), and improved vascular permeability. All of these restrict additional destruction on the wound, facilitate removal of cellular fragments, eliminate live/dead bacteria, and encourage cellular migration. During this inflammatory phase, a cluster of white blood cells called neutrophils enters the wound to remove debris and to prevent infection by attacking pathogens and other harmful reagents. These cells are not often observed in healthy skin, but when recruited during injury, they hit their peak population between 24 and 48 hours. These numbers significantly decrease after three days. As the white blood cells leave, advanced monocyte-differentiated macrophages start to clear debris. Specifically, hemostasis is accomplished via the installation of a provisional fibrin matrix that functions as a foundation for permeating neutrophils and macrophages. Cell types present in the inflammatory response differ with the age of the injury. The schematics of different cells involved in the wound healing process with the time frame are shown in Figure 9.3 and tabulated in Table 9.1.

- **Neutrophils:** these are the most abundant white blood cells and the first inflammatory cells to immigrate to the wound site. These cells act largely during the first 1–2 days.
- **Monocytes:** monocytes replace neutrophils and act predominantly from the 2nd day and lasts two weeks.
- **Macrophages:** Monocytes differentiate into macrophages, and these cells are very long-lived (up to months) and are present during all stages of the tissue repair process. Macrophages are thought to perform multiple roles during wound healing but primarily act in the inflammatory process to help prepare the region for the next phase, i.e., granulation tissue formation.

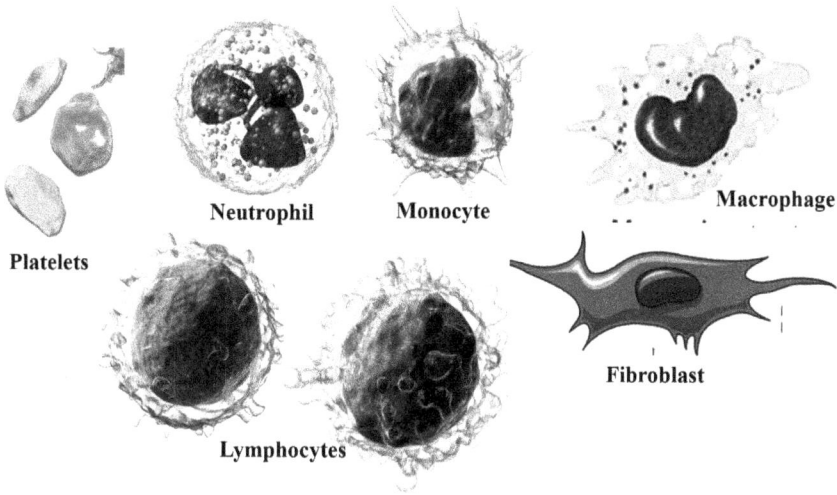

Figure 9.3:   Different kinds of cells involved in the wound healing process with typical morphology (Blaus, 2014).

Table 9.1:   Critical phases and important cells involved in wound healing.

Phase	Important cells involved
Inflammation	Neutrophils, monocytes, and macrophages
Proliferation/repair	Macrophages, fibroblasts, myofibroblasts and keratinocytes
Remodeling	Fibroblasts and macrophages

9.3.1.1 *Proliferative/repair phase*

Once the wound is thoroughly cleaned out, it reaches the next process, i.e., the proliferative phase (approximately 3–10 days after wounding). The main attention is on filling and covering the wound, generating new granulation tissue, and rebuilding the vascular network. The proliferative phase of wound healing overlaps with the inflammatory phase. It is mainly characterized by cellular migration and proliferation, granulation tissue development (dermal repair), re-epithelialization (wound closure), and neo-vascularization (angiogenesis). During this phase, the wound defect is "*rebuilt*" with highly vascular connective tissue, commonly referred to as "*granulation tissue*" comprising collagen and ECM and into which a new network of blood vessels develops. During this phase, the critical aspect of wound closure, i.e., re-epithelialization, occurs where the wound edges are sealed between the underlying wound and the environment. The wound margins are contracted and pulled towards the center of the wound. Basal keratinocytes, the primary epithelial cells, are responsible for re-epithelialization. The process of contracting wound margins is terminated when the migrating cells touch each other.

Finally, neo-vascularization, an essential step in wound healing, takes place. It is a crucial procedure involving the development of vascular networks mainly through angiogenesis. This growth of new capillaries from existing blood vessels is mediated by endothelial cells. Apart from macrophages, cell types present in the proliferative phase are:

- **Keratinocytes:** they are highly specialized epithelial cells that accelerate re-epithelialization by proliferating and migrating across the wounded area to re-establish barrier function. After covering the granulation tissue, the cells meet in the middle. Keratinocytes also regulate fibroblast activities and vice versa.
- **Myofibroblasts:** they are mainly involved in granulation tissue formation.
- **Endothelial cells:** they are mainly involved in neo-vascularization.

9.3.2 *Remodeling phase*

The remodeling phase, also recognized as maturation, occurs in the final stage once the wound is closed and marks the transition from granulation tissue to scar. This phase usually happens from day 21 up to 1 year. This phase is characterized by reduced cellular activity with the abandonment of multiple cell types, including fibroblasts, myofibroblasts, and endothelial cells. During this final remodeling phase, excess macrophages and endothelial cells experience cell death (apoptosis), while fibroblasts and myofibroblasts generate and accumulate a collagenous extracellular matrix. Myofibroblasts are developed from fibroblasts, and mainly contribute to remodeling.

Fortunately, it is possible to manipulate the biomaterial surface properties and increase the chance of effective tissue integration by reducing unwanted protein adsorption and its accompanying inflammatory reactions. Besides, biomaterial surfaces can also be engineered to introduce specific proteins and peptide structures that promote cellular adhesion.

9.4 Surface modification techniques

Several surface modification techniques have been established for all groups of biomaterials (polymer, ceramic and metal) to regulate biological reactions and enhance device performance. This allows for precise cell-material interface configuration that facilitates unique cellular adhesion and performance whilst preventing an unwanted host response. This includes reducing protein adsorption/thrombogenicity, controlling and enhancing cell morphological properties, augmentation, osseointegration, and enhancing wear and corrosion resistance. We have learned from previous chapters that most bulk materials aren't natural biomaterials. This is, they may have excellent mechanical properties but do not interact well with biological tissues and fluids. Hence, a wide variety of surface modifications is usually done on medical implant materials to encourage resistance to corrosion and enhance biocompatibility.

Surface modification of biomaterials can be categorized mainly into two groups; physical-based and chemical-based. Schematic diagrams of various surface modification techniques are shown in Figure 9.4. Physical modification leads to a change in surface topography or morphology without affecting surface chemistry. The modification also covers the coating of the original surface with biomimetic substances and does not change the chemical characteristics of either. Examples include ball milling, etching, grit-blasting, machining, single-layer coatings, or coatings containing

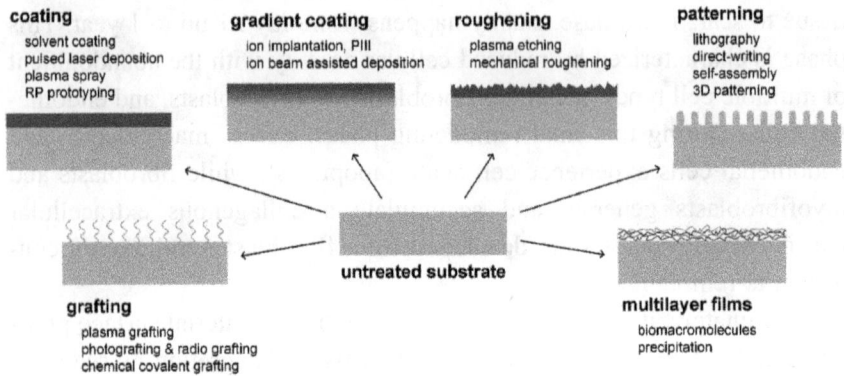

coating
solvent coating
pulsed laser deposition
plasma spray
RP prototyping

gradient coating
ion implantation, PIII
ion beam assisted deposition

roughening
plasma etching
mechanical roughening

patterning
lithography
direct-writing
self-assembly
3D patterning

untreated substrate

grafting
plasma grafting
photografting & radio grafting
chemical covalent grafting

multilayer films
biomacromolecules
precipitation

Figure 9.4:   Schematic diagrams of various surface modification techniques (Qiu *et al.*, 2014).

several layers of distinct compositions. In contrast, chemical modification involves chemical reactions which change existing atoms or molecules on the surface of the material. Oxidizing, nitriding, functionalization, and ion infusion are some of the chemical modifications performed on a material.

Key definitions

Adsorption: It is defined as the accumulation of chemical species (gas, liquid, solid molecules) on a surface.
Absorption: It is simply described as a procedure where one thing becomes part of another thing.

9.4.1 *Surface modification techniques for polymeric biomaterials*

Polymers are the predominant class of biomaterials researched widely for various uses because of their distinctive properties such as moldability and mechanical properties. Details of polymeric biomaterials are discussed extensively in Chapter 5. Given the value of surface engineering, several polymer surface modification procedures have been researched over the years with a primary objective to stop non-specific protein

Polymer surface modification

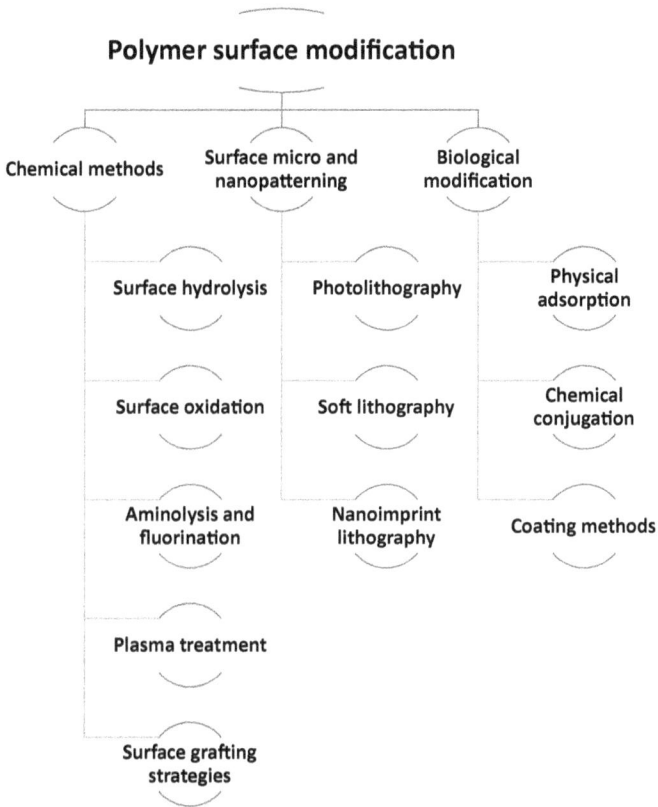

Figure 9.5:   List of various polymer surface modification techniques.

adsorption. The modifications also aim to improve precise cellular adhesion or to facilitate surface-based transfer of bioactive agents. These techniques are presented in Figure 9.5.

9.4.1.1 *Chemical methods*

To modify the polymer surface chemistry, a large number of specific and
non-specific chemical reactions are used. Non-specific reactions establish a
random delivery of several functional groups, for example, those produced
by oxidation or plasma therapy. In comparison, specific reactions alter a
specific functional group with high competence and rare side responses,

such as those produced by radical polymerization. Chemically dependent surface modifications can also range in difficulty from straightforward, to multi-stage surface grafting reactions requiring the modification of a particular functional group, to more than one surface grafting reaction.

a. **Surface hydrolysis:** In the presence of an acidic or basic medium, hydrolysis breaks up the bonding network in the polymer and makes it available for conjugation. A common strategy is to modify aliphatic polyesters like PLA, PGA, and PLGA by fractional surface hydrolysis using acid or base. This leads to the spontaneous breaking of ester bonds in the polymer chain, resulting in surface generation of hydroxyl and carboxylic terminal groups.

b. **Surface oxidation:** Insertion of peroxy organic clusters onto polymer surfaces for immediate grafting can be accomplished either by photo-oxidation (UV radiation) or ozone oxidation. Photo-oxidation in the presence of UV light involves the immersion of polymeric biomaterial into a hydrogen peroxide (H_2O_2) solution. The H_2O_2 groups disintegrate when irradiated by UV light, producing reactive oxygen species such as hydroxyl radicals ($\bullet$OH) on the surface of the material. These new components may be used to initiate polymerization reactions from the revised surface. Ozone (O_3) oxidation is another commonly used method to create reactive groups on polymer surfaces. The exposure of a polymer to O_3 leads to the generation of peroxide, carboxyl (COOH), and carbonyl groups (C=O), which can then be utilized to trigger polymerization of the surface and/or grafting reactions. To enhance conjugation rate, the ozone procedure can sometimes be employed with UV radiation.

c. **Aminolysis and fluorination:** Aminolysis and fluorination are other commonly used forms of chemically dependent functionalization that respectively add reactive amine groups and halogens (fluorine, chlorine) on polymer surfaces, which can be later employed to immobilize biomolecules via conjugation reactions.

d. **Plasma treatment:** A plasma is a partly ionized gas that contains ions, electrons, free radicals, atoms, and molecules that are generally created by ion/electron impact under an applied electric field:

$$A + e^- \rightarrow A^+ + 2\,e^-$$

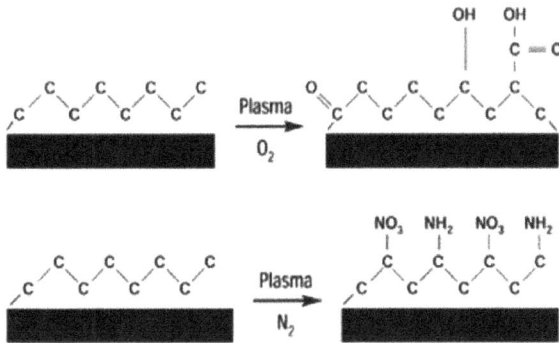

Figure 9.6: Examples of gas plasma treatment.

Plasma treatment can be used to enable surface functionalization on inert polymeric surfaces. The type of functional group placed on the surface of the polymer typically depends on the plasma gas used. For example, reactive NH_3 plasma bestows amine groups, O_2 plasma generates a combination of OH and COOH functional groups, and Ar plasma releases free radicals onto the polymer surface. The schematic illustration of functional group introduction on polymer surfaces by plasma is shown in Figure 9.6.

e. **Surface grafting strategies:** Surface grafting is an attractive surface modification method that adapts a variety of new functional groups onto a polymer surface. It can be generally divided into two categories, i.e., '*grafting-to*' and '*grafting-from*' processes. The technique of "*grafting-to*" initially modifies the solid polymer substrate with the desired functional groups and then grafts a preformed polymer onto the surface through a certain chemical reaction. The chemical response occurs between the chemical group of the solid polymer substrate and the reactive side chains of the preformed polymer to form a *polymer brush*. It should be noted that in the "*grafting-to*" strategy, no monomer polymerization reaction takes place throughout the construction of the *polymer brushes,* and the grafting process typically depends on the chemical reaction between the terminal group of the incoming polymer and the surface group of the polymer solid substrate. In the "*grafting-from*" technique, the polymer chains grow *in situ* from the strongly anchored initiator that has been earlier affixed to the polymer solid surface. The polymer chains

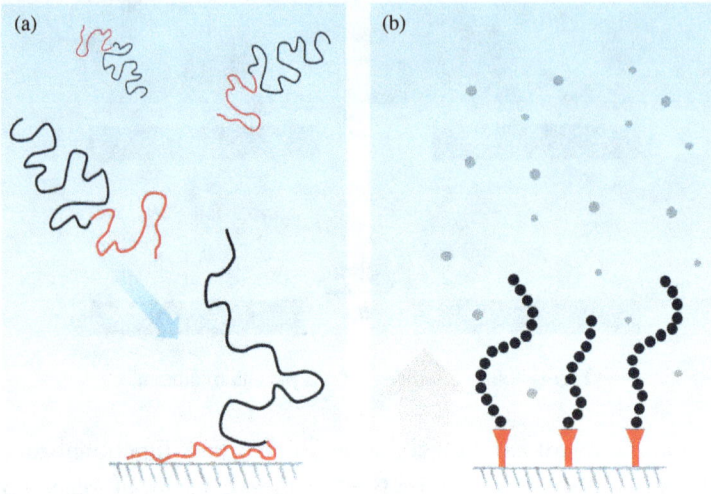

Figure 9.7:   Surface functionalization by (a) grafting-to and (b) grafting-from techniques (Morgese *et al.*, 2017).

progressively mature from the surface and develop gradually to form high-density polymer brushes. The functionalization of substrate via grafting-to and grafting-from approaches is provided in Figure 9.7. In both cases, densely grafted assemblies of polymer chains forming a *"brush"* type of design can be effectively obtained. Among all available hydrophilic polymers, polyethylene glycol and its derivatives have been the most used for grafting purposes. This approach is proved to be effectively employed for the construction and modification of a wide range of biomaterials, comprising scaffolds for tissue engineering, anti-biofouling and antimicrobial surfaces, and biosensors.

9.4.1.2 *Surface micro and nanopatterning*

Polymeric surface characteristics can be altered by implementing a range of techniques that establish novel micro/nanopatterns. Depending on the application, the generated designs can be either random or organized and can be a mixture of physical and chemical techniques. Lithography is a micro- and nano-fabrication technique widely used in the microelectronics industry, employed for polymeric surfaces to enable the formation of precise and complex 2D or 3D micro and nano-patterns at exceedingly small scales. Particularly, photolithography has become one of the prominent methods used to design biomaterials surfaces. For biomedical applications, the unique topographical surface design formed on a silicon wafer is reproduced on the surface of a polymer, including pits, channels with grooves and ridges, and pillars.

a. **Photolithography:** Photolithography is an optical way to transmit a template onto a substrate material. In this procedure, a photoreactive polymer is coated on top of a material, such as a silicon wafer. Previously selected sections of a polymeric substance are subjected to UV radiation, allowing polymerization, cross-linking, or degradation to begin. After the exposure, the substrate is cleaned, and the transferred pattern is etched strongly on the substrate with a suitable solvent. A graphic interpretation of the photolithography process is shown in Figure 9.8.

b. **Soft lithography:** Soft lithography is a group of patterning methods that are fundamentally based on printing, molding, and embossing. It utilizes soft, flexible elastomeric biomaterials to produce or transfer the micron and sub-micron scale structures onto a polymeric surface.

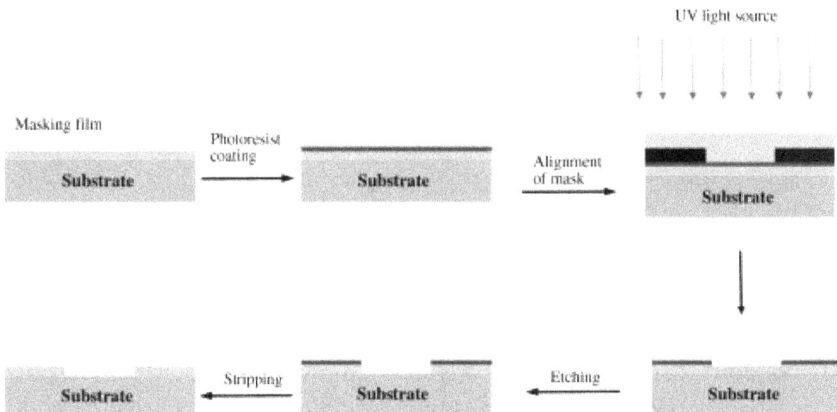

Figure 9.8: Schematic representation of the photolithographic process (Yilbas *et al.*, 2019).

Due to elasticity and ease of fabrication, poly(dimethylsiloxane) elastomer is the most commonly used *"soft"* master for the soft lithography process. Soft lithography includes techniques for creating or replicating structures using elastomeric plates, molds, and photomasks. This technique benefits from relatively lower cost, easier setup, and high throughput. For soft lithography, a universal photolithography procedure is applied to construct a required pattern on a silicon substrate.

c. **Microcontact printing:** Microcontact printing, a subset of soft lithography technique, is yet another significant surface modification technique used for transferring patterns of polymeric biomaterials. In tissue engineering, it is regularly advantageous to design bioactive molecules such as proteins, protein mixtures, peptides, and DNA on the surface of substrates in order to enhance and improve desired cell adhesion and proliferation. During this method, an ink solution is transmitted to a substrate surface from an elastomeric mold or stamp. The stamp is created using previously mentioned soft lithography approaches, and usually the ink solution consists of small bioactive molecules. After pouring the stamping solution onto the stamp, the transition occurs at the paper interface and the target substrate. Graphical diagram of microcontact printing to fabricate a pattern of biological molecules on a polymeric material is shown in Figure 9.9.

d. **Nanoimprint lithography (NIL):** This is a high-resolution nanopatterning method used to manufacture nanoscale characteristics on top of a polymer material. NIL primarily involves the resist layer's direct mechanical deformation and is categorized into thermal-based NIL (T-NIL) and ultraviolet-based NIL (UV-NIL). In the case of T-NIL, a temperature is often applied to soften a thermoplastic polymer resist for imprinting, and before pressing and cooling for solidification. These heat and pressure-induced patterns from a rigid mold are patterned by heating the polymer film above its glass transition temperature. Schematic illustrations of the thermal nanoimprint process on a polymer sheet are shown in Figure 9.10. In UV-NIL, the pattern process uses UV light and a transparent rigid quartz glass or silica mold

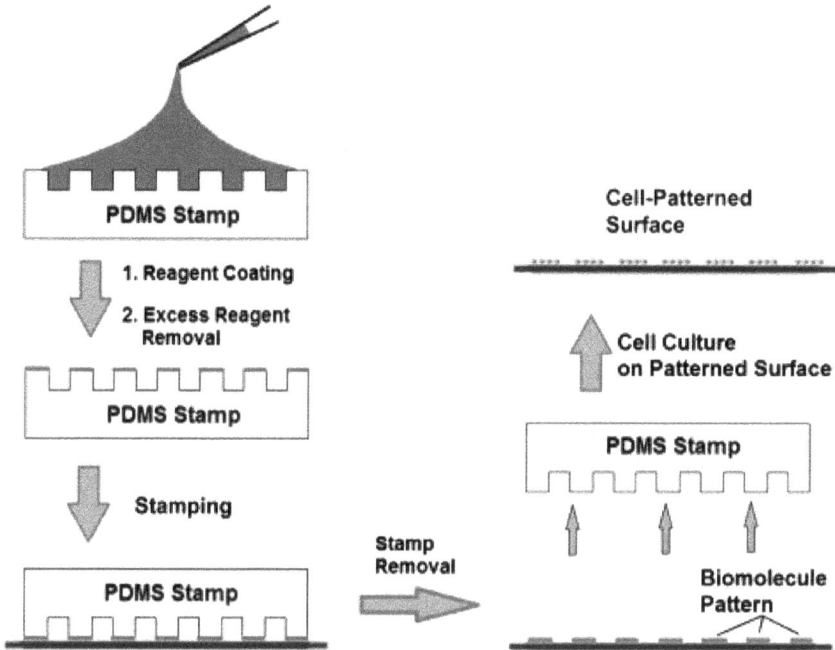

Figure 9.9: Graphical diagram of microcontact printing technology to fabricate a pattern of biological molecules on a polymeric material (Cha *et al.*, 2014).

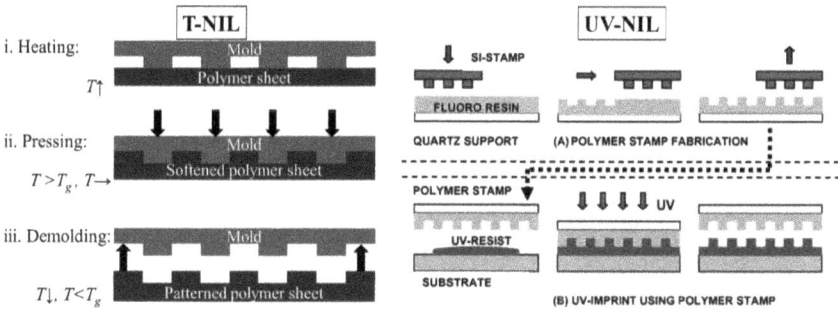

Figure 9.10: (Left) Schematic illustrations of thermal nanoimprint process on a polymer sheet; (Right) schematics of the fabrication procedure of polymer stamp by UV-NIL method (Fu *et al.*, 2019; Haatainen *et al.*, 2009).

to pattern a photoreactive polymer precursor. In brief, a UV-curable resist is spin-coated or drop-dispensed onto the substrate. A transparent template is used for impression, and the printed structures are cured through UV-light treatment, which photo-polymerize the resist. The template is then released from the stamped substrate. Schematics of the fabrication procedure of polymer stamp by UV-NIL method is shown in Figure 9.10. The manufacture of quartz mold for UV-NIL is difficult due to the electron beam exposure.

9.4.1.3 *Biological modification of polymeric surfaces*

a. **Physical adsorption:** Physical adsorption is considered as the easiest way to modify a polymer's surface by incubating the polymer in a biomolecular solution, thereby making the relevant particles attach onto the surface. Adsorption is defined as the adhesion of chemical species onto another solid layer of biomaterial surface by van der Waals or electrostatic forces or weak hydrogen bonding. Physical adsorption can also be used as a technique to alter the surface properties of polymers by immobilizing a bioactive substance pairing of ligand-receptors. However, for effective adsorption, the core structure must have certain functional groups interacting with the coating molecules. Nevertheless, due to weak interactions between the polymer surface and the biomolecules, establishing a long-term stable polymer-biomolecule is difficult.

b. **Chemical conjugation of biomolecules:** As an alternate approach to physical adsorption, through covalent immobilization biomolecules such as cell receptor ligands, enzymes, antibodies, pharmacological agents, lipids, and DNA are made bound to the polymer surface with the help of functional groups like amines, thiols, carboxylic acids, and alcohols. Unlike physical adsorption, in chemical conjugation the binding of chemical groups to the polymer surface is through robust covalent bonding.

c. **Coating methods:** Coating techniques involve thin surface layer deposition of molecule layers of a separate configuration from the original base polymeric material. They consist of non-covalent and covalent coatings. Non-covalent coatings have the potential to cover a range of different polymeric base materials. Langmuir-Blodgett (LB) deposition approach is one of the main non-covalent processes where one or more extremely organized layers of molecules are deposited onto the polymeric base material.

Schematics of different LB deposition stages and deposition of a monolayer of functionalized particles onto a hydrophilic plate using the LB technique are presented in Figure 9.11. To this purpose, water-insoluble polymer substrate is soaked completely in a solution that comprises the desired coating molecules and then gradually withdrawn by lifting. During the process, i.e., dipping and extracting of the material, the transfer of molecules from liquid to solid surface is accomplished at the liquid-air interface. LB films exhibit high order, uniformity, and versatility to integrate a wide variety of chemistries. The molecules employed for deposition have a surfactant structure (a hydrophobic tail and a hydrophilic head). When the molecules of interest are added and dissolved into an aqueous solution containing volatile organic solvents, the molecules scatter rapidly across the water surface. The molecules are rearranged at the air-water interface in such a manner that the polar head groups (hydrophilic) are directed towards the water, while the tail groups (hydrophobic) remain outside. The hydrophobic groups create a repelling impact on each other

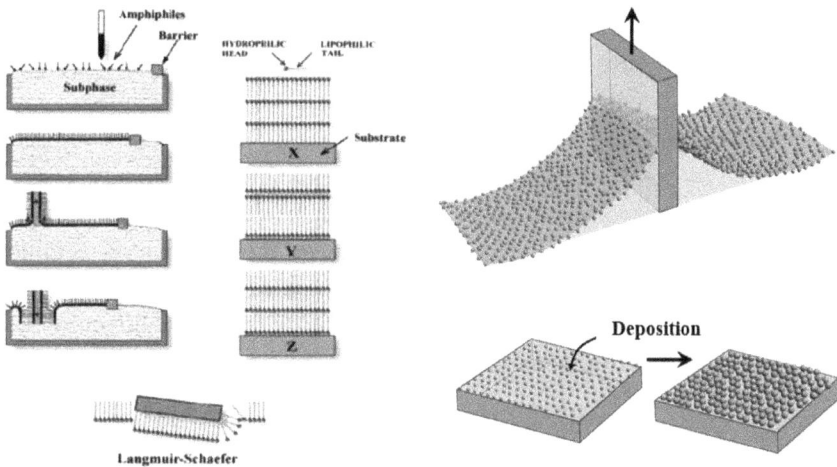

Figure 9.11: (Left) Different stages of LB deposition; (Right) deposition of a monolayer of functionalized particles onto a hydrophilic plate using the LB technique (Giancane *et al.*, 2012; Tahghighi *et al.*, 2018).

which results in a completely ordered floating monolayer at the liquid surface. The stability of the coatings is usually enhanced by cross-linking or polymerizing the surfactant molecules subsequently after film establishment. In contrast, covalent coating procedures directly depend on the immediate hitching of desired molecules onto the polymeric biomaterial.

9.4.2 *Surface modification techniques for metallic biomaterials*

Metallic biomaterials are predominantly used in hard tissue engineering. The desirable mechanical properties of metallic materials such as elastic modulus, ultimate tensile and yield strengths, and ductility have facilitated the establishment of metallic biomedical implants with *in vivo* stability. As mentioned in Chapter 7, the instinctive development of passive surface oxide layers of less than 10 nm (Cr_2O_3 for SS316L and CoCr alloys, and TiO_2 for Ti and its alloys) deliver the required mechanical stability by providing resistance to corrosion. These oxides separate the sensitive base metal from ambient environments and avoid undesirable ion transmission. In fact, the presence of oxide layers makes metal products bioinert, contributing to fibrous capsules that surround implants. Owing to the body's defensive function, such fibrous tissues form against any substance recognized as foreign objects. From this, it is understandable that the response of an implant material towards tissue surroundings is entirely dependent on the surface properties.

Therefore, several innovative surface processing methods have been established to control cascade of cellular events and generate more specific biological responses to boost the performance of metallic biomaterials in biological systems. Surface chemistry and morphology of metallic implants can be altered by mechanical modifications, chemical treatments (acidic or alkaline), and coatings, i.e., deposition and immobilization of biologically active functional molecules.

9.4.2.1 *Mechanical modifications*

Increased surface roughness (micro- or nano-roughness), size, and shape of topographical features of a metallic implant have been established to

Table 9.2: Mechanical modifications on metallic biomaterials.

Mechanical methods	Modification
Grinding	
Polishing	Surfaces are made rough by subtraction process
Machining	
Grit blasting	

result in higher micromechanical retention. Mechanical modification techniques generally come under subtractive techniques, where a layer of the core material is removed to create an un-patterned surface roughness. This includes grinding, machining, or grit blasting, among which grit blasting is a well-researched and most applied technique for metallic implants. Grit blasting or sandblasting is an inexpensive physical modification technique where angular-shaped microscopic hard grit particles are bombarded (by suction blasting or pressure blasting) onto the metallic material at high velocity to enable the formation of the roughed surface. Depending on the application, several particles such as ceramics (Al_2O_3, TiO_2, or $CaCO_3$), steel grit, glass grits, etc., are projected onto the surface through a fluid carrier (compressed air or liquid). The different mechanical modifications performed on metallic biomaterials are shown in Table 9.2.

9.4.2.2 *Chemical modification techniques*

a. **Acid treatment (etching):** Due to issues associated with mechanical modification like substrate damage, surface modification by chemical approaches have been extensively considered as an alternative approach due to its simplicity, cost-effectiveness, and osseointegration capability. Chemical etching functions on the termination of the native oxide layer of metals and enables the formation of a new layer. Strong acids like hydrochloric acid (HCl), nitric acid (HNO_3), sulfuric acid (H_2SO_4), phosphoric acid (H_3PO_4), hydrogen fluoride (HF) and combinations of these acids are commonly utilized for the chemical etching of metallic biomaterials to establish surface roughness and remove contaminants. Also, in a controlled environment, the mixture of these strong acids can create a thin grid of nanopits with diameters ranging from 10–150 nm on the implant surfaces. In the case of titanium implants, acid etching results in the formation of Ti–OH acidic hydroxyl groups.

b. **Alkali treatment:** Alkaline etching is a simple technique to modify metallic materials, especially titanium surfaces. Treatment of titanium surfaces with sodium hydroxide (NaOH) is the most commonly applied technique due to the formation and increase of basic hydroxyl groups. Through NaOH treatment, a sodium titanate gel is created over the Ti substrate, which has the potential for linking up with calcium (Ca) and phosphate (P) groups, thereby enhancing the formation of hydroxyapatite (HA) on the surface.

c. **Electrochemical methods:** Electrochemical processes rely on submerging a metallic biomaterial into a solution of electrolytes (acids, ions, or oxidants) and affixing it to a rod of an electrical circuit. The electrochemical techniques can be divided into anodization, electropolishing, and electroerosion.

1. **Anodization:** Anodization is an electrolytic passivation process where the thickness of the dense natural oxide layer is increased and stabilized. The method changes the metal surface properties by an electrochemical process without altering the core metal composition. This process typically entails electrode reactions in conjunction with the diffusion of electric field-driven metal and oxygen ions, resulting in the development of thin oxide films on the anode surface. In short, the surface of a metallic substance is attached to the anode electrode of an electrochemical cell while the cathode electrode is connected to an inert substance, i.e., either graphite or platinum. When an electric potential is applied between the electrodes, it causes oxidation at the anode surface. Various parameters, including applied current density, electrolyte solution, anodization time, pH, and temperature, can be regulated to obtain desired morphology and alter the physiochemical properties of the oxide film. This technique is used mainly to enhance osseointegration in titanium implants. In metallic biomaterials, this process is also used to fabricate nanophase topographies, such as a self-organized array of nanotubes, by

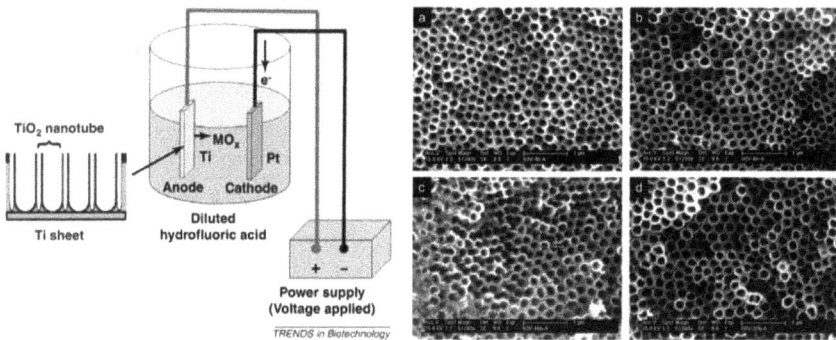

Figure 9.12: (Left) Schematic illustration of the electrochemical anodization process used to fabricate the TiO$_2$ nanotube surface on Ti metal; (Right) SEM images of Ti nanotubes anodized at 60 V for different periods: (a) 4 h, (b) 8 h, (c) 16 h, and (d) 32 h (Brammer *et al.*, 2012; Liu *et al.*, 2016).

changing electrochemical parameters. A schematic illustration of the electrochemical anodization process used to fabricate the TiO$_2$ nanotube surface on Ti metal with corresponding SEM images is shown in Figure 9.12. Some reports also show Co-Cr alloys to possess nanoscale features by anodization. By carefully managing the electrolytes (phosphate solutions), instead of just enhancing topological features, anodizing can also result in the adsorption and incorporation of various inorganic/organic biologically relevant species into the oxide layer.

2. **Electropolishing:** Electropolishing is an industrial process commonly used for the surface polishing of metal parts. A schematic of the electropolishing process is shown in Figure 9.13. The method basically functions as a guided electrochemical destruction of the amorphous pre-existing natural oxide layer to provide the metallic surface a polycrystalline one. It was initially only considered as an eliminating technique of removing unwanted iron and other contaminants from the metal's surface. Nevertheless, metallic materials that are electropolished are shown to have an increase in corrosion resistance.

3. **Electrochemical deposition:** Electrochemical deposition or electrodeposition, is sometimes referred to as electroplating (established on a mixture of ionic species in water) or electrophoretic

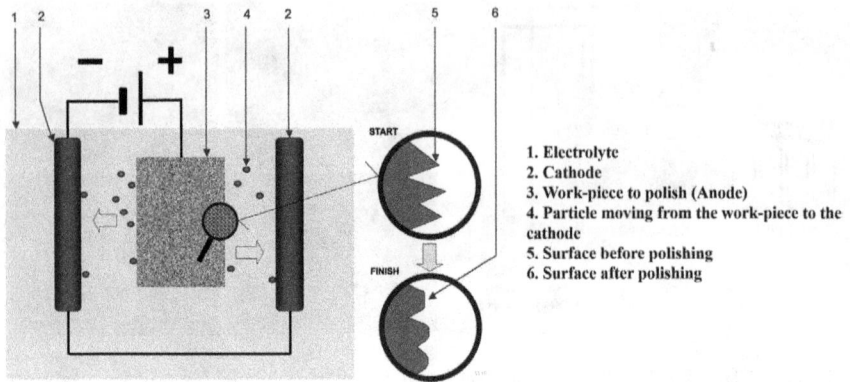

Figure 9.13:   Schematic of the electropolishing process. Image Credit: LaurensvanLieshout.

(established on in-suspension particles) deposition. Even though the process looks similar to anodization, it is exactly the opposite. While both are electrochemical processes, anodizing is an engineered oxidation process powered by electricity, where it typically creates a stable oxide layer of the same base metal. In comparison, electroplating requires depositing a different thin metal layer on the existing metallic surface. By this technique, a conductive nanocoating can be created on a metallic base metal to any thickness from about 10 nm to 100 μm. Two coating preparation procedures are regularly applied: electrophoretic procedure (EPD) and electrolytic procedure (ELD). A graphic illustration of the EPD and ELD techniques is shown in Figure 9.14. The EPD process utilizes ceramic particle suspensions while the ELD process uses solution-based metal salts. This electrochemical deposition is commonly used on titanium substrates for coating.

d. **Ion implantation:** Ion implantation, which is primarily built on ionized particle bombardment, can offer desirable surface layers with preferred characteristics. In particular, this low-temperature process is a material-dominant surface modification technique that inserts ions

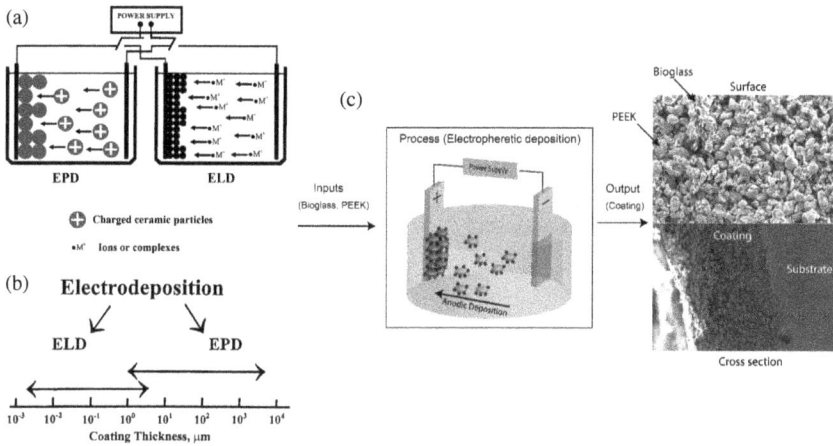

Figure 9.14: (a) A graphic illustration of the EPD and ELD techniques, (b) the range of coating thickness accomplished using EPD and ELD, and (c) example of EPD coatings of PEEK/bioactive glass composite coatings for orthopaedic applications (Atiq Ur Rehman *et al.*, 2017; Maleki-Ghaleh *et al.*, 2012).

of the desired material into another solid material with an energetic ion beam (typically 1 keV to 1 MeV), causing a variation in the physical and chemical surface characteristics of the materials. The fundamental concept behind ion implantation is simple and clear. It includes an ion source, an accelerator, and a target substrate. A beam of desired ions from any source is accelerated at different voltages. It is encouraged to intrude upon a substrate surface such that the ions interact with that surface, and some are embedded in it. For metallic biomaterials, ion implantation has been shown to improve wear resistance (with N_2 ions), surface bioactivity (with Ca and P ions), and corrosion resistance (with C ions). The schematic diagram before and after ion implantation is shown in Figure 9.15.

Plasma immersion ion implantation (PIII) is an advanced technique compared to traditional ion implantation, which can more efficiently process samples with a complicated structure. In PIII, the samples are enveloped by a high negative potential relative to the chamber wall via plasma and pulse biases. The schematic illustration of PIII is shown in Figure 9.15.

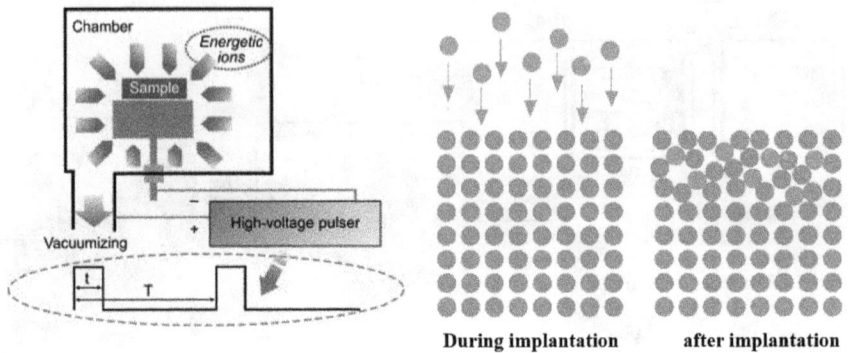

During implantation   **after implantation**

Figure 9.15: (Left) Graphic illustration of plasma immersion ion implantation (PIII); (Right) schematics before and after ion implantation (Chu *et al.*, 2015).

e. **Sol-gel techniques:** Sol-gel processes are simple wet chemical processes that represent a chemical route for forming inorganic (ceramic) adhesive layers on a given metallic substrate. They are based primarily on hydrolysis and condensation reactions of metal alkoxides. As a surface modification technique, sol-gel coatings offer several advantages: accurate command on the chemistry and composition at the molecular level, and porosity at the nanoscale level. Sol-gel hybrid coatings not only maximize adhesion by developing chemical bonds between metals and hybrid coatings, but also enhance robustness by offering suitable resistance against corrosive elements. Due to ease of the process, various organic polymers or organic functionalities can be incorporated into a gel network to maximize the potential and achieve desired properties like hydrophilicity, bioactivity, etc. For metallic implants, sol-gel processes are widely used to achieve biomimetic coatings. CaP coatings are organized onto a metallic substrate by soaking the material in Ca (typically nitrate salt) solution and P gels for a suitable time. The biological efficiency of biomimetic coatings achieved by sol-gel is usually better than other surface modification techniques, especially when compared to ion implantation and chemical etching. Thin-film deposition using the sol-gel method is shown in Figure 9.16. Through this process, the development of rough and porous coatings supports the movement of physiological fluids and promotes the transportation of nutrients and

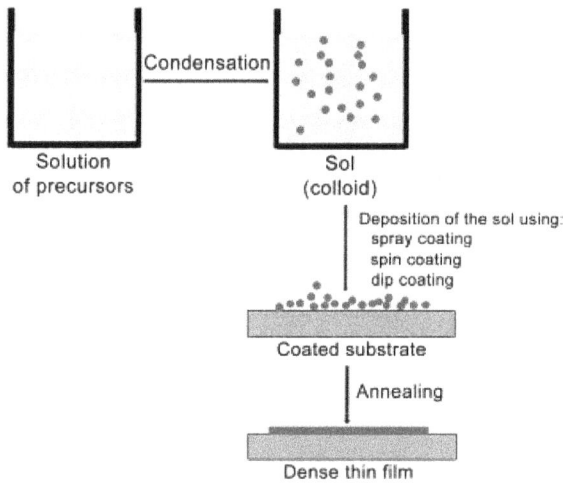

Figure 9.16: Thin film deposition using the sol-gel method (Neacşu *et al.*, 2016).

tissue growth. The involvement of hydroxyl groups in the sol-gel system facilitates the precipitation of Ca and P and thus increases osteoblast interactions. Sol-gel-derived coatings thus offer remarkable solutions to materials involved in orthopedic and dental implants.

f. **Dip coating:** Dip coating (coating with withdrawal) is a well-known technique to establish a thin and uniform coating onto a flat or cylindrical substrate (Figure 9.17). This technique involves immersing a substrate in a desired low viscosity precursor solution at a constant speed and then lifting it upright with a steady speed from the solution, usually with the help of a motor. In this way, a wet homogeneous liquid film of some thickness is drawn upwards. By gravitational draining and solvent evaporation, a deposition of a solid film is formed on the substrate.

g. **Spin coating:** Spin coating is a commonly used method for applying uniform thin film liquid-based coatings using centrifugal force on a solid spinning substrate. A typical spin-coating method comprises four basic phases: deposition, spin up, spin off, and evaporation (Figure 9.18). During the deposition stage, the desired liquid coating material is added to the surface of the substrate. The volume of liquid added depends on the liquid's viscosity and the thickness of the

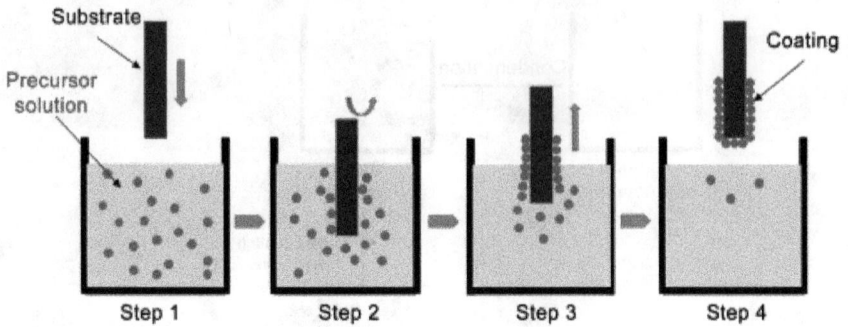

Figure 9.17:   Graphical representation of the dip-coating technique (Neacşu *et al.*, 2016).

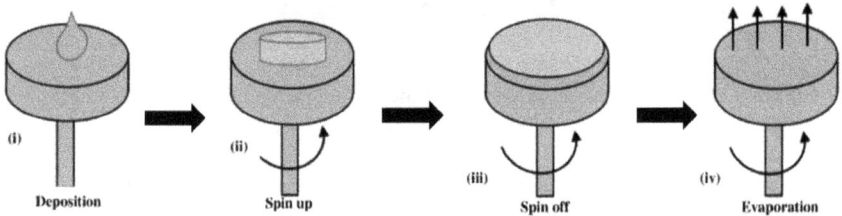

Figure 9.18:   Stages of spin coating (Yilbas *et al.*, 2019).

coated substrate. The process can produce uniform coatings with a thickness of 1–10 μm. Final thickness of the film depends on the nature of the coating parameters such as solution viscosity, rotation speed, evaporation rate, percent solids, surface tension, etc.

9.4.3 *Surface modification techniques for ceramic biomaterials*

Highly efficient bioceramics, such as zirconia, alumina, and their composites, are the most attractive materials for the manufacture of load-bearing implant applications (orthopaedic and dental) due to their exceptional mechanical properties, biocompatibility, corrosion resistance, and aesthetic value. One of the fundamental properties of these high-engineering ceramics is bioinertness, which means they have a biologically inert surface, so they do not cause unnecessary immune system reactions with surrounding tissues. This particular property makes bioceramics an excellent candidate in circumstances where minimum or no interactions with surrounding tissues are wanted, such as dental braces, crowns, and bridges. In comparison, ceramic surface inertness is often an obstacle in cases where good tissue contact is necessary, as is the case with bone implants. For instance, the porous and non-adherent fibrous coating forms around the implant and at the bone-implant interface, which later contributes to implant loosening and, thereby, the implant's failure. Nevertheless, extensive research on these ceramics is still required before their full potential can be utilized as implant materials, particularly in surface optimization.

In line with polymeric and metallic biomaterials, several specific studies have also explicitly associated the clinical effectiveness of ceramic biomaterials with their surface properties, i.e., surface topography and chemical composition. It is important to note that several methods utilized to modify the topography of metallic biomaterials such as machining, sandblasting, plasma spraying, electrochemical etching, etc., have also been applied on high-performance ceramics. Such surface modifications demonstrated that surface topography has a strong influence on the biological response of ceramics as well. Given this, detailed sub-sections on surface modification techniques on ceramic biomaterials shall not be elaborated.

As discussed in an earlier chapter, because of its biocompatibility and favourable mechanical properties, alumina and zirconia are extensively used as ceramic biomaterials for implant applications, especially in orthopaedic and dental. Surface modification by chemical treatments on bioceramic materials is intended to add bioactive functional groups such as $-OH$, $-COOH$, PO_4H_2, and $-NH_2$ to alter surface chemistry for desirable optimization. Physical deposition methods, such as ion implantation, UV treatment, CO_2 irradiation, and laser treatment, have also been applied to modify the surface chemistry of bioceramics to improve their biological properties.

9.5 Antibacterial coatings on implants

Implanted biomaterials play a significant role in the current success of orthopaedic and trauma surgeries. However, biomedical materials, including sutures, implants, and scaffolds, carry the risk of implant-associated infections caused by various kinds of bacteria. Healthcare-associated infections, surgical site infections, and hospital-acquired infections are some of the common infections associated with public healthcare. Bacteria have an extremely successful and diversified approach to conforming to nearly any natural and synthetic surface and to endure on it. The adherence of planktonic bacteria (free-floating or free-living bacteria) and recruitment of additional planktonic bacteria onto a surface leads to the formation of "*biofilm*".

Biofilms are tightly packed three-dimensional microbial cell colonies that grow or expand over living or inert surface areas and develop inherent resistance to antimicrobial agents. They have damaging effects on the surrounding tissues and lead to poor functional outcomes and chronic infections. The bacterial infections, once adapted, do not react to/ acknowledge any traditional systemic antibiotic therapy. Therefore, a deep understanding of biofilm development on surfaces is necessary for a comprehensive analysis of techniques aimed at eliminating or preventing its formation. Biofilm formation is a complex process that involves distinct stages. A schematic of the four distinct stages in biofilm formation is depicted in Figure 9.19. It is important to note that adhered biofilm

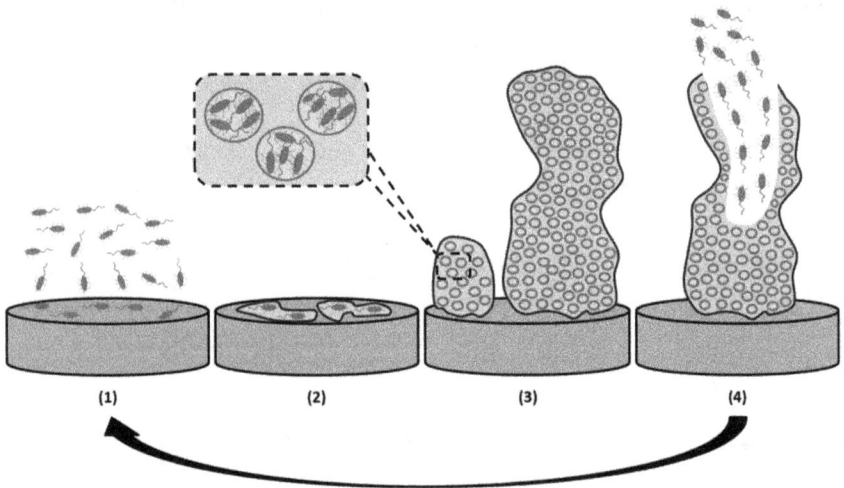

Figure 9.19:   Graphical illustration of the four main phases of biofilm development. (1) Reversible attachment of bacteria cells, (2) irreversible attachment due to extracellular polymeric matrix (EPM) secretion, (3) development of biofilm structure and maturation, and (4) dispersion or detachment of bacteria from biofilm to colonize in newer areas (Olmo *et al.*, 2020).

Table 9.3: Brief list of infection rates, infection routes, and infectious species responsible for colonizing some standard in-dwelling medical devices (Zare et al., 2021).

Biomedical device	Infectious species	Time taken to cause infection	Rate of infection	Biomaterials used	Routes of infection
Central venous catheters	*S. epidermidis, S. aureus, C. albicans, P. aeruginosa, K. pneumoniae*	Within 10 days	3–14%	Silicone, polytetrafluoroethylene, polyurethane, polyvinyl chloride	1. Wound created to insert the catheter 2. Contaminated catheter hub 3. Bloodstream infection 4. Contaminated infuscate
Prosthetic heart valves	*S. aureus, Streptococcus,* gram-negative bacilli, *Candida, Enterococcus,* diphtheroids	Immediate	1–4%	Polytetrafluoroethylene, pyrolytic carbon	1. Bloodstream infections 2. Heart valve infections are common in patients with a repetitive history of endocarditis or frequent surgeries
Contact lenses and corneal implants	*S. epidermidis, E. coli, P. aeruginosa, S. aureus*	Immediate to several weeks	2.5–6%	Silicone hydrogel, polymethyl methacrylate	1. Direct contact with lenses or via lens cases 2. It is also mediated by other risk factors such as age, gender, extended wear, etc.
Peri-implantitis and periodontitis dental implants	*Veillonella, F. nucleatun, A. naeslundii, Streptococcus, C. albicans,*	Immediate to 14 years	10–56%	Acrylic resin, titanium and its alloys, zirconia	1. Dental plaque 2. Dental caries 3. Oral microbiome

(Continued)

Table 9.3:　(*Continued*)

Biomedical device	Infectious species	Time taken to cause infection	Rate of infection	Biomaterials used	Routes of infection
	S. sanguinis, P. gingivalis, E. timidum, E. brachy, P. anerobicus				
Orthopaedic implants	Staphylococcus (20–50%), Streptococcus, Enterococcus, P. mirabilis, E. coli, P. aeruginosa, P. acnes, MRSA	• Early infection: 3 months or less • Late infection: 3–24 months • Secondary infection: After 24 months	5–40%	High molecular weight polyethylene, polymethyl methacrylate, ceramics, cobalt, chromium, titanium, stainless steel, other metals and its alloys	1. At the time of implantation through direct inoculation or from airborne contamination of wound or device 2. Bloodstream infections or adjacent focus of infection
Breast implants	S. aureus, Enterococcus, S. epidermidis, P. acnes, diphtheroids	20–280 days	1–35%	Silicone gel within silicone rubber envelope, inflatable saline	Skin microflora during surgery is the most common origin of infection, while other routes include: 1. Contaminated implant or surgical environment 2. Skin-penetrating accidents 3. Local soft tissue infections 4. Breast trauma and seeding of an implant from remote infections

develops an improved bacterial metabolism and can often be stronger than free-floating bacteria. These kinds of infections are persistant and one of the main reasons for implant failure causing high economic and social costs, morbidity, and mortality.

Staphylococcus, the group of gram-positive, non-motile, and non-spore-forming bacteria, is the most widespread pathogen and causes the highest number of implant-associated infections. Under this genus, *Staphylococcus aureus* (*S. aureus*) is highly accountable for early bacterial infections. In contrast, the more idle, coagulase-negative *Staphylococcus epidermidis* (*S. epidermidis*) is commonly responsible for late-onset infections. A brief list of infection rates, infection routes, and infectious species responsible for colonizing some standard in-dwelling medical devices is tabulated in Table 9.3.

9.5.1 *Biofilm prevention strategies*

Over the last few decades, numerous studies have explored various surface modifications that can potentially reduce bacterial adhesion and subsequent biofilm formation on the implanted surface to ensure successful implantation. Most of the strategies, as presented in Figure 9.20, are closely related to surface design. The primary mechanism is based on the prevention of biofilm formation. In contrast, the secondary mechanism corresponds to the creation of bactericidal surfaces, which can potentially disrupt bacterial cell walls on contact. Due to the involvement of many

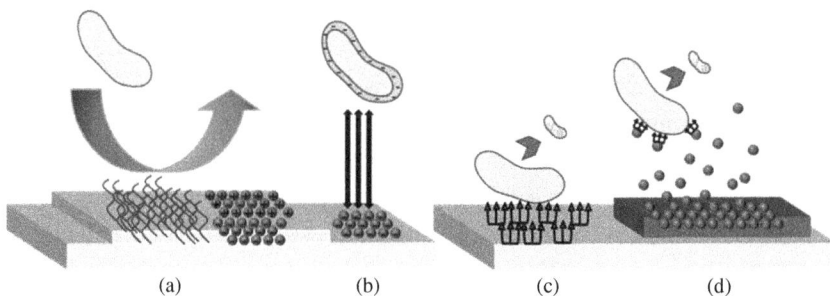

Figure 9.20:   General strategies for the development of antibacterial surfaces based on: (a) bacteria repelling, (b) electrostatic, (c) contact killing, and (d) biocide release effects (Olmo *et al.*, 2020).

bacterial and material parameters, there is no single, widely agreed surface modification technology and standardized testing method.

Implanted surface characteristics such as surface roughness, overall hydrophobicity, and electrostatic charge play crucial roles in bacterial attachment. The selection of a suitable antimicrobial treatment technique is a vital factor in achieving satisfactory results. Generally, bacterial infections are commonly treated and inhibited by the local and systemic application of antibacterial agents and antibiotic drugs. Antibiotic drugs or agents produce antibacterial surfaces by releasing antibacterial components from their core in a controlled manner. However, bacteria responsible for infections, especially methicillin-resistant *Staphylococcus aureus* (MRSA), can develop resistance against antibiotic drugs at a faster pace, and many antibiotic drugs have a narrow spectrum of activity. Antibacterial techniques mainly comprise methods that release ions with antimicrobial activity such as silver and povidone-iodine. The details of both methods are described in brief in corresponding sections.

9.5.1.1 *Bacteria-repelling surfaces*

Due to the nature of biofilms, strategies to reduce initial bacterial adhesion are extremely necessary to prevent surface infection. As previously mentioned, raw fresh wounds or surgical areas are susceptible to bacterial penetration in greater depth, therefore implant surfaces with anti-adhesive capacity are important. Surface nanostructuring, i.e., developing unique micro/nano-topographies on the implant surfaces, is acknowledged as a promising method for long-term inhibition of bacterial attachment. The continuous irregular or regular nano-topography morphologies establish anti-fouling or anti-adhesive properties. Such nanostructures act as bacteria-repelling surfaces and are not considered toxic because there is no release of chemical compounds or restricting agents from the system. Another approach, hydrophilic polymeric coatings, is where a thin layer of inert anti-adhesive polymers such as polyethylene glycol or polyethylene oxide is employed for inhibiting bacterial adhesion. Additionally, albumin, the high-affinity protein, is also studied on minimizing the number of bacteria attaching to an implant.

9.5.1.2 *Bacteria-killing surfaces*

Bactericidal agents are competent to destroy bacteria by disturbing bacterial cell membranes, hindering its DNA replication, hampering cell respiration, or negatively interfering in protein synthesis. Surface nanostructuring, which is primarily developed to inhibit bacterial adhesion, is also employed to kill a certain type of bacteria by having unique nano-scale pillar formation. The bacteria that attach to these kinds of unique surfaces get their cell wall ruptured, resulting in death. Inorganic metal nanoparticles such as silver (Ag), copper (Cu), and zinc (Zn) have been well-researched and documented sufficiently in the literature for their antibacterial activity. The ion equivalent of Ag^+, Cu^+, and Zn^{2+} are incorporated on the implant surface by various methodologies. The antibacterial activity is studied by the release of ions from the metal surface into adjacent tissues. In addition, antimicrobial performance of TiO_2 nanoparticles on gram-positive and gram negative bacteria, yeast, and green algae has been studied widely. The bacteria-killing effect of TiO_2 photocatalysts is frequently ascribed to the formation of OH• free radicals and other reactive oxygen species. On the other hand, acute and chronic bacterial orthopaedic diseases are frequently diagnosed and avoided by the local and intrinsic application of antibiotic drugs such as gentamicin, vancomycin, tobramycin, rifampicin, and ibuprofen. Many studies have also illustrated antimicrobial peptide-based implant surface functionalization approaches to reduce implant failure associated with bacterial infections.

9.6 Viricidal coatings

A pandemic is a global outbreak that occurs when a new strain (bacterium or virus) emerges and has the potential to spread from person to person widely and rapidly. Viruses are infectious agents constituted by a group of heterogeneous organisms with a size range of 100–300 nm. Most viruses have either RNA or DNA as their genetic material, encircled by a protective protein coating known as a capsid. The last two decades have seen a rampage of several viral pandemics, such as:

Table 9.4: Persistence of coronaviruses on different types of inanimate surfaces (Kampf *et al.*, 2020).

Type of surface	Virus	Temperature	Persistence
Steel	MERS-CoV	20°C	48 h
	HCoV	21°C	5 days
Aluminium	HCoV	21°C	2–8 h
Metal	SARS-CoV	RT	5 days
Wood	SARS-CoV	RT	4 days
Paper	SARS-CoV	RT	4–5 days
Glass	SARS-CoV	RT	4 days
Glass	HCoV	21°C	5 days
Plastics	HCoV	RT	2–6 days
PVC	HCoV	21°C	5 days
Silicon rubber	HCoV	21°C	5 days
Surgical glove (latex)	HCoV	21°C	≤8 h
Disposable gown	SARS-CoV	RT	24 h
Ceramic	HCoV	21°C	5 days
Teflon	HCoV	21°C	5 days

- Severe acute respiratory syndrome coronavirus (SARS-CoV1) in 2002–2003
- Swine flu influenza (H1N1) in 2009–2010
- Middle East Respiratory Syndrome Coronavirus (MERS-CoV) in 2012
- Coronavirus disease 2019 (SARS-CoV-2)

While viruses do not grow on non-living surfaces, recent studies have shown that they can remain effective or infectious for several hours or days regardless of material such as metal, glass, wood, fabrics, and plastic. The details are presented in Table 9.4.

Humans may have little or no immunity against a new virus. Hence, efforts have been turned to putting up preventative measures. The development of viricidal coatings has received growing attention in recent years to prevent the propagation of pathogenic microbes. Various strategies such as chemical disinfectants, surface modification (hydrophobic coatings), and

Table 9.5:   Comparison of the typical metal-based nanoparticles as antiviral materials.

Type	Synthesis	Size (nm)	Summary
Ag	Electrochemical	7.1	Infected cells cultured in 100 ppm Ag nanoparticles for 48 h, cell survival rate reached 98%
ZnO	Sonochemical	<100	Inhibited viral attachment to host cells
Ag@OTV	Surface modifier	3	Cell survival rate remains 90%
Ag_2S	Chemical reduction	<5	Inhibited Porcine epidemic diarrhea virus by more than 99%
Au	Chemical reduction	10	Reduced viral infections
CuO	Surface modifier	<100	Improved five levels in virus killing compared to N95 control
Cu_2O	Chemical reduction	50	Decrease in viral infections
TiO_2	Sonochemical	8	Exceptional antiviral presentation against Newcastle disease virus at specific concentrations

various metals and metal oxides like zinc ions, silver ions or copper are being developed and have shown very promising results to inactivate viruses (Table 9.5). Some of these nanocoatings demonstrated up to 99.9998% effectiveness against bacteria, formaldehyde, mold, and viruses.

9.7 Multiple choice questions

1. Select the TRUE statement(s) regarding surface modifications of biomaterials.
   (a) to improve the performance of bioimplants
   (b) to enhance the relation of material towards biocompatibility and bondability
   (c) to increase material core properties such as melting point
   (d) to improve tribological properties of the material

2. Arrange the wound healing phases in increasing order of occurrence.
   (a) proliferative; inflammatory; hemostasis; remodeling
   (b) inflammatory; proliferative; remodeling; hemostasis
   (c) hemostasis; inflammatory; proliferative; remodeling
   (d) inflammatory; remodeling; proliferative; hemostasis

3. The first incident that occurs during blood-material interaction is
   (a) cellular attachment
   (b) platelet interaction
   (c) adsorption of plasma proteins
   (d) absorption of plasma proteins

4. Treatment of the implant surface by acid etching and grit blasting
   (a) increases surface roughness and increases cell adhesion
   (b) decreases surface roughness and increases cell adhesion
   (c) increases surface roughness and decreases cell adhesion
   (d) decreases surface roughness and decreases cell adhesion

5. Which of these factors influences the healing of a wound?
   (a) vascular insufficiency
   (b) diabetes mellitus
   (c) site of wound
   (d) all of the above

6. Rough surface of the implant material usually
   (a) does not have any effect on cellular properties
   (b) is avoided because it has a negative effect on cellular properties
   (c) is desirable as it enhances cellular adhesion and proliferation properties
   (d) all of the above

7. Which of the following is/are NOT true regarding acid treatment on substrate?
   I. produces a clean and uniform surface
   II. eliminates the oxide layer and contamination
   III. improves osteoconductive properties
   IV. provides unfavourable growth conditions for cells
   (a) only I
   (b) only II and III
   (c) only I and IV
   (d) only IV

8. The main reason to perform alkali treatment on substrates is to
   (a) enhance the bioactivity and increase cell adhesion and proliferation
   (b) increase melting temperature of the sample

(c) decrease osteoblast cell adhesion and proliferation
(d) increase or decrease Young's modulus

9. What is the end stage of the healing process after biomaterial implantation?
(a) fibrous encapsulation
(b) coagulation and hemostasis
(c) proliferative phase
(d) epithelialization

10. Plasma-sprayed coatings on metallic implants such as Co-Cr and Ti, and bioceramics such as Al_2O_3
(a) increase surface roughness and bone bonding; no effect on hardness
(b) increase surface roughness and bone bonding; increase hardness
(c) no effect on surface roughness; decrease hardness
(d) no effect on bone bonding; increase hardness

11. Which of the following is/are TRUE about microporosity and particle size?
  I. higher microporosity induces better protein adsorption
 II. smaller particle size induces better protein adsorption
III. lower microporosity induces better protein adsorption
IV. larger particle size induces better protein adsorption
   (a) only I and IV
   (b) only II and III
   (c) only III and IV
   (d) only I and II

12. Coating the surface of hip implants
(a) significantly reduces failure rates
(b) increases wear rates
((c) decreases implant-bone bonding
(d) none of the above

References & Further Reading

Atiq Ur Rehman, M., Bastan, F. E., Haider, B., & Boccaccini, A. R. (2017). Electrophoretic deposition of PEEK/bioactive glass composite coatings for orthopedic implants: A design of experiments (DoE) study. *Materials & Design, 130*, 223–230. doi:10.1016/j.matdes.2017.05.045.

Blaus, B. (2014). Medical gallery of Blausen Medical 2014. *WikiJournal of Medicine, 1*(2). doi:10.15347/wjm/2014.010.

Brammer, K. S., Frandsen, C. J., & Jin, S. (2012). TiO_2 nanotubes for bone regeneration. *Trends in Biotechnology, 30*(6), 315–322. doi:10.1016/j.tibtech.2012.02.005.

Cha, C., Piraino, F., & Khademhosseini, A. (2014). Chapter 9 — Microfabrication Technology in Tissue Engineering. In C. A. V. Blitterswijk & J. De Boer (Eds.), *Tissue Engineering (Second Edition)* (pp. 283–310). Oxford: Academic Press.

Chu, P. K., & Wu, G. S. (2015). Chapter 3 — Surface design of biodegradable magnesium alloys for biomedical applications. In T. S. N. S. Narayanan, I.-S. Park, & M.-H. Lee (Eds.), *Surface Modification of Magnesium and its Alloys for Biomedical Applications* (pp. 89–119): Woodhead Publishing.

desJardins-Park, H. E., Mascharak, S., Chinta, M. S., Wan, D. C., *et al.* (2019). The Spectrum of Scarring in Craniofacial Wound Repair. *Frontiers in Physiology, 10*(322). doi:10.3389/fphys.2019.00322.

Fu, X., Chen, Q., Chen, X., Zhang, L., *et al.* (2019). A Rapid Thermal Nanoimprint Apparatus through Induction Heating of Nickel Mold. *Micromachines, 10*(5), 334. doi:10.3390/mi10050334.

Giancane, G., & Valli, L. (2012). State of art in porphyrin Langmuir–Blodgett films as chemical sensors. *Advances in Colloid and Interface Science, 171–172*, 17–35. doi:10.1016/j.cis.2012.01.001.

Haatainen, T., Mäkelä, T., Ahopelto, J., & Kawaguchi, Y. (2009). Imprinted polymer stamps for UV-NIL. *Microelectronic Engineering, 86*(11), 2293–2296. doi:10.1016/j.mee.2009.04.020.

Kampf, G., Todt, D., Pfaender, S., & Steinmann, E. (2020). Persistence of coronaviruses on inanimate surfaces and their inactivation with biocidal agents. *Journal of Hospital Infection, 104*(3), 246–251. doi:10.1016/j.jhin.2020.01.022.

Liu, G., Du, K., & Wang, K. (2016). Surface wettability of TiO_2 nanotube arrays prepared by electrochemical anodization. *Applied Surface Science, 388*, 313–320. doi:10.1016/j.apsusc.2016.01.010.

Maleki-Ghaleh, H., Khalili, V., Khalil-Allafi, J., & Javidi, M. (2012). Hydroxyapatite coating on NiTi shape memory alloy by electrophoretic deposition process. *Surface and Coatings Technology, 208*, 57–63. doi:10.1016/j.surfcoat.2012.08.001.

Morgese, G., & Benetti, E. M. (2017). Polyoxazoline biointerfaces by surface grafting. *European Polymer Journal, 88*, 470–485. doi:10.1016/j.eurpolymj.2016.11.003.

Neacşu, I. A., Nicoară, A. I., Vasile, O. R., & Vasile, B. Ş. (2016). Chapter 9 — Inorganic micro- and nanostructured implants for tissue engineering. In A. M. Grumezescu (Ed.), *Nanobiomaterials in Hard Tissue Engineering* (pp. 271–295): William Andrew Publishing.

Negut, I., Grumezescu, V., & Grumezescu, A.M. (2018). Treatment Strategies for Infected Wounds. *Molecules, 23*(9), 2392. doi:10.3390/molecules23092392.

Olmo, J. A.-D., Ruiz-Rubio, L., Pérez-Alvarez, L., Sáez-Martínez, V., *et al.* (2020). Antibacterial Coatings for Improving the Performance of Biomaterials. *Coatings, 10*(2), 139. doi:10.3390/coatings10020139.

Qiu, Z.-Y., Chen, C., Wang, X.-M., & Lee, I.-S. (2014). Advances in the surface modification techniques of bone-related implants for last 10 years. *Regenerative Biomaterials, 1*(1), 67–79. doi:10.1093/rb/rbu007.

Rezvani Ghomi, E., Khalili, S., Nouri Khorasani, S., Esmaeely Neisiany, R., *et al.* (2019). Wound dressings: Current advances and future directions. *Journal of Applied Polymer Science, 136*(27), 47738. doi:10.1002/app.47738.

Sridharan, R., Cameron, A. R., Kelly, D. J., Kearney, C. J., *et al.* (2015). Biomaterial-based modulation of macrophage polarization: A review and suggested design principles. *Materials Today, 18*(6), 313–325. doi:10.1016/j.mattod.2015.01.019.

Tahghighi, M., Mannelli, I., Janner, D., & Ignés-Mullol, J. (2018). Tailoring plasmonic response by Langmuir–Blodgett gold nanoparticle templating for the fabrication of SERS substrates. *Applied Surface Science, 447*, 416–422. doi:10.1016/j.apsusc.2018.03.237.

Walker, J. T., Kim, S. S., Michelsons, S., Creber, K., *et al.* (2015). Cell-matrix interactions governing skin repair: matricellular proteins as diverse modulators of cell function. *Research and Reports in Biochemistry, 5*, 73–88. doi:10.2147/RRBC.S57407.

Yilbas, B. S., Al-Sharafi, A., & Ali, H. (2019). Chapter 3 — Surfaces for Self-Cleaning. In B. S. Yilbas, A. Al-Sharafi, & H. Ali (Eds.), *Self-Cleaning of Surfaces and Water Droplet Mobility* (pp. 45–98): Elsevier.

Zare, M., Zare, M., Butler, J., & Ramakrishna, S (2021). Nanoscience-Led Antimicrobial Surface Engineering to Prevent Infections. *ACS Applied Nano Materials*, under review (as of 15 April 2021).

Chapter 10
Tissue engineering and regenerative medicine

10.1 Introduction

From Chapter 3, we have studied the importance of cells for tissue regeneration. In addition to its genome, we have also acknowledged that a cell must be assessed in the context of its ECM, growth factors, and other biomolecules responsible for regulating its functions, resulting in the fundamental development of an organ, and in effect the entire organism. It is also discussed that the primary objective of tissue engineering is to build conditions that effectively facilitate cell growth without losing the functionality of the damaged tissue. The ultimate success and effectiveness of tissue engineering depend largely on the function of scaffolds that serve as the synthetic ECM. In tissue engineering, scaffolds with porosity, especially with interconnective pores, are often required for superior infiltration of cells (cellular ingrowth). These kinds of pore structures can be adjusted by various fabrication methods and proved to be ideal for tissue ingrowth. In the current chapter, we discuss and learn about various methods to fabricate scaffolds that closely mimic the natural ECM. The potential applications of tissue engineering and regenerative medicine (section 10.8) are presented in Figure 10.1.

Disease, injury, and trauma may result in tissue loss/damage and deterioration of the human body. This condition often needs treatment to boost repair, recovery, reconstruction, or regeneration. Given this, can we think of curing diseases by simple cell programming? Or is it possible to construct an entire living creature by using fundamental cells? Or is it

246

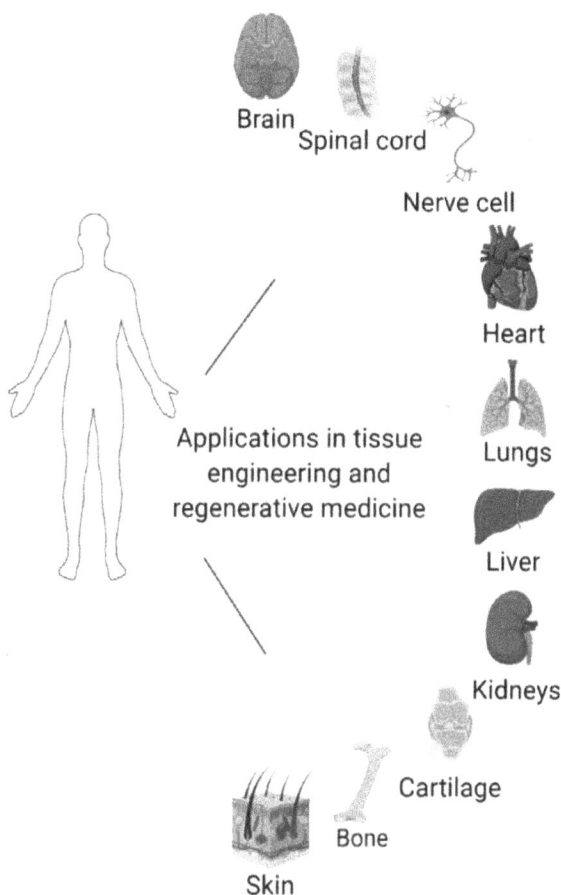

Figure 10.1: Potential applications in tissue engineering and regenerative medicine (Tsiapalis *et al.*, 2020).

possible to use cells as living materials to engineer organs and tissues? The partial answer to these questions is YES!

Over the last few decades, there has been increasing interest in developing biomedical methodologies to restore the function of damaged tissue or replace organs. This has led to the introduction or beginning of the new area known as tissue engineering. Tissue engineering intends to restore the damaged tissue by combining body cells with biocompatible materials and signalling molecules (Figure 10.2). The laboratory-developed

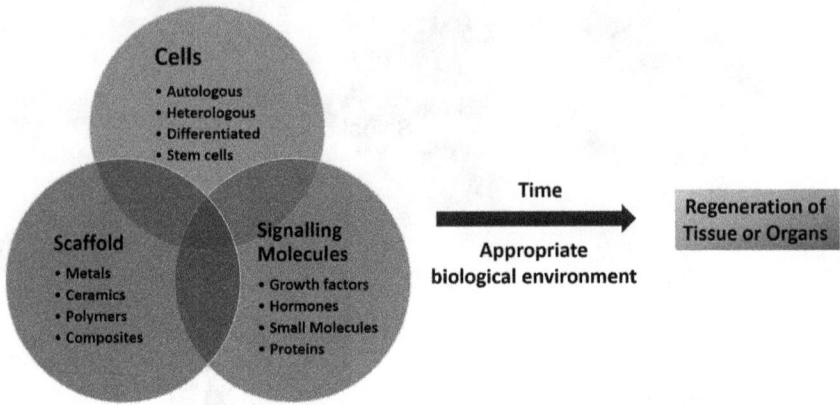

Figure 10.2:   Tissue engineering triad.

materials serve as models for tissue regeneration and appropriately guide the development of new tissue. The reach of tissue engineering is vast and has an exemplary impact on society: thousands of medical procedures are completed every day to substitute or restore tissues that have been injured due to disease or trauma. Strategies to build tissues *in vitro* (in the laboratory or outside the body) have grown exponentially due to a patient population experiencing an increasing need for tissue and organ implantation. As of today, several attempts have been made *in vitro* to engineer nearly every tissue and organ in the body, such as liver, nerve, kidney, intestine, pancreas, and even heart muscles and their valves. In fact, maximum success rates were achieved in skin, bladder, and bone, where patients successfully used tissue-engineered constructs.

Tissue engineering is a specific branch under biomedical engineering (bioengineering) that integrates biology, chemistry, material science, and engineering. It is often described as *"an interdisciplinary field that applies the principles of engineering and life sciences towards the development of biological substitutes that seek to repair, restore, replace, or enhance biological tissue and organs"*. The underlying universal principles of tissue engineering involve the integration of living cells with a natural/synthetic structure or scaffold to create a construct that is physically, structurally, mechanically, and fundamentally similar to or superior to the tissue being replaced (Figure 10.3). Developing such construction requires a cautious assessment of four primary materials: 1) scaffold; 2) growth factors; 3)

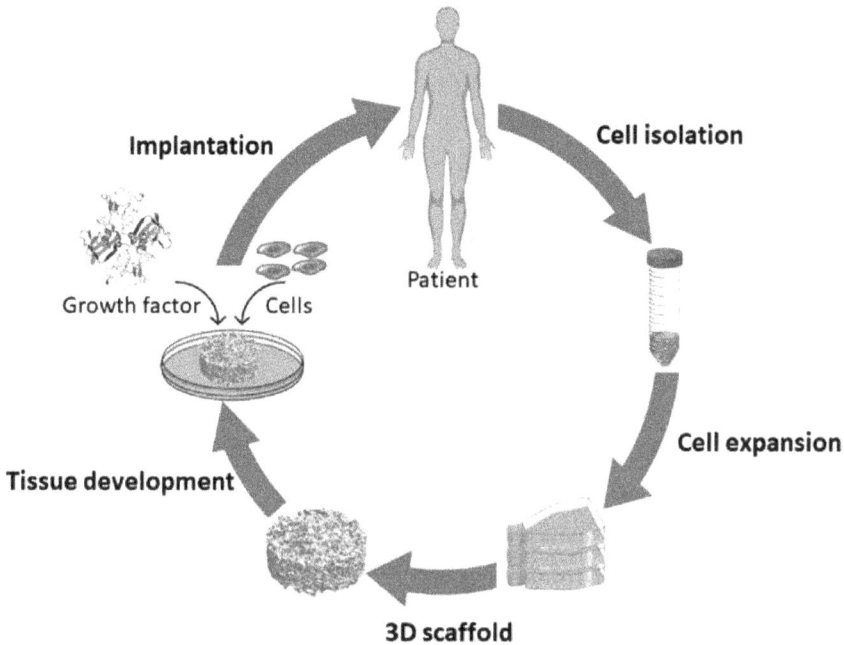

Figure 10.3: Schematic of the scaffold-based tissue engineering approach (Asadian *et al.*, 2020; Lei *et al.*, 2020).

extracellular matrix; and 4) cells. These fundamentals are covered in detail in this chapter.

10.2 Main objectives of tissue engineering

(a) Tissue Regeneration
- Replacement of lost tissue with tissue itself
- Instigate regeneration of tissue where it is normally not observed
- E.g., Cartilage or bone regeneration

(b) Tissue Repair
- Replacement of lost tissue with a functional substitute
- Enhance the rate of repair where it is seen
- E.g., All tissues

(c) Tissue Replacement
- Replacement of missing cell population
- E.g., Red blood cells in blood transfusion

As mentioned, this interdisciplinary field of combining engineering and biological science has significantly developed since its beginnings in the late 1980s. The regeneration of tissues, scaffolds, and complex organs from a very simple cell was almost a dream to mankind. Nevertheless, over the past few decades, major developments have occurred in this area, and promising solutions to many existing biological problems emerged. This vision of imitating nature has become possible in regenerative medicine through modern technology, and even found its way to organ transplantation. Researchers have moved the idea of producing new tissues from fantasy to reality in today's world.

10.3   Fundamentals of tissue engineering

10.3.1   *Tissue engineering before 1993*

Just a little over 27 years ago in 1993, a research article on tissue engineering was submitted to the journal *Science* by Robert Langer and Vacanti. This article laid a strong foundation for humanity's research in pursuit of this new field and contributed significantly to the advancement of tissue engineering. The paper gave us a clear view of various human health issues and the ways in which tissue engineering can address these problems. The authors mentioned three approaches:

- Using isolated cells or cell substitutes
- Using tissue-inducing constituents
- Randomly arranging cells within the matrices

The authors discussed their advantages, drawbacks, and possible applications in ectodermal, endodermal, and mesodermal tissues systems. Langer and Vacanti concluded by describing the significance of each scientific field which will contribute to tissue engineering and the areas where researchers will need to concentrate on in the future. Some highlighted disciplines include cell biology (cell differentiation and development, how ECM affects cell function), immunology and molecular genetics (cell design), and material sciences (what sort of materials to use).

10.3.2 *Tissue engineering progress from 1993–2002*

Griffith and Naughton wrote an article in the same journal *Science* over a decade later (2002). In this article, the authors addressed the significant tissue engineering advancements that have been established. The need for the Food and Drug Administration (FDA)'s premarket approval for various tissue-engineered products was discussed for the first time. Griffith and Naughton noted that there were three specific therapeutic methods available to treat injured tissue or disease:

- Implanting freshly isolated cells
- Implanting of tissue culture *in vitro*
- *In situ* tissue regeneration

10.4 Scaffolds

Excluding blood cells and other specific cells, many normal cells in human tissues rely on the ECM, meaning they are anchorage-residing. The ECM exemplifies the mother nature platform for tissue development and repair. One of the key challenges of tissue engineering is to replicate exactly what occurs in nature. In other words, theoretically, the best platform for an engineered tissue should be the same ECM of the target tissue in its natural state. However, the numerous functions, intricate structure, and dynamic nature of ECM make it challenging to imitate accurately. Hence, the idea of scaffolding in tissue engineering came into existence with the key aim to mimic or imitate the specific tasks of native ECM to some extent. Isolated cells (from an autologous/allogeneic/xenogenic source) need supporting structures to expand on and to develop new tissues. The supportive arrangements or platforms are regularly referred to as "*scaffolds*", in which biomaterials are used to simulate a particular microenvironment. It is important to stress to our readers that the area of scaffold-based tissue engineering is still evolving under experimental study with several different approaches. Examples of different forms of scaffold structures made from different materials are presented in Figure 10.4. However, till today, what constitutes as an ideal scaffold or scaffold construction, even for a particular type of tissue, is not defined.

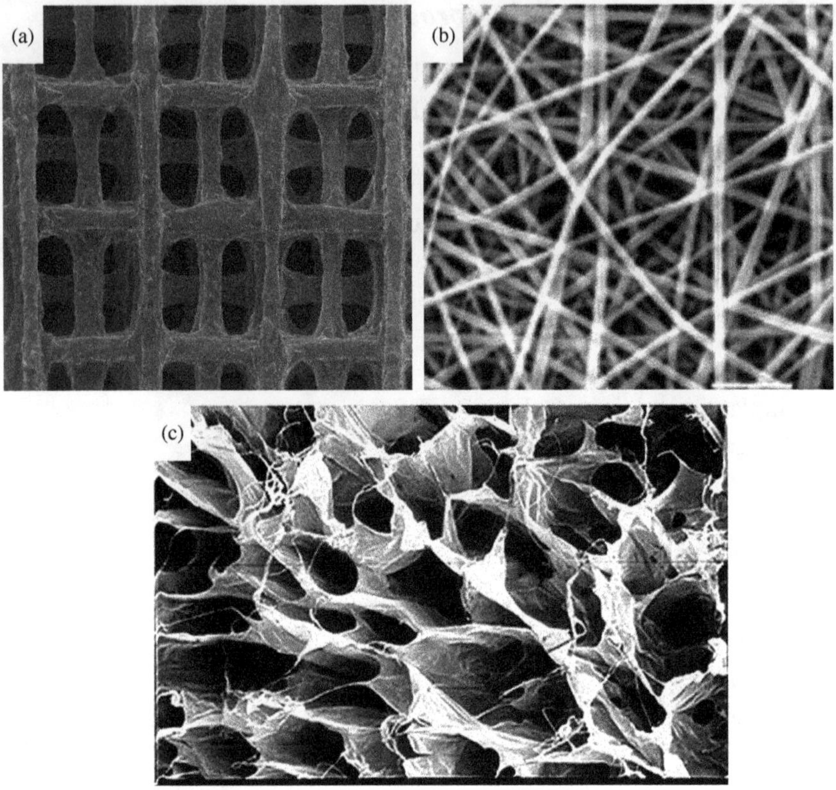

Figure 10.4: Examples of different forms of scaffolds (a) 3D printed scaffold; (b) electrospun nanofibers; (c) high porous scaffold (Cheng *et al.*, 2017; Ramakrishna *et al.*, 2006; Serra *et al.*, 2013).

The ideal tissue-engineered scaffold should act as cellular structures that direct cellular growth, serve as their microenvironment, provide adequate mechanical support, incorporate growth factors, and operate as optimal carriers for the delivery of cells for tissue regeneration or repair. It should be proficient in reproducing the intrinsic properties and inhabiting the host cell to meet the needs of regeneration and repair. As mentioned in the previous chapter, the developed scaffolds or material for tissue reconstruction and replacement must satisfy stringent requirements such as biocompatibility, non-toxicity, non-immunogenicity, suitable surface characteristics, biodegradability (if designed), and permeability.

For example, physical properties such as fibrous structure (random or oriented), foam or sponge, and surface properties (hydrophobic or hydrophilic) are crucial. The basic characteristics of scaffolds for tissue engineering applications are presented in Table 10.1.

10.4.1 *Requirements of engineered scaffolds*

- Should be non-toxic, non-carcinogenic and possess high cell/tissue biocompatibility
- Should provide adequate physical support for cells to inhabit and permit cell adhesion, proliferation, and migration
- Should provide bioactive signals for cells to react to their microenvironment and allow the diffusion of vital nutrients and expressed products into cells
- Should provide an adaptable physical environment where cells and biochemical components can be distributed and maintained
- Should exert mechanical and biological pressures to change cell phase behavior

10.4.2 *Component consideration for designing scaffolds: Design criteria*

The choice of materials for tissue engineering scaffolds is a huge factor and impacts heavily on scaffold efficiency. It is not only necessary to consider the material properties, but optimizing and adjusting the cellular properties with respect to tissue response is also crucial. In view of this, a myriad of scaffolding-friendly biomaterials has been developed and produced, which includes polymers, ceramics, and metals. Details of each of these materials have been discussed in the previous chapters. Among these, tissue-based scaffolds consisting of naturally developed biomaterials and synthetic biopolymers have been widely used since they can be modified to optimize physicochemical efficiency. For polymers, the effect of scaffold pore size and interconnectivity, as well as porosity, are undoubtedly critical. The ECM scaffold is largely obtained from allogeneic and/or xenogenetic whole tissues and organs and devised through decellularization and other manufacturing processes.

Table 10.1: Basic characteristics of scaffolds for tissue engineering applications.

Property	Description	Examples
Mimic natural ECM	Should replicate exactly what occurs in nature.	Polymeric scaffolds
Bioresorbable	Able to be absorbed into living tissue without leaving any residual content, thereby avoiding a continual inflammatory reaction.	Natural polymer (collagen), calcium phosphate ceramics
Biodegradable	Able to be broken down into multiple single entities through various processes (in the case of polymers it is through hydrolytic or enzymatic degradation). The products of degradation should be generally unreactive, non-toxic, non-immunogenic, and chemically inert.	Polymer-based scaffolds, Mg-based alloys
Porosity Pore surface Pore size Pore structure (interconnection)	Interconnecting pores enable or accelerate cell viability and proliferation into scaffold material more efficiently. They also promote tissue infiltration, oxygen, and nutrient supply.	All biocompatible polymers for soft tissue engineering and their composite materials
Interface adherence	Should enhance the adhesion and proliferation of cells to facilitate cell contact and migration.	
Modifiable surface	Should enable chemical or biomolecular modifications to enhance cell-material interactions.	All polymeric, ceramic, and metallic materials
High surface-area-to-volume ratio	Allows high rates of mass transfer, better cell ingrowth, and improved vascularization.	Polymers and composite nanofibers, hydrogels

Table 10.1: (*Continued*)

Property	Description	Examples
Matching mechanical strength	Mechanical properties (stiffness and strength) should match the replaced natural tissue to withstand *in vivo* environment and loads. These properties should be optimal; an over-designed matrix can cause instability, while an under-designed matrix may collapse.	All polymeric, ceramic, metallic, and alloy-based materials
Sterilizable	For clinical use, to remove or avoid toxic contaminations, the designed scaffold surfaces must be quick to respond to the sterilization process positively.	
Reproducible and processable	Should be reproducibly produced in a wide range from flexible manufacturing techniques.	

10.5 Growth factors

Growth factors are unique protein signalling molecules that have a vital responsibility in regulating several critical cellular processes such as cellular growth, differentiation, proliferation, and cell division. They also act as growth stimulators (mitogens) and inhibitors, chemotactic agents, and participants in angiogenesis (growth of new blood vessels) and apoptosis (cell death). Growth factors include both cytokines and hormones, and can form crucial parts of a scaffold implanted for tissue regeneration. Growth factors that are employed in a cell-scaffold structure are found to stimulate tissue regeneration in contrast to non-use of growth factors. They exhibit several effects through the activation of signal transduction pathways by attaching their receptors onto the surface of target cells. Signals triggered by growth factors mediate inter-cell contact in all developmental organs.

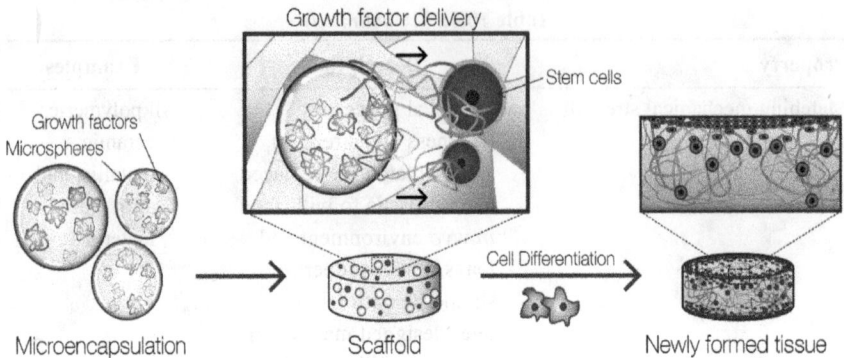

Figure 10.5:   Schematic representation of the delivery of growth factors using micro-spheres. During the microencapsulation process, growth factors are entrapped within spheres (Caballero Aguilar *et al.*, 2019; Khan *et al.*, 2020).

Table 10.2:   Some important growth factors and their functions.

Growth factor	Function
BMPs	Known as cytokines and metabologens; regulate bone organogenesis
EGF	Stimulates the growth of epithelial cells
FGF	Regeneration of tissues
NGF	Stimulates the growth of neuronal cells
PDGF	Stimulates the growth of muscle cells and connective tissue cells
VEGF	Simulates the formation of blood vessels (angiogenesis) and endothelial cell proliferation
IGF-1	Controls cell growth and survival
TGF	Has an impact on cell growth, development, and differentiation, and plays a crucial role in wound repair and immune responses
Erythropoietin	A hormone naturally produced in the liver and also known as hematopoietin; regulates red blood cell levels

While these are protein molecules made by the body, genetic engineering can also create them *in vitro* for use in biological therapy. A schematic representation of the delivery of growth factors using microspheres is shown in Figure 10.5.

Examples of important growth factors (Table 10.2) are bone morphogenetic proteins (BMPs), epidermal growth factor (EGF), fibroblast growth factor (FGF), nerve growth factor (NGF), platelet-derived growth factor (PDGF), vascular endothelial growth factor (VEGF), insulin-like growth factor-1 (IGF-1), transforming growth factor (TGF), and erythropoietin. Most growth factors attach to specific receptors on the cell surface and regulate only certain types of cells and tissues. For instance, PDGF acts on several mesenchymal cells, but VEGF acts only on endothelial cells. However, their brief biological half-lives restrict the consumption of most of these growth factors and necessitate repeated applications.

10.6 Scaffold fabrication methods

As we know by now, cells and tissues within the body are arranged in a three-dimensional architecture. To design or repair these operational tissues and organs, scaffolds must be constructed by unique methodologies to accelerate cell migration, growth, and differentiation into three-dimensional space. Therefore, the development of an effective scaffold framework for both *in vitro* and *in vivo* implant applications is crucial for efficient cell growth. However, because of complications such as material selection (type, degradation), architecture (porous, non-porous, size of pores, interconnection), mechanical stability, and surface reactions, it remains a major challenge to design an exact scaffold. The research in this field is still evolving, and different methods are being tested experimentally.

In view of this, there are several fabrication technologies that have been developed to engineer a 3D scaffold that fulfils all standards and criteria to a certain level. Many distinct synthetic and natural polymers are subjected to a range of processing methods in an effort to imitate natural ECM. From the perspective of scaffolding design and operation, each processing approach differs immensely in its practicality, scalability, and capabilities and has its own advantages and drawbacks. When designing tissue scaffold, choosing an effective manufacturing method that is well-suited with the native biological conditions is as important as choosing the proper biomaterial. The design of such scaffold manufacturing technologies has been an extremely hot area of research over the past decade. This chapter aims to provide an overview of the currently most relevant scaffold fabrication techniques. The principal manufacturing techniques for

Table 10.3:   Scaffold fabrication methods.

Conventional	Rapid Prototyping
Solvent casting	Fused deposition modeling
Particulate leaching	Three-dimensional printing
Solvent casting/particulate leaching (SCPL)	Selective laser sintering
Melt molding	Laminated object manufacturing
Gas foaming	
Freeze drying	
Phase separation	
Self-assembly	
Electrospinning	

designing the scaffolds are typically classifiable into (i) conventional fabrication techniques and (ii) rapid prototyping. The details of each manufacturing technique are presented in Table 10.3. Due to the huge potential of rapid prototyping (or additive manufacturing) techniques, it is treated as a separate chapter in this book.

10.6.1 *Solvent casting*

Solvent casting or solution casting method is often used to synthesize polymeric or composite membranes. Based on the evaporative property of the solvents, solvent casting is a very basic, quick, and inexpensive route for preparing scaffolds. This process does not need any huge or expensive machinery and is entirely established on the evaporation of solvents. Fabricating of scaffolds by solvent casting is based on either of two ways:

- Approach 1: To form a polymeric membrane sheet, immerse the mold into a polymer solution and allow adequate time to extract the solvent.
- Approach 2: Insert the polymer solution into a mold and offer the solvent sufficient time to evaporate. Following evaporation, a layer of membrane is left behind, adhering to the mold. A schematic of the preparation of nanocomposite membranes is illustrated in Figure 10.6.

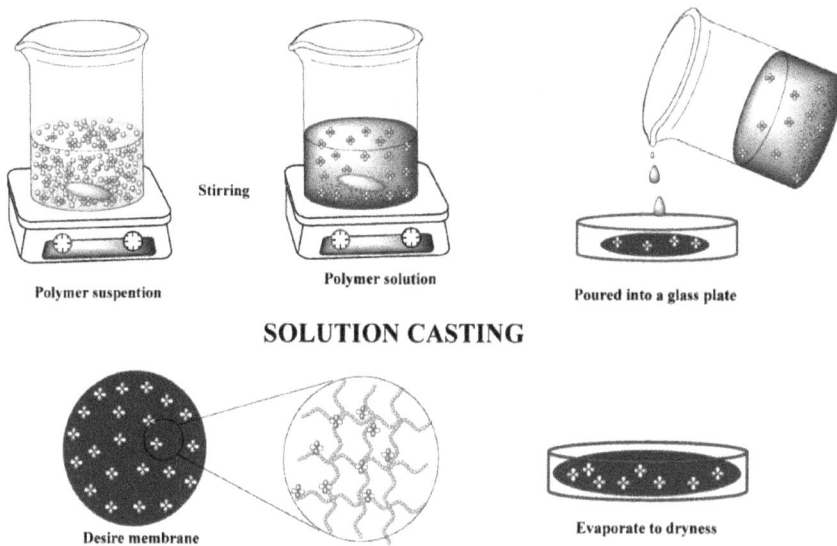

Figure 10.6:   Preparation of nanocomposite membranes by solution casting method (Roy *et al.*, 2017).

The residual toxic solvent which can affect the subsequent *in vitro* and *in vivo* studies would be one of the major questions of this strategy. To address this, subsequent steps were added to the process to extract harmful solvents by doing lyophilization in vacuum conditions. Nonetheless, due to unpredictable mechanical properties in the scaffold structure and extra processing measures, recent studies have combined solvent casting with particulate leaching techniques, with encouraging results.

10.6.2 *Particulate leaching*

Particulate leaching or porogen leaching is one of the oldest standard techniques that is extensively employed to construct scaffolds for tissue engineering applications. This process is based on dispersing chemically or physically incompatible porogen particles within a polymeric or mono-meric solution. Once the scaffold construct materializes via solvent evaporation, chemical or physical cross-linking, the porogen is selectively removed by freeze-drying. Porogen agents such as salt or wax are commonly used to build pores or channels in the architecture. One of the major advantages of this fabrication technique is the achievement of large pore size (~500 μm) and a high degree of porosity (typically in the range of 90–95% or higher). However, due to this high level of porosity, the mechanical properties are severely compromised. Particulate leaching is classified into particle leaching, ball leaching, and fibre leaching, according to the type of porogen used.

10.6.3 *Solvent casting and particulate leaching*

Solvent casting/particulate leaching (SCPL), which is basically solvent casting followed by porogen leaching, is one of the most frequent methods used for polymeric scaffold fabrication. The principle of this procedure largely relies on the dispersion of particulates (porogens) into a polymer solution. A schematic diagram of the SCPL technique is shown in Figure 10.7. In brief, this technique involves mixing a homogenous polymeric solution into an organic solvent containing particulates, which is usually not soluble in the solvent, to produce a semi-liquid mix. This blend (polymeric solution + porogen) is then cast into a membrane. Over a period, the liquid portion is evaporated under homogenized conditions to create a stable

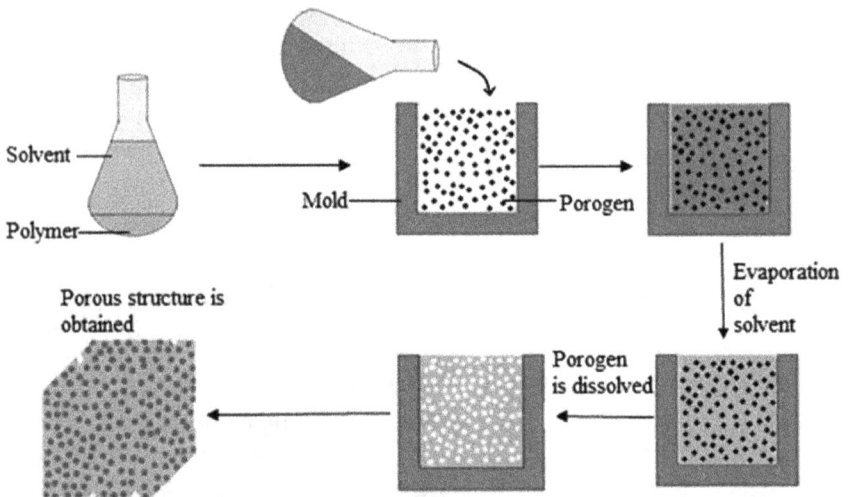

Figure 10.7: A schematic diagram of the solvent casting and particulate leaching (SCPL) technique (Sampath *et al.*, 2016).

composite of polymer and porogen. Subsequently, the porogen is filtered out of the structural composition through submersion in an aqueous leaching solution, thereby creating a solid membrane with an open pore structure. Salt particles are significantly used in SCPL as the porogen agents.

Nevertheless, other complexes such as sugar and gelatin particles have also been used. SCPL scaffolds are usually portrayed as materials with poor mechanical properties and lacking uniform arrangement. There also have been concerns with residual solvent and porogen cytotoxicity.

10.6.4 *Gas foaming*

Gas foaming, originally intended for drug delivery applications, was once extensively used to create tissue engineering scaffolds. It was employed to resolve residual porogen and/or solvent-based problems in solvent casting and SCPL. The inclusion of gas-foaming agents in a solid sample of polymers to form pores is the main factor in the gas foaming process. Briefly, at elevated pressures, molded biodegradable polymers are pressurized with gas foaming agents like CO_2, N_2 or fluoroform. Once the polymer is saturated, the release of pressure (depressurization) leads to the nucleation and growth of gas bubbles in polymers with sizes ranging from 100–500 μm. A schematic representation of scaffold fabrication by the gas foaming method is presented in Figure 10.8. Compared to other traditional scaffolding methods, the main benefit of this approach is that it does not

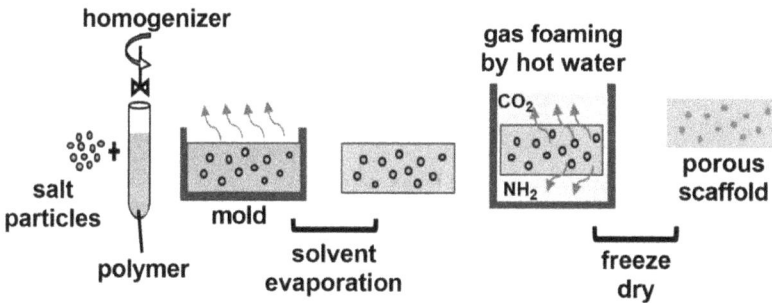

Figure 10.8: Schematic representation of scaffold fabrication by gas foaming method. This technique includes both melt molding and particulate leaching aspects (Abbasi *et al.*, 2020).

depend on solvents or porogens (organic solvent-free operation). Porosity as high as 90% with pore sizes from 200–500 μm can be achieved by employing this method. However, some of the major drawbacks are non-homogenous porosity, limited pore interconnectivity, and an external non-porous surface.

10.6.5 *Emulsion freeze-drying*

Based on the principle of sublimation, freeze-drying is a thermodynamic method used in the fabrication of porous scaffolds using organic solvents. The process involves creating an emulsion by homogenizing a polymer solution in a solvent mixture and rapidly bringing it into a thermodynamically unstable state by decreasing the emulsion system's temperature. The material is then frozen into the solid-state structure, and the solvent is separated via lyophilization by using high vacuum conditions. A schematic diagram of the emulsion freeze-drying process is shown in Figure 10.9.

The scaffolding structure obtained from this process can have two types of pores, macropores and micropores. Micropores are obtained by eliminating the aqueous solvent sequentially, while macropores are produced during homogenization due to the amalgamation of micropores. In addition, the solution's quenching rate also plays a significant role in determining the scaffold pore size. Fast quenching rates have been found to

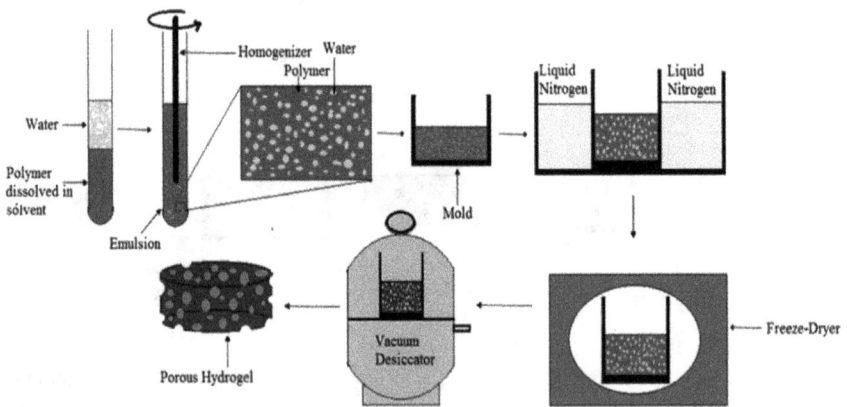

Figure 10.9:   Schematic diagram of the emulsion freeze-drying process (Sampath *et al.*, 2016).

produce scaffolds with a small average pore size. Due to faster cooling, the initial two-phase structures are frozen at quicker rates, allowing small pores (micropores) to be sublimated by the solvent. On the other hand, phase amalgamation occurs at slow cooling rates due to decreased interfacial energy, which ultimately leads to the creation of larger pores (macropores). Depending on the polymer-solvent system, the engineered scaffolds exhibit leaflet or capillary-like microfeatures. Typically, a freeze-dryer unit comprises a cooling system, vacuum system, control panel, storage chamber, and condenser. The procedure usually involves four stages: pretreatment or preparation, freezing, primary drying, and secondary drying. The freeze-drying technique can fabricate 3D porous scaffolds with porosity of more than 90% and pore diameters ranging from 20–400 μm.

10.6.6 *Melt molding*

Melt molding technique is one of the alternate approaches to obtain scaffolds by cushioning a mold with polymer powder/porogen particles and heating above the glass transition temperature (amorphous polymers) or melting temperature (crystalline polymers). After the polymer's restructuring, the composite is removed from the mold, cooled to room temperature, cleaned, and lyophilized (freeze-dried) under vacuum conditions. The structure of the scaffold is obtained from the exact shape of the mold. Melt molding is generally divided into (i) compression molding and (ii) injection molding.

Compression molding is based on blending gelatin microspheres in a Teflon mold with a biocompatible polymer powder. The mixture is then heated beyond the polymer glass transition temperature (T_g) while constantly applying pressure to the blend simultaneously. This procedure results in the powder particles attaching or bonding together. Once the mold is removed, the gelatin portion is drained out by dipping into water, and then the structure is dried and retained. Due to the lower T_g, PLGA is the most suited polymer for melt molding. Other well-recognized melt-based techniques used for 3D porous scaffold fabrication are extrusion and injection molding combined with blowing agents. Schematic illustration of the PCL tissue scaffold fabrication using a microcellular injection molding method is presented in Figure 10.10.

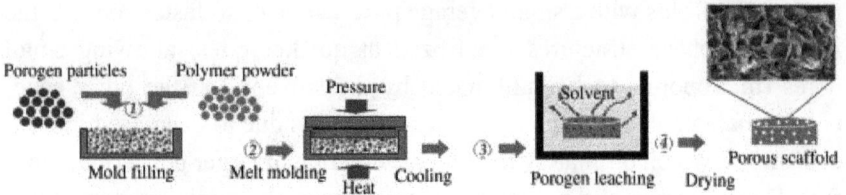

Figure 10.10: Schematic diagram of compression molding/particulate-leaching (CM/PL) scaffold fabrication technique (Huang *et al.*, 2017; Allaf, 2018).

10.6.7 *Fiber bonding*

Fiber-based manufacturing techniques for scaffold fabrication have been very attractive, owing to the large surface-area-to-volume ratio property they offer. The fiber bonding method involves heating of two separate non-woven fibers just above their melting point and binding them at the point of intersection. The interconnection of these fiber networks gives a structural form for a scaffold. The commercially available PGA suture material in the form of long fibers is developed by this technique. However, the application of fiber bonding-designed structures *in vivo* is very much restricted by the mechanical instability, lack of control over porosity, unavailability of suitable solvents, and immiscibility of two polymers in the melt state.

10.7 Nanofibrous scaffolds for tissue regeneration

10.7.1 *Phase separation*

Phase separation is one of the methods used to fabricate porous membranes, foams, and interwoven nanofibrous scaffolds by precipitation of polymers from a polymer-rich domain (solvent-poor domain) and a polymer-poor domain (solvent-rich domain). The structural characteristics obtained by this technique can be constructed to mimic the intrinsic ECM or offer a platform that can induce different cellular responses. A schematic representation of the phase separation method is shown in Figure 10.11a. Thermally-induced phase separation (TIPS), a subset of the phase separation method, is a thermodynamic process involving a phase separation of two or multi-phase systems due to their physical incompatibility. The entire process of engineering a scaffold through TIPS involves five crucial steps: polymer dissolution, liquid-liquid phase separation, gel formation, withdrawal through a solvent, and freeze-drying.

During this process, the required biocompatible polymer is dissolved in a high boiling or low molecular weight liquid to make a homogeneous polymeric solution. The polymeric solution is then casted or molded into the preferred shape. The phase separation into polymer-rich (solvent-poor) and polymer-poor (solvent-rich) phases is stimulated by changing quenching temperature of the polymer solution. The mixture is then brought down to the required quenching temperature to produce a gel-like

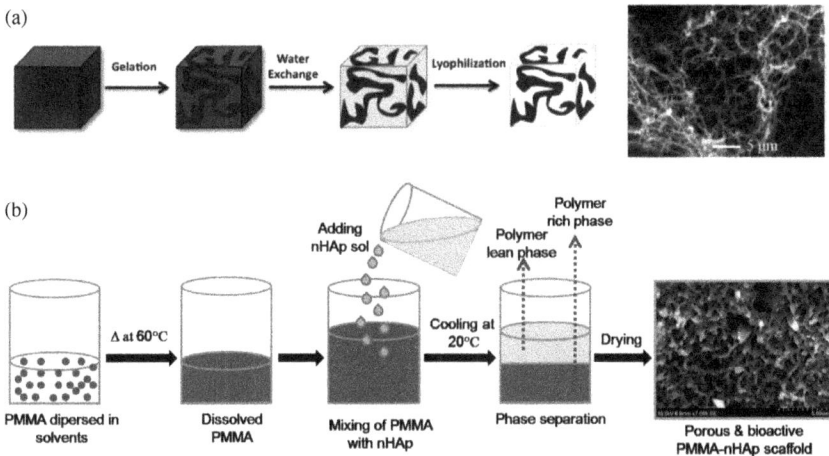

Figure 10.11: (a) Schematic representation of the phase separation method; (b) schematic representation of nHAp-PMMA scaffolds prepared by conjugated TIPS and wet-chemical route (G *et al.*, 2017; Wade *et al.*, 2012; Wang *et al.*, 2018).

substance. The diluent is typically extracted by lyophilization and evaporated by freeze-drying or freeze-extraction to generate a microporous structure. One of the most relevant advantages of this technique is that it is comparatively simple, inexpensive, scalable, compatible with a broad selection of materials, and requires minimal apparatus. The properties of scaffolds can be simply monitored by modifying the parameters such as polymer concentration, quenching temperature, quenching time, solvent/ non-solvent ratio, and surfactant addition. Also, scaffolds obtained by this process display an extremely interconnected porous design. Several biocompatible polymers such as PLLA, PMMA, and PCL are employed for the phase separation technique. A schematic representation of nHAp-PMMA scaffolds prepared by conjugated TIPS and the wet-chemical route is presented in Figure 10.11b.

10.7.2 *Self-assembly*

Self-assembly, also referred to as self-organization, involves naturally arranging individual components into an organized, stable structure with pre-programmed covalent bonds. It is a reversible method of fabricating organized scaffold structures from pre-existing system components that are not aligned with structure/order. Self-assembly has issues such as complicated laboratory procedures, low yield, and restrictions in polymer configurations (deblock and triblock copolymers, dendrimers). One of the benefits associated with the self-assembly process is that it can be conducted under physical conditions without the need for any toxic organic solvents, thus making the procedure more suitable for *in vivo* applications. A schematic representation of the self-assembly method is shown in Figure 10.12.

10.7.3 *Electrospinning*

Electrospinning, a simple electrohydrodynamic process, is the most efficient and widely used modern technique to fabricate a nanofibrous scaffold for tissue engineering. This versatile technique has also been widely acknowledged as a convenient approach for producing

Self-Assembly

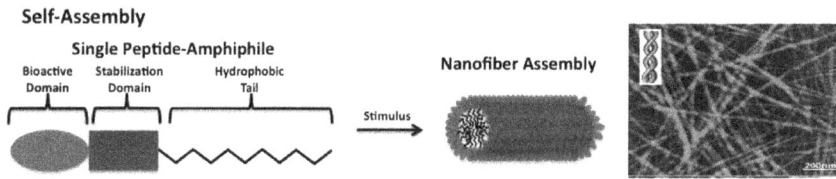

Figure 10.12:   Schematic representation of the self-assembly method (Wade *et al.*, 2012; Zhao *et al.*, 2010).

Electrospinning

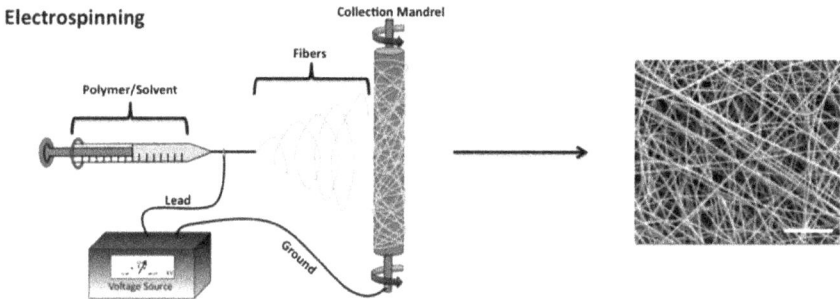

Figure 10.13:   Schematic illustration of the electrospinning apparatus and working mechanism (Wade *et al.*, 2012).

functional nanofibrous biomaterials. This system exploits an electro-static field for advancing and stretching a charged polymer to generate ultrafine fibers with dimensions stretching from 10 nm to quite a few micrometres. Electrospun materials possess many desirable properties suitable for the effective growth of cells and tissues, such as a large surface-to-volume ratio, fine nano diameter, and a three-dimensional interconnected porous network. To date, over 200 natural (silk fibroin, chitosan, gelatin, collagen, etc.) and synthetic polymers (PVA, PVP, PLLA, PCL, etc.) and their composites have been fabricated by electrospinning.

The experimental arrangement of an electrospinning setup consists of four important sections: a glass syringe holding polymeric solution, a blunt metallic needle, a high voltage source (up to 50 kV DC output), and a grounded metallic collector. A schematic illustration of the electrospin-ning apparatus and the working mechanism is presented in Figure 10.13.

In brief, under constant flow rate, the liquid droplet of the polymer solution emerges from a nozzle and is held at its tip by surface tension. When a sufficiently high voltage is applied to the liquid spherical droplet, the liquid body is charged and deformed into a conical shape (Taylor cone). Once the electrical field achieves a critical threshold value at which the electrostatic repulsion counteracts the surface tension, the droplet is stretched until it reaches the grounded collector and deposits as a non-woven fibrous layer. During this process, the polymer solution experiences a process of whipping instability and stretching, during which the solvent evaporates. For desired morphology and properties of electrospun materials, parameters such as solution characteristics (polymer M_w, concentration, viscosity, charge density, conductivity), process variables (flow rate, voltage, tip-target distance, needle tip diameter and design, collector geometry), and environmental considerations (temperature, humidity, air perturbation) can be easily manipulated.

It is worth mentioning that the scaffold properties could be controlled by choosing the proper fabrication technique. For instance, if the application in soft tissue needs greater flexibility, better surface-to-volume ratio, and decent porosity, electrospinning would be the perfect fabrication method. On the other side, hard tissue application necessitates load-bearing material with high mechanical properties and appropriate bioactivity. In such cases, 3D printing techniques or freezing of inorganic/organic composites would provide adequate scaffolding. The various scaffold fabrication methods with advantages, drawbacks, and applications are tabulated in Table 10.4. As presented in Figure 10.14, polymeric biomaterials and polymeric/ceramic composites play a central role in tissue engineering.

10.8 Regenerative medicine

Adults have the potential for regeneration. For example, if a portion of the liver is damaged because of injury or illness, it can grow back to its original size. Our skin is another part of our body that can fix and rebuild itself. Some tissues and organs in the human body do not have that ability to grow back naturally, but it can be engineered to do so by using stem cells.

Table 10.4: Scaffold fabrication methods with advantages, drawbacks, and applications.

Fabrication method	Advantage	Drawback	Application	Form and dimension of the scaffold
Solvent casting / particulate leaching	Controlled porous scaffold; less material required	Limited mechanical properties; residual solvent may induce toxicity; non-interconnected porosity	Bone and cartilage tissue engineering	Film, can be designed as a patterned or smooth structure
Freeze-drying	Interconnective pores can be achieved	Lower porosity when compared to other 3D fabrication techniques; pore size limitations	Tissue engineering scaffolds	Foam or sponge
Gas foaming	No use of solvents or porogens	Non-homogeneous porosity; limited pore interconnectivity; an external non-porous surface	Drug delivery; limited in tissue engineering	Foam
Fiber bonding	High surface-to-volume ratio	Poor mechanical properties	Tissue engineering scaffolds, especially PGA fiber-based scaffolds	Nano or microfibers
Melt molding	Flexible geometry: composite materials are easily prepared	High temperature is required; limited polymers; no pore interconnectivity	Tissue engineering scaffolds	Nano or microfibers
Electrospinning	High surface-to-volume ratio; exact mimic of ECM	Reduced control over fiber deposition; no control over porosity; poor mechanical properties	Tissue engineering scaffolds	Nano or microfibers
Phase separation	Minimum apparatus; inexpensive; highly interconnected porous architecture	Difficult shapes for tissue engineering applications can be fabricated	Tissue engineering	Film
Self-assembly	No use of solvents or porogens	Complex laboratory procedure; low yield; few suitable polymer configurations	Peptide-amphiphile membranes	Film

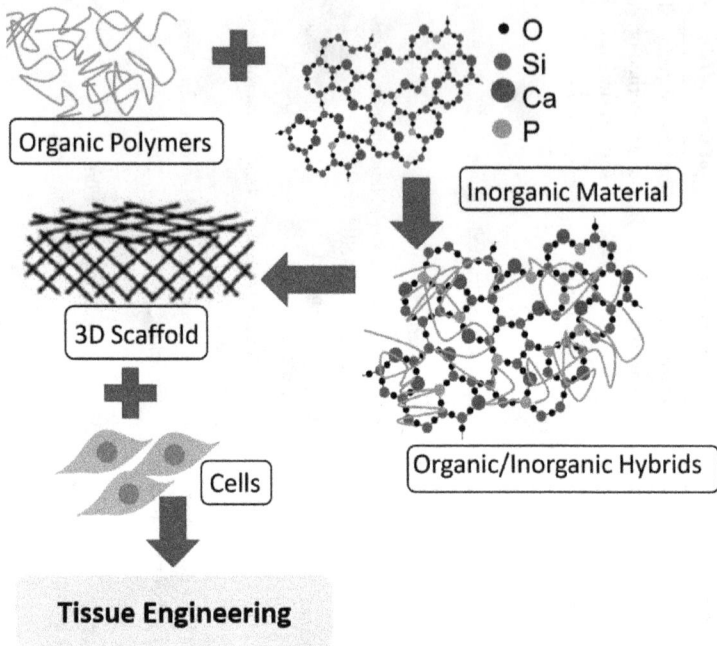

Figure 10.14:   Polymeric biomaterials and polymeric/ceramic composites play a central role in tissue engineering (Aslankoohi *et al.*, 2019).

Regenerative medicine is a branch of tissue engineering and molecular biology that applies principles of engineering and life sciences to regenerate human tissues and organs that have been damaged by disease and trauma and to restore their functions. Since the inception of the field several decades ago, regenerative medicine has enabled researchers to grow several tissues and organs in the research laboratory and securely implant them when the body is unable to heal itself. Since *"tissue engineering"* and *"regenerative medicine"* concentrate on replacing or repairing the damaged tissue and organs, they are almost used interchangeably at times. However, both have separate approaches with a unique difference between them. Tissue engineering merges cells, scaffolds, and growth factors to induce and promote regeneration in damaged tissue outside the human body (*in vitro*). In contrast, regenerative medicine unites tissue engineering with other strategies, such as cell-based therapy, gene therapy, and immunomodulation, to induce tissue/organ regeneration in the body itself (*in vivo*).

Tissue engineering is more reliant on the type of cells, scaffold architecture, and growth factor stimulation, whereas regenerative medicine depends on the qualities and mechanism of stem cells. Stem cells are undifferentiated and have the capability to differentiate into many types of special tissues and be engineered to restore or regenerate tissues. The aspects of stem cells are discussed in detail in Chapter 4. Although regenerative medicine is still in its evolution stage, major progress has taken place in the last few years, with close to 100 regenerative FDA-approved products in the market. More than 300 open trials are registered for regenerative medicine in the US National Institutes of Health clinical trials database (http://clinicaltrials.gov).

10.8.1 *Applications of regenerative medicine*

One of the main goals of regenerative medicine is to generate new parts of the body from a patient's own cells and tissues. This will relieve not only organ demand but also problems caused by organ denial. The overall model of organ bioengineering presented in Figure 10.15 is entirely based on the production of whole-organ scaffolds by perfusion decellularization. These organ scaffolds can then be further recellularized with various cell types under suitable biological conditions in a perfusion bioreactor.

From Chapter 3, we have learnt that embryonic stem cells are short-lived pluripotent cells isolated from the undifferentiated inner cell mass of

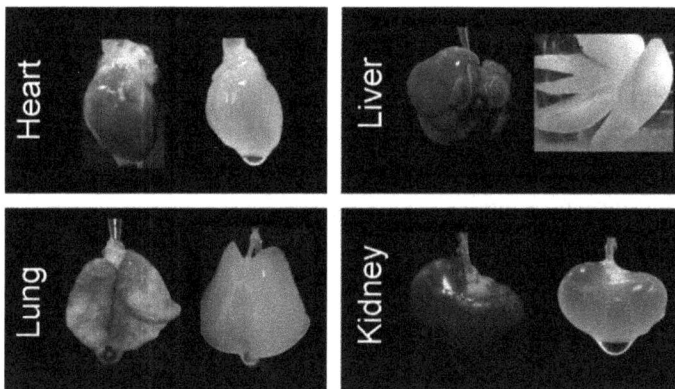

Figure 10.15: Different organs decellurized. Probably from mice. Source: miromatrix. com. (Hickerson *et al.*, 2020; Moran *et al.*, 2014).

a very early stage embryo and have the capacity to develop (i.e., differentiate) into any sort of cell and build any cell type in the body, for example, skin cells, brain cells, muscle cells, etc. When tissue or organs are injured, these cells are used to repair. Additionally, stem cells may also serve to diagnose several diseases and genetic disorders such as blood disorders (type 1 diabetes), neurological disorders (Parkinson's and Alzheimer's diseases), bone disorders (multiple sclerosis and rheumatoid arthritis), leukemia, and Crohn's disease.

10.9 Multiple choice questions

1. Imagine you have prepared electrospun nanofibers, and you are optimizing parameters. How do you image and measure the porosity quickly?
    (a) by doing basic image analysis using a microscope
    (b) by doing image analysis using transmission electron microscopy
    (c) by using X-ray diffraction analysis
    (d) none of the above

2. Which of the following is considered *least* when designing a scaffold for bone tissue engineering?
    (a) biodegradation properties
    (b) mechanical properties
    (c) pore size and pore morphology
    (d) none of the above

3. An ideal scaffold should have the following properties:
    (a) biodegradable properties irrespective of the application
    (b) mechanical stability, non-toxicity and suitable biodegradation
    (c) toxicity and non-biodegradability
    (d) immunogenic and low strength

4. A scaffold material should
    (a) remain longer than needed in the body and provide mechanical support even after tissue is regenerated
    (b) potentially stress-shield the tissue
    (c) have mechanical properties more than required
    (d) gradually degrade with time as new tissue formation increases

5. Issues with conventional fabricated scaffolds for tissue engineering include
    I. pore size control
   II. toxicity induced by biodegraded products
  III. weak mechanical properties
   (a) only I
   (b) only II and III
   (c) all of the above
   (d) only I and II

6. In solvent casting and particulate leaching, internal architecture is determined by
   (a) polymer matrix
   (b) solvent
   (c) embedded salts in the dissolved polymer matrix
   (d) none of the above

7. Pore diameter in solvent casting and particulate leaching is controlled by
   (a) size of the salt particles
   (b) molecular weight of polymer matrix
   (c) size of the mold
   (d) none of the above

8. Select the main issue(s) with conventional fabrication techniques:
   (a) no or less control in pore geometry
   (b) no or less control in precise pore size
   (c) difficulty in construction of the internal architecture
   (d) all of the above

9. Which of the following is NOT true about the electrospinning technique?
   (a) it yields a three-dimensional scaffold that mimics the ECM matrix
   (b) evaporation of solvent does not happen during the electrospinning process
   (c) rotating mandrel yields aligned nanofibers
   (d) the process involves the use of a high-voltage power supply

References & Further Reading

Abbasi, N., Hamlet, S., Love, R. M., & Nguyen, N.-T. (2020). Porous scaffolds for bone regeneration. *Journal of Science: Advanced Materials and Devices, 5*(1), 1–9. doi:10.1016/j.jsamd.2020.01.007.

Allaf, R.M. (2018). Chapter 4 — Melt-molding technologies for 3D scaffold engineering. In Y. Deng & J. Kuiper (Eds.), *Functional 3D Tissue Engineering Scaffolds: Materials, Technologies and Applications* (pp. 75–100): Woodhead Publishing.

Asadian, M., Chan, K. V., Norouzi, M., Grande, S., *et al.* (2020). Fabrication and Plasma Modification of Nanofibrous Tissue Engineering Scaffolds. *Nanomaterials, 10*(1), 119. doi:10.3390/nano10010119.

Aslankoohi, N., Mondal, D., Rizkalla, A. S., & Mequanint, K. (2019). Bone Repair and Regenerative Biomaterials: Towards Recapitulating the Microenvironment. *Polymers, 11*(9), 1437. doi:10.3390/polym11091437.

Caballero Aguilar, L. M., Silva, S. M., & Moulton, S. E. (2019). Growth factor delivery: Defining the next generation platforms for tissue engineering. *Journal of Controlled Release, 306*, 40–58. doi:10.1016/j.jconrel.2019.05.028.

Cheng, X., Shao, Z., Li, C., Yu, L., *et al.* (2017). Isolation, Characterization and Evaluation of Collagen from Jellyfish Rhopilema esculentum Kishinouye for Use in Hemostatic Applications. *PLOS ONE, 12*(1), e0169731. doi:10.1371/journal.pone.0169731.

G. R., S. B., Venkatesan, B., & Vellaichamy, E. (2017). A novel nano-hydroxyapatite — PMMA hybrid scaffolds adopted by conjugated thermal induced phase separation (TIPS) and wet-chemical approach: Analysis of its mechanical and biological properties. *Materials Science and Engineering: C, 75*, 221–228. doi:10.1016/j.msec.2016.12.133.

Hickerson, D., Somara, S., Martinez-Fernandez, A., Lo, C., *et al.* (2020). Chapter 9 — The Next Wave: Tissue Replacement and Organ Replacement. In A. A. Vertès, D. M. Smith, N. Qureshi, & N. J. Dowden (Eds.), *Second Generation Cell and Gene-based Therapies* (pp. 243–268): Academic Press.

Huang, A., Jiang, Y., Napiwocki, B., Mi, H., *et al.* (2017). Fabrication of poly (ε-caprolactone) tissue engineering scaffolds with fibrillated and interconnected pores utilizing microcellular injection molding and polymer leaching. *RSC Advances, 7*(69), 43432–43444. doi:10.1039/C7RA06987A.

Khan, I., Neumann, C., & Sinha, M. (2020). Chapter 24 — Tissue regeneration and reprogramming. In D. Bagchi, A. Das, & S. Roy (Eds.), *Wound Healing, Tissue Repair, and Regeneration in Diabetes* (pp. 515–534): Academic Press.

Lei, Y., Goldblatt, Z. E., & Billiar, K. L. (2020). Chapter 2.6.4 — Micromechanical Design Criteria for Tissue-Engineering Biomaterials. In W. R. Wagner, S. E. Sakiyama-Elbert, G. Zhang, & M. J. Yaszemski (Eds.), *Biomaterials Science (Fourth Edition)* (pp. 1335–1350): Academic Press.

Moran, E. C., Dhal, A., Vyas, D., Lanas, A., *et al.* (2014). Whole-organ bioengineering: current tales of modern alchemy. *Translational Research, 163*(4), 259–267. doi:10.1016/j.trsl.2014.01.004.

Ramakrishna, S., Fujihara, K., Teo, W.-E., Yong, T., *et al.* (2006). Electrospun nanofibers: Solving global issues. *Materials Today, 9*(3), 40–50. doi:10.1016/S1369-7021(06)71389-X.

Roy, S., & Singha, N. R. (2017). Polymeric Nanocomposite Membranes for Next Generation Pervaporation Process: Strategies, Challenges and Future Prospects. *Membranes, 7*(3), 53. doi:10.3390/membranes7030053.

Sampath, U. G. T. M., Ching, Y. C., Chuah, C. H., Sabariah, J. J., *et al.* (2016). Fabrication of Porous Materials from Natural/Synthetic Biopolymers and Their Composites. *Materials, 9*(12), 991. doi:10.3390/ma9120991.

Serra, T., Planell, J. A., & Navarro, M. (2013). High-resolution PLA-based composite scaffolds via 3-D printing technology. *Acta Biomaterialia, 9*(3), 5521–5530. doi:10.1016/j.actbio.2012.10.041.

Tsiapalis, D., & O'Driscoll, L. (2020). Mesenchymal Stem Cell Derived Extracellular Vesicles for Tissue Engineering and Regenerative Medicine Applications. *Cells, 9*(4), 991. doi:10.3390/cells9040991.

Wade, R. J., & Burdick, J. A. (2012). Engineering ECM signals into biomaterials. *Materials Today, 15*(10), 454–459. doi:10.1016/S1369-7021(12)70197-9.

Wang, W., Nie, W., Zhou, X., Feng, W., Chen, L., Zhang, Q., You, Z., Shi, Q., Peng C., & He, C. (2018). Fabrication of heterogeneous porous bilayered nanofibrous vascular grafts by two-step phase separation technique. *Acta Biomaterialia, 79*, 168–181. doi:10.1016/j.actbio.2018.08.014.

Zhao, Y., Tanaka, M., Kinoshita, T., Higuchi, M., & Tan, T. (2010). Nanofibrous scaffold from self-assembly of β-sheet peptides containing phenylalanine for controlled release. *Journal of Controlled Release, 142*(3), 354–360. doi: 10.1016/j.jconrel.2009.11.016.

Chapter 11
Drug delivery

11.1 Introduction

Historically, physicians have sought to tailor their treatments directly to areas of the body that are at risk or impacted by a disease. It is essential to find treatments with efficient and optimized approaches that enhance current methods without side effects and without damaging the surrounding tissues. The procedures should effectively diagnose pathological conditions at their initial or premature stages and enhance patients' health conditions. Medicines (drugs) have been used for a long time to prolong life.

Drug delivery represents one such localized and widely accessible method in scientific and technical fields. It refers to the transport of foreign pharmaceutically active material within the body to accomplish a therapeutic effect. Drug release is characterized as the transfer of trapped biologically active compounds from their location to the outer surface and then to the release medium. Different elements regulate this process, including the products' physicochemical characteristics, the material structures of delivery systems, the release medium's properties, and a combination of all these variables. Before reading this chapter, one should familiarise with the most important terms used in drug delivery systems. The therapeutic window of administered drugs and drug release kinetics is shown in Figure 11.1.

- **Therapeutic effect:** Intended effect of the drug.
- **Therapeutic index:** The index between the minimum amount at which the drug is effective and the maximum amount beyond which the drug is toxic. Concentrations above or below therapeutic index

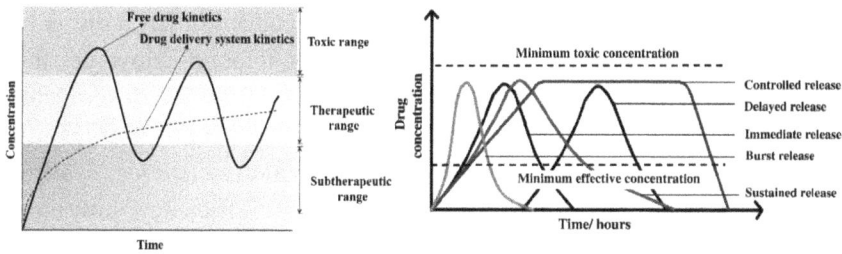

Figure 11.1: Therapeutic window of administered drugs and drug release kinetics (Goonoo *et al.*, 2014; Janssen *et al.*, 2014).

can produce adverse effects to the body or provide no therapeutic benefit at all, respectively.

- **Delayed release:** A dosage type which delivers a selective portion or portions of the drug at a time other than promptly after administration. In other words, the commencement of the drug release action starts at a later phase. The delayed time release of the drug can be achieved by a barrier coating or by stimulation.
- **Sustained release:** A dose which results in a slow release of the drug over a long period.
- **Controlled release:** A dosage which also attains slow discharge of drug for a long time, while maintaining a *constant* level of drug in blood and tissue for a long time.

11.2 Conventional drug delivery systems

Conventional/traditional drug delivery systems are designed to offer an immediate release of drugs. The delivery of the drug is difficult to control, and the successful concentration at the desired target site cannot be regulated for an extended period. In fact, such systems are used more frequently when the purpose is to absorb a drug quickly. Such drug releases usually result in a sudden/rapid increase in concentration, followed by an immediate decrease in concentration. This sudden-increase-and-decrease drug release methodology may cause an unsafe toxic threshold or sometimes fall below its effective therapeutic level. Besides, at any given period, these mechanisms cannot maintain the drug concentration at a fixed and constant level.

One approach to solve the drug instability concentration issue is by offering several doses (repeated doses) at periodic intervals. However, this approach is not only profligate but also contributes to overdose-related side effects due to frequent infusion of a significant excess of drugs in a short period. Therefore, in a nutshell, conventional drug delivery systems are illustrated by inadequate biodistribution, low efficiency, unwanted side effects, and absence of selectivity. Given this, a more reliable distribution strategy of drug delivery is needed that can overcome these limitations and dole out the active drug agents at a required concentration in the desired target medium at a slow rate. Many technological advancements have recently been made that brought about the development of modern drug delivery techniques.

11.3 Controlled-release drug delivery systems

The novel drug delivery systems, also known as controlled-release drug delivery systems, blend cutting-edge techniques and innovative dosage forms. These systems effectively monitor drug release, provide more protection, and precisely guide medication to the targeted tissue. The word *"controlled release"* suggests a process or mechanism that delivers the drug with consistent and reproducible kinetics at a predetermined rate of time with a defined release mechanism. Such systems have several advantages over conventional drug delivery systems, such as temporal and/or spatial control over the drug release mechanism, protection of delicate drugs, predictability, and long-term regulation. Depending on the design, different forms of mass transport methods can be involved in regulating the release of drugs from an enclosed component. These methods include water diffusion into the system, drug diffusion out of the system, drug breakdown, polymer swelling, matrix erosion, and osmotic effects.

All these methods have a controlled release system by which the drug is released at constant or variable rates. Generally, controlled-release medications can be grouped into pulse-release, extended-release, and delayed-release drugs. Some of the advantages and disadvantages of controlled drug delivery systems are presented in Table 11.1.

Table 11.1: Advantages and disadvantages of controlled drug delivery systems.

Pros	Cons
Localized drug delivery	Degraded products may be harmful if not controlled
Reduced dosing frequency and greater compliance with patients	High cost due to fabrication
Less or no side effects by local administration	
Maintaining concentration of the drug within the therapeutic range	
Less wastage of drug	

11.4 Methods of achieving controlled release

11.4.1 *Diffusion-controlled systems*

Diffusion, a mass transport mechanism, is by far the most significant method used to regulate the release of drugs from pharmaceutical products. Water-insoluble polymer films using a diffusion mechanism allow aqueous fluids from the surroundings to pass into the layered core. The drug is then absorbed, and the drug molecules are diffused across the polymeric membrane and into the body.

In a diffusion-based control system, the release of a drug is primarily affected by the diffusion properties of the drug in the matrix and its membrane but not by the rate of dissolution. The associated release kinetics mainly rely on the size and shape of the dosage type. The desired release profiles can be easily manipulated by changing the geometry and device dimensions. In diffusion-controlled designs, the encapsulated drug particles diffuse through a polymeric membrane via pores in the polymer matrix or through polymer chains. These systems can be separated into two subsystems, (i) membrane-controlled reservoir systems and (ii) monolithic matrix systems. In both reservoir and monolithic matrix systems, the drug core is surrounded or coated by a rate-regulating membrane. The physiological factors, such as pH and the existence of hard substances in the gastrointestinal tract, may affect drug release of diffusion-controlled systems. The advantages and disadvantages are presented in Table 11.2.

11.4.1.1 *Membrane-controlled reservoir systems*

In this reservoir system, a bioactive drug is either dissolved (liquid form) or dispersed (powdered form) within a device known as the core or reservoir. The device is then covered with a layer of a non-biodegradable polymer material known as a membrane or capsule. The drug slowly diffuses through the polymeric membrane, and its release rate is regulated by the polymer's chemical structure, molecular weight, membrane thickness, and porosity. The physicochemical properties of the enclosed drug such as solubility, stability, and particle size may also affect diffusivity. It is important to note that the presence of an outer membrane typically offers an improved release profile. Schematics based on physical structure (porous or non-porous membrane) for diffusion-controlled systems are presented in Figure 11.2. Considering the diffusion in a single direction, x, Fick's first law of diffusion is given by

$$J = -D \frac{dC}{dx}$$

where D is diffusion coefficient (diffusivity) ($\frac{m^2}{s}$), J is rate of transfer per unit area ($\frac{kg}{m^2 s}$), and $\frac{dC}{dx}$ is the concentration gradient ($\frac{kg}{m^4}$).

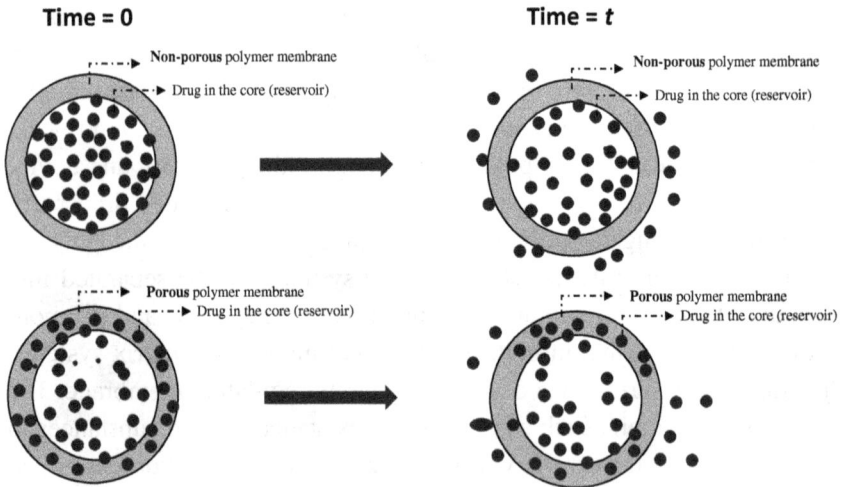

Figure 11.2:   Schematics based on physical structure (porous or non-porous membrane) for diffusion-controlled systems.

11.4.1.2 *Monolithic matrix systems*

Monolithic matrix systems (Figure 11.3) include a drug to be encapsulated or dispersed in a matrix. The outer membrane present in the reservoir system is absent in monolithic matrix systems. From an engineering perspective, the word *"matrix"* refers to a three-dimensional network, most frequently a polymeric network produced for an application and contains drugs and other substances such as solvents. These matrix systems get exposed to solution first, dissolve, and allow slow diffusion of the drug out of the polymeric matrix material. They also offer a sustained release of the drug over a long period. These systems may be used to shape hydrophobic and/or hydrophilic matrices to enable control or prediction of the release of drugs.

Various factors affect the release pattern:

- If the drug is dissolved: Fick's second law
- If the drug is dispersed: Fick's first law
- If the polymer is a porous matrix: Higuchi's theory for porous form
- If the polymer is a hydrophilic matrix: Gelation or diffusion

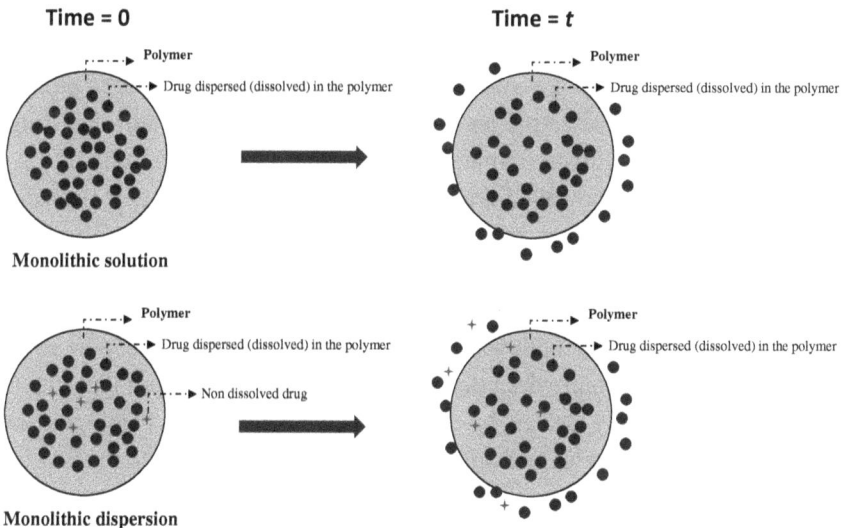

Figure 11.3:   Schematics based on initial drug loading (dissolved and non-dissolved) for monolithic matrix drug delivery.

Table 11.2: Advantages and disadvantages of diffusion-controlled drug delivery systems.

	Pros	Cons
Membrane-controlled reservoir system	Easier to achieve zero-order kinetics	High uniformity of thickness needs to be maintained for consistent drug release rates
	Drug inactivation by contact with the polymeric matrix can be avoided	Polymer membrane should be removed after release of the drug (non-biodegradable polymers); biodegradable systems with polymers are difficult to design.
		Accidental rupture of the membrane will lead to a large amount of drug dumped at once
Monolithic matrix system	No membrane; uniform drug distribution is possible	Challenging to achieve zero-order kinetics
	No danger in rupture and accidental dumping	Limitations of drugs

11.4.2 *Water penetration-controlled systems*

11.4.2.1 *Osmotically controlled drug delivery systems*

Osmotically controlled drug delivery systems employ osmotic pressure principles for controlled delivery of embedded drug molecules. Osmotic pumps represent one of the effective and reliable techniques for controlled drug delivery for oral administration and implantation. One of the main advantages of osmotically controlled drug delivery systems is that almost constant or zero-order drug release is preserved until complete exhaustion of the drug packaged in the reservoir. Pharmaceutical delivery from these techniques is largely independent of the gastrointestinal tract's factors, such as pH. These systems can be used for both systemic and targeted drug delivery. A schematic of the osmotic pump drug delivery system is illustrated in Figure 11.4. As osmosis is mainly driven by a difference in membrane-wide solvent concentrations, drug release from osmosis-based systems is controlled by many formulation aspects such as core component solubility, osmotic strain, size of the delivery hole, and function of the rate-controlling membrane.

Osmosis is a special type of diffusion characterized by the spontaneous movement of solvent molecules (example water) through a semipermeable membrane in response to unequal concentrations of solutes (drug

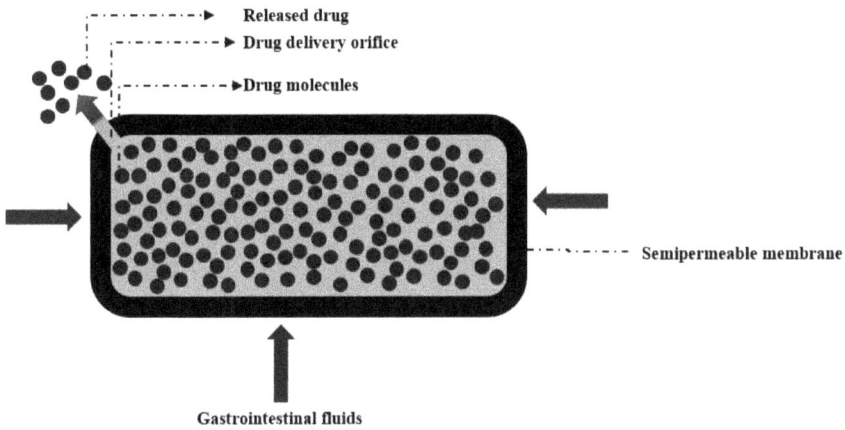

Figure 11.4: Elementary osmotic pump drug delivery system.

molecules) on either side of the membrane. It is a biophysical manifestation that naturally occurs in all biological systems. Specifically, the term osmotic pressure is defined as the minimum hydrostatic pressure required to prevent the inward flow of water movement across the semipermeable membrane. It is important to note that osmosis allows only water to diffuse through the semipermeable membrane but excludes most solutes or ions. Due to this, osmosis is an ideal method for the delivery of therapeutic agents. The delivery of a therapeutic agent from oral osmotic systems is controlled by the influx of solvent passing through the semipermeable membrane. The basic equation which applies to osmotic systems is

$$\frac{dM}{dt} = \frac{dV}{dt}c$$

where $\frac{dM}{dt}$ is mass release rate, $\frac{dV}{dt}$ is water influx rate, and c is the concentration of the drug.

The volume of solvent (water) passing across the semipermeable membrane is defined by

$$\frac{dv}{dt} = \frac{A}{h}Lp[\sigma \Delta\pi - \Delta P]$$

where A is membrane area, h is membrane thickness, Lp is mechanical membrane permeability, σ is reflection coefficient, $\Delta\pi$ is osmotic pressure difference, and ΔP is hydrostatic pressure difference.

When $\Delta\pi \gg \Delta P$,

$$\frac{dv}{dt} = \frac{A}{h} Lp[\sigma \Delta\pi]$$

Let K be the membrane permeability, given by $Lp[\sigma]$, then the above equation becomes

$$\frac{dv}{dt} = \frac{A}{h} K\pi$$

The underlying equation for all osmotically driven pumps is therefore

$$\frac{dM}{dt} = K\left(\frac{A}{h}\right)\pi C$$

where K is the permeability of the semipermeable membrane, A is the surface area of the semipermeable membrane, and C is the drug concentration of the dispensed solution.

11.4.2.2 *Swelling-controlled drug delivery system*

Swelling-controlled drug delivery systems are three-dimensional networks built upon polymeric chains that are chemically or physically cross-linked. A schematic of the swelling-controlled mechanism is shown in Figure 11.5. Polymers that are employed for swelling-controlled drug delivery systems can be (i) water-insoluble hydrogels and (ii) hydrophilic polymers. The polymer system is initially in the dry, glassy, non-swollen state, where the movement of polymer chains is very much restricted. The drug molecules are entrapped in this state. Upon contact with aqueous solutions or any biological fluids, the solvent infiltrates into the available areas on the surface between the macromolecular chains. When sufficient water enters the inner areas, the network rehydrates and "relaxes". This relaxing allows an increase in the system's net volume and mobility of the entrapped drug molecules, thereby releasing the entrapped drugs by dissolution and diffusion. For hydrophilic

Time = 0   **Time = *t***

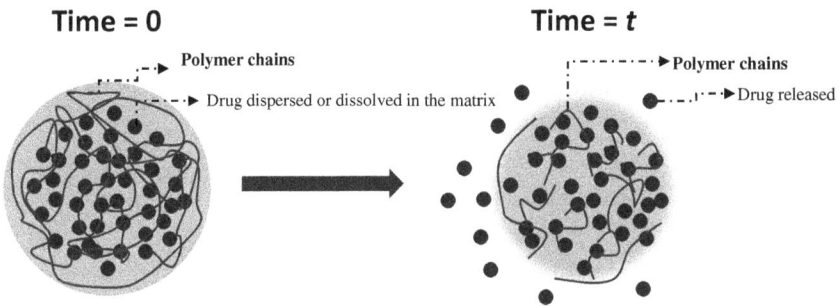

Figure 11.5:   Swelling-controlled mechanism.

polymers, a sufficient water concentration is required to trigger the relaxation mechanism.

Key definitions

Bioavailability: It is a subcategory of absorption and is defined as the amount of drug that reaches the systemic circulation.

pK_a: $= -\log_{10}K_a$. Apart from pH, pK_a is one of the other parameters used to signify the strength of an acid. The lower the pK_a value, the stronger the acid.

11.4.3 *Chemically controlled systems*

Chemically controlled drug delivery systems are self-regulated. They are skilled in obtaining input information from its surroundings and modifying/acting in response to that information. The drug stored within is released based on a series of chemical reactions. Two radically different approaches are possible in the design of these systems. In one method, the feedback signal modulates the percentage of drug discharge from the delivery system, and in another system, the feedback signal activates drug release from the system.

11.4.3.1 *Polymer-drug dispersion system*

In a polymer-drug dispersion system, the drug is released from the polymer matrix either by bioerosion (surface erosion) or biodegradation (bulk degradation or bulk erosion). The difference between these two models is based on how degradation occurs. In both systems, matrix disturbance of the polymeric chains is liable for the drug release. The disruption occurs either by water or enzymatic hydrolysis. The time taken to hydrolyze surface polymer chains into insignificant soluble constituents (T_e) can be used to evaluate the suitable mode of degradation. The time taken for diffusion of water into a polymer (D_T) depends on the polymer's properties such as molecular weight, density, etc. Bulk degradation is distinguished by a superior rate of water diffusion to hydrolysis ($D_T \gg T_e$), and surface erosion occurs when $T_e \gg D_T$.

Dispersion through bioerosion or surface erosion: Bioerosion occurs when the size, mass or magnitude of the system shrinks. A schematic of drug delivery by bioerosion or surface erosion is shown in Figure 11.6. The polymer should be bio-erodible, meaning that after use, the product can degrade and need not be removed from the body. A bioerosion-controlled drug delivery system thus comprises a drug-encapsulated bio-erodible polymer matrix, usually poly(vinyl methyl ether).

Dispersion through biodegradation or bulk erosion: Biodegradation is a chemical decomposition of materials by the action of living organisms, which typically occurs via chain cleavage and results in a decrease in the molecular weight of the polymers. By the action of surrounding biological activity, most biodegradable polymers are intended to decay or breakdown into biologically acceptable smaller compounds (CO_2, H_2O, and salts), leading to a significant change in their mechanical and chemical properties. The biodegradation may occur due to bulk hydrolysis of the

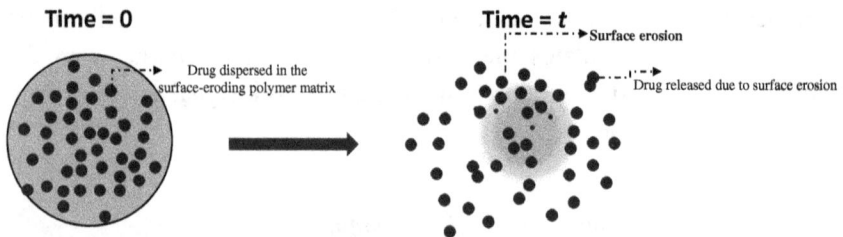

Figure 11.6:   Drug delivery by bioerosion or surface erosion.

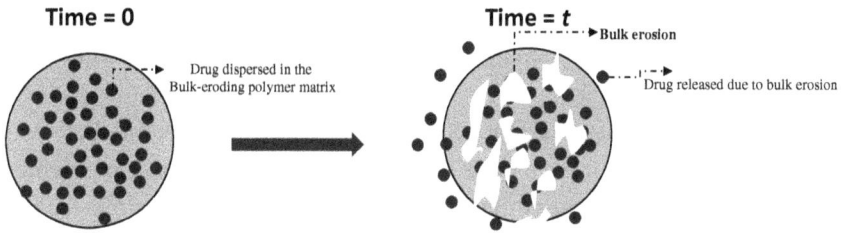

Figure 11.7: Drug delivery by biodegradation or bulk erosion.

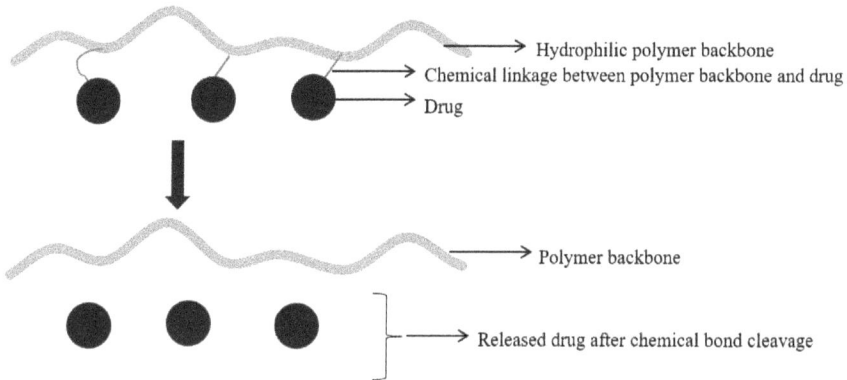

Figure 11.8: Schematic of the polymer-drug conjugate system (Larson *et al.*, 2012).

polymer chains or enzymatic reactions. A schematic of drug delivery by biodegradation or bulk erosion is shown in Figure 11.7.

11.4.3.2 *Polymer-drug conjugate systems*

In the polymer-drug conjugate system, the active drug particles are covalently bonded to a hydrophilic polymer often by means of a spacer molecule that is biologically active. A schematic of the polymer-drug conjugate system is shown in Figure 11.8. This method allows for high drug loadings with the polymer. Once within the body, either hydrolysis or enzyme cleavage terminates the connection between the polymer carrier and the drug. Compared to other drug encapsulated methods, the polymer-drug conjugate system offers several significant advantages such as aqueous solubility and stability, high drug loading efficacy, and sustained release of drug over long periods. Various types of biodegradable polymers, including PEG and N-(2-hydroxypropyl)methacrylamide (HPMA), are used to bind drugs.

It is important to note that adverse interaction or reactions between drugs and polymer can be resolved by conjugating the drug to the polymer via bonding. This technique has a decisive edge over other drug-loaded nano/microparticles, as it allows for accurate monitoring of the drug dosage being introduced. It is also ideal for providing high matrix stability of the drug and preventing drug accumulation, burst release, and drug loss at later stages of sterilization or scaffold purification, such as removal of cross-link agents. Besides, when compared with physical loading methods, drug conjugation significantly reduces the release levels of medications.

11.4.4 *Stimulus-responsive systems*

In an attempt to improve precision and effectiveness, experts from various disciplines continue to investigate easier and safer ways to dispense drugs locally to specific sites of action. Stimulus-responsive drug delivery systems are one such method that has increasingly gained attention as '*smart*' drug delivery systems. Such systems have the ability to transport drugs in a controlled manner to a specific target site by altering their physico-chemical characteristics upon exposure to external or internal stimuli. Also, stimulus-responsive drug delivery has become the most appealing drug delivery technique for its efficiency in minimizing damage to healthy tissues/organs and decreasing side effects by optimizing them to patient-centric care. This technique was extensively investigated to accomplish tumor targeted delivery, where internal or external triggers may be used to activate the controlled release of carried drugs. Many endogenous (internal) responsive triggers such as (i) pH, (ii) ROS (reactive oxygen species), (iii) redox, (iv) enzymes, (v) temperature, and exogenous (external) triggers such as (i) light, (ii) temperature, (iii) magnetic field, (iv) electrical signals, and (v) ultrasound were explored to address intracellular delivery barriers and attain release of drugs on demand.

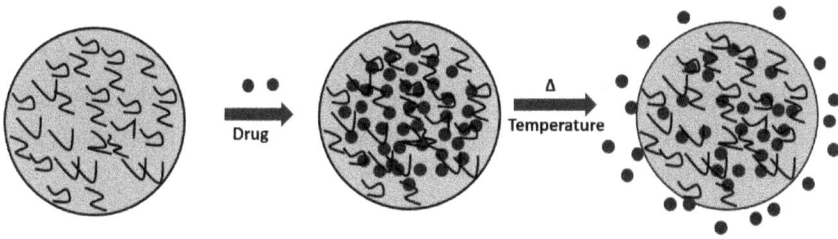

Figure 11.9: Schematic of temperature-responsive drug delivery systems.

11.4.4.1 *Temperature-responsive drug delivery systems*

Temperature-sensitive drug delivery systems (Figure 11.9) are the most widely studied class of environmentally responsive systems due to their phase-transition behaviour concerning variations in temperature. In general, injured tissues have higher temperatures and greater sensitivity than healthy tissues. This is exploited in the design of temperature-responsive drug delivery systems, where a majority of the temperature-responsive polymers are synthesized according to *lower critical solution temperature (LCST)* values. Thermosensitive polymers exhibit this occurrence where they swell and become hydrophilic below LCST, and shrink and display intramolecular hydrophobic interactions above LCST. The swelling changes or patterns of the polymers are regulated by the hydrophilic/hydrophobic stability. If the local temperature around the drug is marginally greater than that of the LCST, the polymer chain gets dehydrated and becomes more hydrophobic and collapses, allowing the delivery of the encapsulated compound. To control the properties (solubility, hydrophilic/hydrophobic balance) of the thermoresponsive polymers, the temperature can be applied externally in a non-invasive manner (e.g., the body is subjected to localized heat outside) or generated internally due to a pathological condition (e.g., tumor or inflammation).

11.4.4.2 *pH-responsive drug delivery systems*

Drug delivery systems can be engineered to react to variations in ecological/ambient conditions, especially pH values. Different organs, tissues, and cellular parts of the human body have specific pH values. For example, pH value for skin is 4–6.5, gastric is 1.35–3.5, blood is 7.35–7.45, interstitial fluid is 7.2–7.4, pancreatic juice is 7.5–8, etc. Also, the pH of infected regions such as malignant tumor and damaged tissues has long been considered to be naturally acidic (pH 6.5), which is nearly one complete pH unit lower than that of healthy blood (pH 7.4). These differences in the pH value at different locations have attracted attention to design 'smart' drug delivery systems where pH values are used to trigger an effective controlled release of drug molecules and facilitate therapeutic delivery into the desired location. In particular, for oral drug delivery, the noticeable changes in pH along the gastrointestinal tract from acidic in the stomach (pH 1.0–3.0) to basic in the small intestine (pH 5.5–6.8) has become a prominent factor while designing drugs. Graphic illustrations of the potential mechanisms for drug release from a pH-responsive drug delivery system with polymeric nanocarriers as an example are presented in Figure 11.10.

The selection of ionizable biocompatible polymers with a pK_a value between 3 and 10 is a prerequisite for designing pH-responsive drug delivery procedures. pH-sensitive polymers comprise polyacids and/or polybases that can receive and/or contribute multiple protons and go through conformational variations upon stimulation to provide on-demand

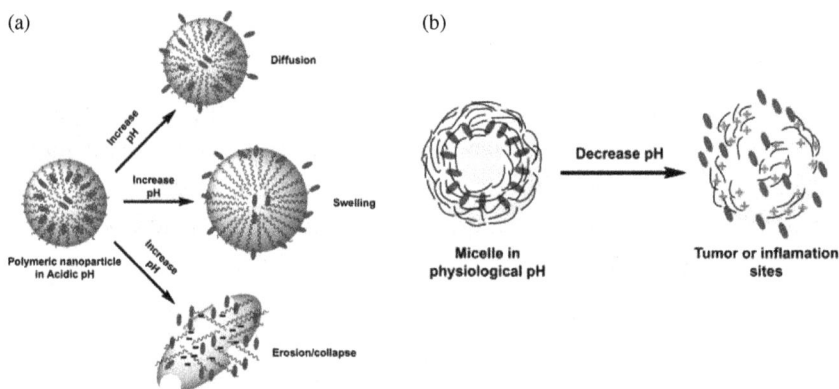

Figure 11.10:   (a) Graphic illustrations of the potential mechanisms for drug release from a pH-responsive drug delivery system with polymeric nanocarriers and (b) drug release from a micelle (Li *et al.*, 2019; Ratemi, 2018).

drug release. These polymers contain either pendant acidic groups such as -COOH and -SO$_3$H that grow/swell in basic pH or basic groups such as -NH$_2$ that grow/swell in acidic pH.

pH-responsive acidic polymers

- *Carboxylic acid groups*: At basic pH values, carboxylic acid groups undergo deprotonation (removal of a proton) and become carboxylate anions. Polymers like poly(acrylic acid) (PAA), poly(methacrylic acid) (PMAA), poly(ethyl acrylic acid) (PEAA), poly(propyl acrylic acid) (PPAA), and poly(butyl acrylic acid) (PBAA) were researched and employed for the expansion of pH-sensitive drug delivery systems.

- *Boronic acid*: Under normal conditions, polymers with boronic acid groups in the backbone are extremely hydrophobic. However, they become extremely hydrophilic when it is negatively charged at pH values above its pK$_a$, providing a pH-responsive mechanism for drug delivery. An example is the phenylboronic acid moiety (–PhB(OH)$_2$).

- *Sulfonamide*: The acidic protons of sulfonamide groups are instantly dissociated when there is an increase in the pH.

pH-responsive basic polymers

- Polybases which go through protonation (addition of proton) at pH 5–11 are employed as pH-responsive basic polymers. The amine groups accept protons by forming cationic ammonium groups at low pH values and then release them under basic conditions. Examples include polymethacrylate-based polymers and methacrylamide.

pH-responsive natural polymers

- Due to its strong biocompatibility and effective modifications by basic chemistry, natural biodegradable polymers have also gained considerable interest in recent years. Hyaluronic acid, alginate, and gelatine are amongst the few widely used natural polymers for drug delivery applications. In particular, chitosan is extensively used for tumor-targeted drug and gene delivery. It is insoluble at neutral pH but soluble and positively charged at acidic pH values (pH 4.0 and 6.0).

11.4.4.3 *Light-responsive drug delivery systems*

Light-responsive drug delivery systems have been given importance in biomedical applications due to their non-invasiveness, convenience for on-demand drug release, greater spatiotemporal resolution, and cost-effectiveness. Furthermore, the drug's release rate can be effortlessly monitored by simply adjusting the light intensity and duration. Light-sensitive drug delivery systems alter their stability and release their entrapped drugs under different wavelengths of an external light source, including ultraviolet (UV), visible, and near-infra-red (NIR) light. Most of the established light-sensitive drug delivery systems react to UV light (10–400 nm). However, this system has a drawback of not only poor tissue penetration depth but is also harmful to cells and tissues. Alternatively, the NIR light technology with a wavelength of 650–900 nm has excellent tissue penetration capacity, undergoes less scattering and absorption, and causes minimal tissue damage. Furthermore, with the aid of various photothermal materials, NIR light can be converted into heat. There are three reported mechanisms for NIR drug release:

- Photothermal effect (PTE)
- Two-photon absorption (TPA)
- Up-converting nanoparticles (UCNPs)

11.4.4.4 *Ultrasound-responsive drug delivery systems*

Ultrasound energy at a frequency of 0.8–3 MHz serves as a local stimulation to regulate therapeutic targeting at the appropriate locations non-invasively. Various biodegradable and non-biodegradable polymers have been used for drug-releasing structures that are sensitive to ultrasound. The design of ultrasound-responsive systems for utilization in targeted drug delivery is primarily centered on the accretion of dose at the preferred location and stimulating the release of the drug with the ultrasound field, whether through cavitation, thermal, and/or mechanical effects. Physically trapped drugs can be released either by destruction of the carrier or by breaking the chemical connection between carrier and drug. For biodegradable polymers, the use of ultrasound will increase the rate of biodegradation, and for non-biodegradable polymers, the use of ultrasound will improve the diffusion rate of drugs.

11.4.4.5 *Magnetic field-sensitive drug delivery systems*

Magnetic field-reactive devices are not only used in drug delivery applications but also extensively in imaging and diagnosis. It is due to their non-invasive nature, high penetration depth, and lack of energy dissipation. The main feature of magnetic drug delivery systems is their use of a series of permanent magnets to create a magnetic field for stimulation. Many drug delivery devices with magnetic sensitivity have been comprehensively investigated for cancer treatment and therapy. After intravenous or intraarterial injection, intense accretion of drugs at a target location in the body can be accomplished with an elevated external magnetic field gradient provided by rare earth magnets.

Blood hemoglobin is an iron-containing protein that is magnetic in nature. Due to the reasonable biocompatibility, low toxicity and ease of synthesis, magnetic materials such as magnetite Fe_3O_4 or maghemite γ-Fe_2O_3 in the form of nanoparticles or nanocapsules have been considerably used in magnetic field-sensitive drug delivery systems. In theory, under an external magnetic field, these magnetic nanoparticles or nanocapsules typically undergo a physical shape or size distortion reversibly. In principle, because of non-interference with the body physically, the use of a material's magnetic property is safer and preferable to light irradiation, ultrasound, or electrical fields.

11.4.5 *Nanocarrier-based drug delivery systems*

The use of nanotechnology is expected to expand rapidly in the field of medicine. It is anticipated to bring significant advances in drug delivery systems, and more precise diagnosis and treatment of diseases. Nanomaterials possess many unique properties, such as large functional surface area, high surface-to-volume ratio, and ability to adsorb and carry other complexes with it. Due to these unique properties, nanoparticles as drug carriers have demonstrated tremendous potential by offering ease of transportation of drugs, probes, proteins, and imaging agents to target locations across the bloodstream. The engineered structures with dimensions ≤100 nm have proved to minimize drug loss ability, reduce toxicity, provide higher loading efficiency, and demonstrate better biodegradability and longer shelf life. Different types of nanocarriers and their benefits in nanomedicine are shown in Figure 11.11.

Given this, various drug-encapsulated materials such as micelles, liposomes, dendrimers, nanocapsules, and nanospheres have been developed and researched extensively for the treatment, prevention, and diagnosis of diseases.

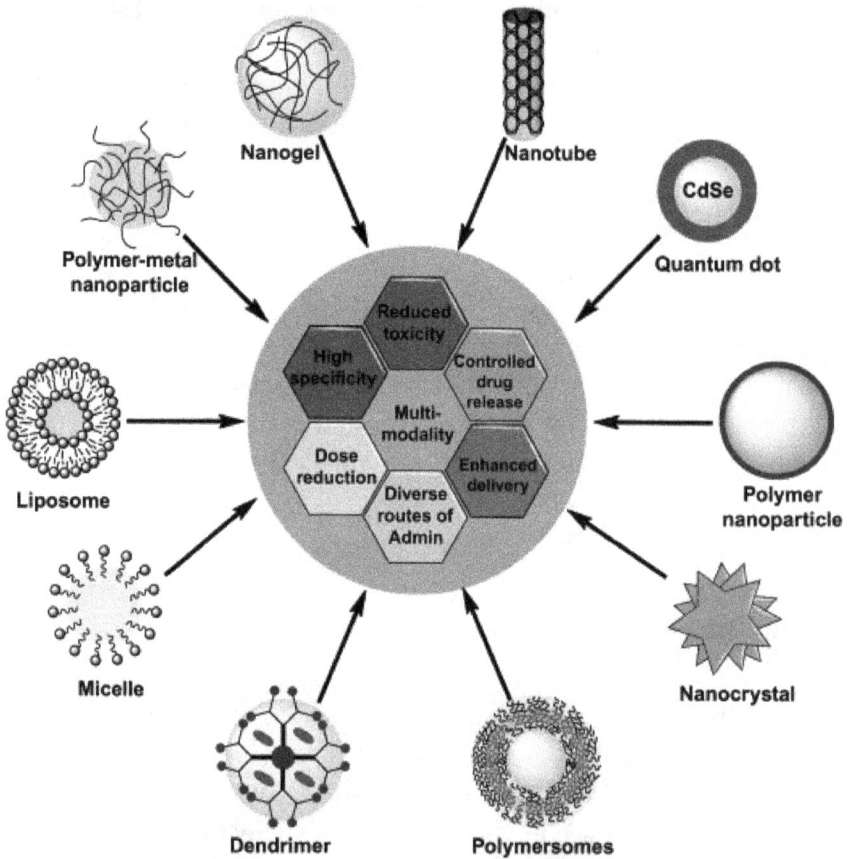

Figure 11.11: Different types of nanocarriers and their benefits in nanomedicine (Faheem *et al.*, 2020; Kumar *et al.*, 2014; Ratemi, 2018).

11.4.5.1 *Polymeric micelles*

Nanosized polymeric micelles (PMs), self-assembling nano-constructs with an approximate size of 10–100 nm, serve as a novel drug delivery system and are widely used to facilitate the delivery of hydrophobic drugs in medicine. PMs are formed spontaneously in aqueous solutions above critical micelle concentration (CMC) by the arrangement of amphiphilic block copolymers. The key functionality of PMs depends on its unique core-shell structure. The hydrophobic core functions as a nano-chamber for hydrophobic drugs, and the hydrophilic shell/corona secures the hydrophobic core from the surrounding aqueous environment. A schematic of PM demonstrating these features is shown in Figure 11.12.

PMs are most ideal for therapeutic applications because of many exciting features like controlled drug release, non-toxicity, core-shell structure, unique morphology, nano-size features, and relatively high stability. The properties can be easily controlled by altering the chemical configuration, polymeric M_w, and co-block dimension ratios. PMs are known for solubilizing water-insoluble drugs in their cores while maintaining intact. The micelle inner shell structure protects the entrapped drug from hydrolysis and enzymatic degradation. Several morphologies of PMs such as star, flower, worm, vesicle, torus, and helix were identified, but spherical PMs are the most commonly observed and studied.

Polymeric micelle

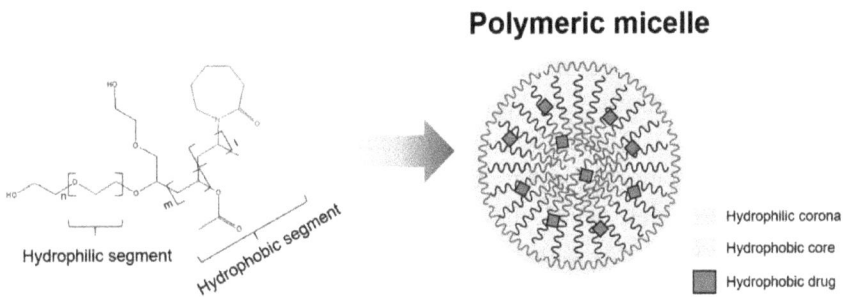

Hydrophilic segment

Hydrophobic segment

Hydrophilic corona

Hydrophobic core

Hydrophobic drug

Figure 11.12: Polymeric micelle prepared with a triblock-copolymer of polyvinyl caprolactam, polyvinyl acetate, and polyethylene glycol (Noh *et al.*, 2018).

Based on the kind of material used, PMs can be subdivided into two common types:

- **Block copolymer micelles:** These are used as carriers for hydrophobic drugs. The morphology of block copolymer micelles is nearly completely spherical when in dilute solution.
- **Polyion complex micelles:** These are used as potential carriers for charged molecules such as small interfering enzymes, proteins, RNA (siRNA), or DNA. Numerous efforts have been made to use polyion complex micelles for siRNA and the transmission of genes. However, their medical and therapeutic application still poses many challenges and thus are still under extensive research.

Several amphiphilic copolymers including di-block (A-B), tri-block (A-B-A), and graft copolymers were employed to form micelles. The most frequently studied hydrophilic block is PEG with an M_w of 2–15 kDa. In contrast, the hydrophobic blocks are usually polyesters, polyethers, or polyamino acids, such as PLA, PCL, and poly(propylene oxide) (PPO).

11.4.5.2 *Liposomes*

Liposomes are the first-generation versatile drug nanocarriers. They are unilamellar or multilamellar sphere-shaped vesicular structures composed of single or multiple concentric phospholipid layers enclosing an aqueous core. The hydrophobic sections (tails) of liposomes are repelled by water molecules, which results in liposome self-assembly. The general structure of liposomes is shown in Figure 11.13. Notably, the striking resemblance of liposomes to the eukaryotic cell membrane made them a prospective carrier for drug delivery applications. Liposome demonstrates the unique ability of an ideal drug carrier for both hydrophilic and lipophilic entities. Hydrophilic water-soluble drugs can be encapsulated in the aqueous core, while hydrophobic water-insoluble drugs can be solubilized in the lipid bilayer. This unique structure is exploited in several nanomedicine

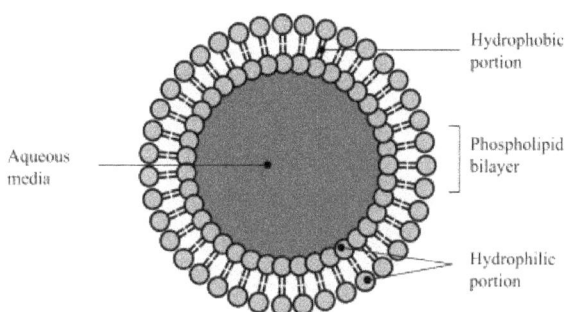

Figure 11.13: The general structure of liposomes (Deb *et al.*, 2019; Rooijen, 1998; Sercombe *et al.*, 2015).

formulations, mostly for encapsulation of chemotherapeutic drugs for anticancer activity.

However, the high phagocytic capacity (i.e., recognized by phagocytic cells) of tissues removes about 50–80% of the liposomes from the blood circulation by attaching them to opsonins, which prevents them from reaching their targets. To reduce the recognition and achieve long circulation, i.e., slow elimination from the blood, liposomes are surface-modified with inert, biocompatible polymer PEG (known commonly as PEGylation of liposomes) to form a protective steric barrier around the liposome.

11.4.5.3 *Dendrimers*

Dendrimers are a relatively new class of compounds that are distinguished by special molecular architecture and dimensions. These are globular three-dimensional, highly branched, well-organized synthetic polymeric structures characterized by high physical and chemical stability. Dendrimers have gained significant attention in biological applications because of their high water solubility, biocompatibility, flexibility, and specific molecular weight. The highly efficient water solubility and stability (more than micelles and liposomes) make dendrimers an excellent drug delivery agent. Dendrimers possess a unique molecular architecture that comprises three different topological parts:

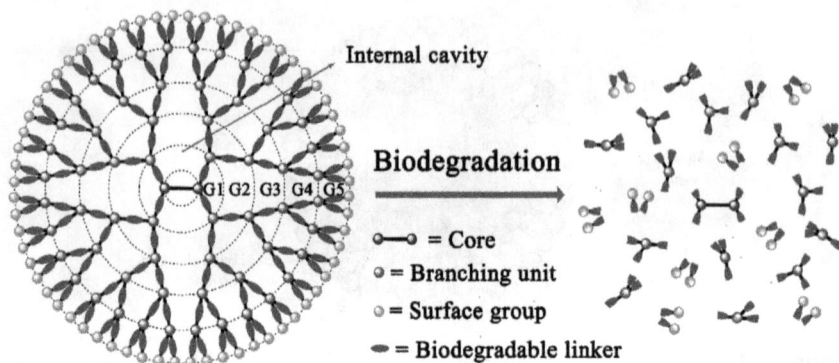

Figure 11.14:   Schematic illustration of biodegradation of dendrimers (Huang *et al.*, 2018; Kumar *et al.*, 2014).

- **A central core:** this contains two or more reactive groups.
- **Interior layers:** these are branching repetitive units that are covalently attached to the core. Each layer is called one "*generation*".
- **Outer surface functional groups:** these are located on the exterior of the macromolecule groups and play a key role in dendrimer properties. The terminal groups show higher chemical reactivity and are engineered to accommodate weak water-soluble drug molecules by interacting with the external environment.

With these unique structures, drugs are either non-covalently encapsulated in the dendrimer's internal core structure, covalently conjugated to the end functional groups, or physically adsorbed on the dendrimer surface. The option of the immobilization approach usually hinges on the drug properties. Non-biodegradable polymers such as polypropylene imine (PPI), poly(amido amine) (PAMAM), and poly(L-lysine) (PLL) are extensively used dendrimers for drug delivery applications. Biodegradable dendrimers such as polyester dendrimers and polyacetal dendrimers have also been found as interesting candidates for drug delivery (Figure 11.14). In addition, the ability to release the hydrophilic or hydrophobic drugs in a controlled manner is independent of the drug holding capacity of dendrimers, whether physically or chemically bonded.

11.4.6 *Other classification of nanomaterials which are used in drug delivery*

Carbon nanomaterials: Carbon nanocarriers that are employed in drug delivery systems are divided into carbon nanotubes (CNTs) and carbon nanohorns (CNHs). CNTs are cylindrical-shaped low-dimensional sp^2 hybridized carbon nanomaterials formed from single or multiple layers of graphene sheets. For various therapeutical agents, such as anti-cancer and anti-inflammatory drugs, CNTs are used as drug carriers as they are able to impede cell membranes and display blood circulation half-lives in the order of hours. CNHs with a diameter of 80–100 nm have also been exploited as a drug carrier to treat tumor tissues. The drugs can be immobilized onto nanohorns by adsorption or nanoprecipitation. Drug release from CNTs and CNHs can be controlled externally by electricity and internally by the chain of chemical reactions. However, much work is still underway on using carbon nanomaterials for drug delivery as it has been shown that these materials induce necrosis (cell death) or apoptosis (programmed cell death) of macrophage cell lines.

Silica materials: Silica materials are employed in controlled drug delivery systems because of their large surface area, biocompatibility, and ease of synthesis. Based on their chemical and physical stability, silica materials are classified as fumed nanoparticles, mesostructured spheres, and xerogels. Importantly, silica xerogels have an amorphous arrangement with high porosity and large surface area. Drugs are loaded onto silica materials by chemical and physical adsorption.

Quantum dots: Quantum dots are fluorescent semiconductor nanoparticles (2–10 nm in core size diameter) with unique optical and electronic properties, and they represent a versatile platform for design and engineering of drug delivery. Drugs can be loaded into quantum dots by means of dissolving, dispersing, adsorption, and coupling.

Gold nanoparticles: Colloidal gold nanoparticles are commonly utilized in controlled drug release, particularly in anti-cancer therapy. The release of drug molecules from gold nanoparticles is usually performed by external stimuli, i.e., by absorbing heat and raising kinetic energy to release drug molecules.

11.5 Multiple choice questions

1. Drug delivery is significant as conventional methods result in
   (a) low bioavailability
   (b) no side effects
   (c) high efficacy
   (d) all of the above

2. Typical properties of carrier-mediated drug transport include
   I. non-saturability
   II. active transport
   III. chemical specificity
   (a) only I
   (b) only I and II
   (c) only II and III
   (d) all of the above

3. Which of the following is/are TRUE for using nanocarriers in drug delivery?
   I. have improved solubilization and can be delivered non-invasively
   II. deliver to site-specific targets
   III. induce damage to the surrounding tissue considerably
   (a) only I
   (b) only I and III
   (c) only I and II
   (d) only III

4. Which of the following is/are NOT true about drugs?
   I. drugs can only be hydrophobic but not hydrophilic
   II. hydrophobic drugs are easily wetted
   III. hydrophobic drugs have low solubility in water
   IV. hydrophilic drugs can easily pass through membrane bilayers

(a) only I, II and III

(b) only I and II

(c) only II, III and IV

(d) only III

5. Which of the following is NOT true about drug release?

(a) drug release pattern can be altered by changing geometry and the device

(b) sustained drug release is possible in monolithic matrix systems

(c) drug release from reservoir systems normally follows zero-order kinetics

(d) in membrane-controlled reservoir systems drug is either in liquid or powdered form

6. Which of the following about burst release of drug is/are TRUE?

I. has short half-life *in vivo*

II. patient does not require frequent dosing

III. unpredictable and difficult to control

IV. high release rates can be reached in the initial stages after activation

(a) only I

(b) only I, III and IV

(c) only I, II and IV

(d) only I, II and III

7. Which of the following is not a route of drug administration?

(a) intravenous

(b) subcutaneous

(c) intramuscular

(d) dissolution

8. Which of the following is TRUE for implantable drug delivery devices?

I. requires invasive surgery

II. possibility of dose dumping

III. low bioavailability

IV. high concentration of drug is delivered at the implantation site

(a) only I, II and IV
(b) all of the above
(c) only III and IV
(d) only II and IV

9. From which type of diffusion-controlled device will release rate decrease with time?
(a) monolithic diffusion device
(b) membrane-controlled reservoir systems
(c) all of the above
(d) none of the above

10. Which of the following is most extensively utilized by the drug industry in forming drug salts for water solubilization?
(a) sodium
(b) magnesium
(c) calcium
(d) phosphorus

11. Encapsulation of a drug usually involves
(a) suspensions
(b) association colloids and emulsions
(c) micelles
(d) liposomes

12. Polymeric micelles are extensively used for
(a) delivery of poorly water-soluble drugs
(b) delivery of highly water-soluble drugs
(c) any kind of drug, irrespective of solubility
(d) all of the above

13. In polymeric micelles, drugs are loaded
(a) on the external surface
(b) into the hydrophilic cores
(c) into the hydrophobic cores
(d) into the hydrophilic tails

References & Further Reading

Deb, P. K., Al-Attraqchi, O., Chandrasekaran, B., Paradkar, A., *et al.* (2019). Chapter 16 — Protein/Peptide Drug Delivery Systems: Practical Considerations in Pharmaceutical Product Development. In R. K. Tekade (Ed.), *Basic Fundamentals of Drug Delivery* (pp. 651–684): Academic Press.

Faheem, A. M., & Abdelkader, D. H. (2020). Chapter 1 — Novel drug delivery systems. In A. Seyfoddin, S. M. Dezfooli, & C. A. Greene (Eds.), *Engineering Drug Delivery Systems* (pp. 1–16): Woodhead Publishing.

Goonoo, N., Bhaw-Luximon, A., Ujoodha, R., Jhugroo, A., *et al.* (2014). Naltrexone: A review of existing sustained drug delivery systems and emerging nano-based systems. *Journal of Controlled Release, 183*, 154–166. doi:10.1016/j.jconrel.2014.03.046.

Huang, D., & Wu, D. (2018). Biodegradable dendrimers for drug delivery. *Materials Science and Engineering: C, 90*, 713–727. doi:10.1016/j.msec.2018.03.002.

Janssen, M., Mihov, G., Welting, T., Thies, J., *et al.* (2014). Drugs and polymers for delivery systems in OA joints: Clinical needs and opportunities. *Polymers, 6*(3), 799–819. doi:10.3390/polym6030799.

Kumar, N., & Kumar, R. (2014). Chapter 2 — Nano-based drug delivery and diagnostic systems. In N. Kumar & R. Kumar (Eds.), *Nanotechnology and Nanomaterials in the Treatment of Life-threatening Diseases* (pp. 53–107): William Andrew Publishing.

Larson, N., & Ghandehari, H. (2012). Polymeric conjugates for drug delivery. *Chemistry of Materials: A Publication of the American Chemical Society, 24*(5), 840–853. doi:10.1021/cm2031569.

Li, C., Wang, J., Wang, Y., Gao, H., *et al.* (2019). Recent progress in drug delivery. *Acta Pharmaceutica Sinica B, 9*(6), 1145–1162. doi:10.1016/j.apsb.2019.08.003.

Noh, G., Keum, T., Seo, J.-E., Choi, J., *et al.* (2018). Development and evaluation of a water soluble fluorometholone eye drop formulation employing polymeric micelle. *Pharmaceutics, 10*(4), 208. doi:10.3390/pharmaceutics10040208.

Ratemi, E. (2018). Chapter 5 — pH-responsive polymers for drug delivery applications. In A. S. H. Makhlouf & N. Y. Abu-Thabit (Eds.), *Stimuli Responsive Polymeric Nanocarriers for Drug Delivery Applications, Volume 1* (pp. 121–141): Woodhead Publishing.

Rooijen, N. V. (1998). Liposomes. In P. J. Delves (Ed.), *Encyclopedia of Immunology (Second Edition)* (pp. 1588–1592): Elsevier.

Sercombe, L., Veerati, T., Moheimani, F., Wu, S. Y., *et al.* (2015). Advances and challenges of liposome assisted drug delivery. *Frontiers in Pharmacology, 6*(286). doi:10.3389/fphar.2015.00286.

Chapter 12
Biosensors

12.1 Introduction

Have you ever wondered how does the glucometer that detects our body glucose levels work? How do diagnostic centres accurately quantify or detect the exact number or amount of ions present in our body? How are electronics and biology related to medicine?

Clinical diagnosis is a crucial component in the modern healthcare system, allowing (early) rapid disease identification, timely initiation of appropriate treatment, and monitoring of therapeutic progression. Since a disease state is often synonymous with the abnormality or deviation of certain molecular assemblies from normal conditions, precise and systematic evaluation of these abnormal chemical changes can provide a timely diagnosis. Quantification or calculation of redox reactions and biochemical processes is of utmost value in medical and biological procedures. However, due to the complexity involved, converting biological reactions into readable data is very challenging. Nevertheless, in recent decades, such highly responsive, accurate, and economic instruments that can contribute to medical diagnosis, remote sensing, and personalized medicine has witnessed tremendous demand.

The term "biosensor" was coined by Karl Cammann, and its definition was instituted by the International Union of Pure and Applied Chemistry. In simple terms, a biosensor is a portable high technology biological sensor device that is used in connection with a biological/ biochemical detection system. This monitoring and analytical device combines a biological component with a physicochemical component to detect a specific analyte. Such instruments benefit from the high

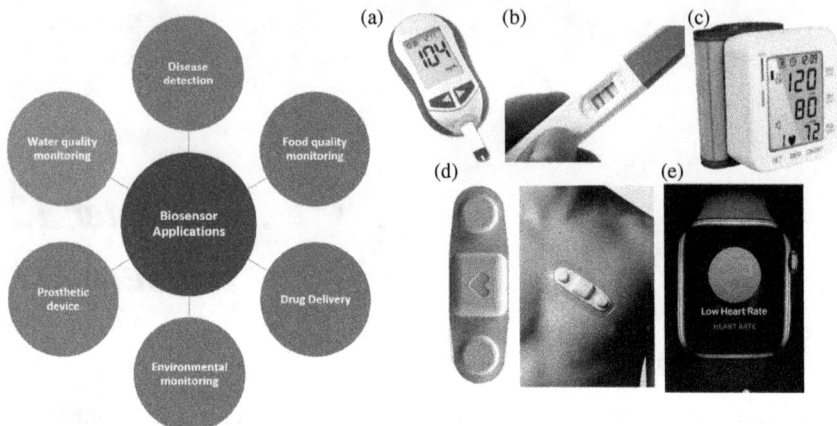

Figure 12.1: Different applications of biosensors and some examples: (a) blood glucose monitor (detects insulin levels); (b) pregnancy test (detects human chorionic gonadotropin hormone in urine or blood); (c) blood pressure measuring device; (d) cardiac sensor patch (generates a continuous stream of ECG rhythm); (e) watch (detects irregular heartbeats and records ECG) (Ensafi, 2019; Metkar *et al.*, 2019).

degree of selectivity and sensitivity of a biologically active material and provide highly accurate quantitative or semi-quantitative analytical information in the form of signals. Different applications of biosensors and some examples are shown in Figure 12.1. These devices are independent of physical parameters, including pH and temperature, and are reusable. Biosensors are now being employed for rapid diagnostics because of their *point-of-care* use capability with minimal operator input requirements.

Typically, a biosensor is composed of a biologically sensitive/recognition material immobilized in close contact with a transducer device that converts the biochemical signal into measurable or processable electrical or optical signals. Visual description of the various steps involved in the signal processing of any biosensor is shown in Figure 12.2. In the biological sensing device, a specific biological molecule is detected by a reaction, adsorption, or other physical/chemical mechanisms. The transducer translates this information into functional signals that can be further measured and analyzed. The biologically sensitive material can be enzymes,

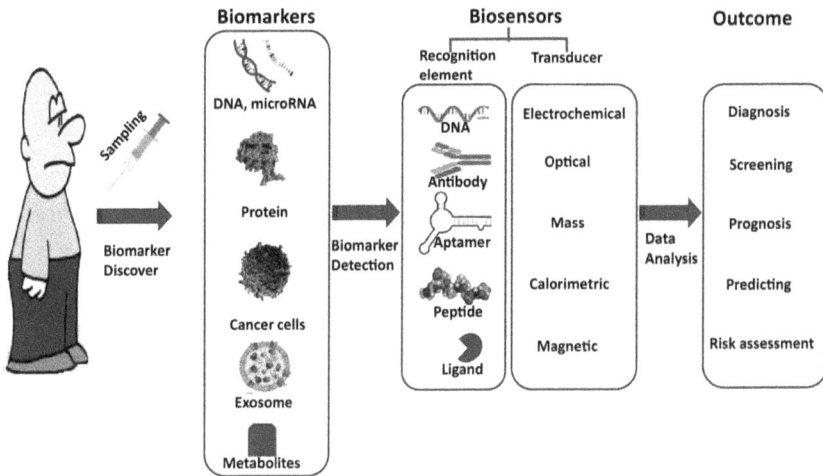

Figure 12.2: Graphic narrative of the various steps involved in the signal processing of any biosensor (Qian *et al.*, 2019; Parkhey *et al.*, 2019).

antibodies, lipid layers, DNA probes, RNA probes, tissues, cell receptors, and aptamers. The transducer device can be a piezoelectric, optical, or physicochemical material. Hence, designing a smart sensing material to enhance biorecognition and transduction functions is crucial in the construction of biosensors.

Biosensor-associated work is therefore comprehensive and includes different scientific and technical expertise involving electrochemistry, surface chemistry, biochemistry, solid-state physics, etc. Based on the sensitive material and transducer used, biosensors can have applications in various fields like diagnostics, disease monitoring, food industry, and environmental monitoring, etc. (Figure 12.1).

- **Analyte:** It is an element, chemical species, chemical constituent, or a substance of interest that needs to be detected. For example, glucose is an '*analyte*' in a biosensor designed to detect glucose. A list of common analytes targeted by biosensors is tabulated in Table 12.1.
- **Bioreceptor:** Without the influence of external factors, a molecule that explicitly recognizes the analyte is known as a bioreceptor.

Table 12.1:   List of common analytes targeted by biosensors.

Type	Specific analytes
Ions	H^+, Li^+, K^+, Na^+, Ca^+, phosphates, heavy metal ions
Respiratory gases	O_2, CO_2
Metabolites	Glucose, urea
Microorganisms	Viruses, bacteria, parasites
Antigens and antibodies	Human Ig, anti-human Ig
Proteins and nucleic acids	DNA, RNA
Toxic gases	H_2S, Cl_2, CO, NH_3

A bioreceptor is integrated into a biosensor to specifically recognize and bind the desired analyte. Bioreceptors can be enzymes, antibodies, lipid layers, DNA probes, RNA probes, tissues, cell receptors, aptamers, etc. When bioreceptors interact with the analyte, a signal will be generated based on the change in heat, potential, current, mass, pH, etc. Depending on the reaction between analyte and bioreceptor, they can be classified as:

→ *Affinity sensor*: In these kinds of sensors, the bioreceptor binds to the analyte.
→ *Metabolic sensor*: The bioreceptor and analyte produce chemical changes in these metabolic sensors, which may measure the concentration of a substrate affected by those chemical changes.
→ *Catalytic sensor*: The bioreceptor interacts with the analyte in these sensors and transforms it into an auxiliary substrate.

• **Transducer:** A transducer is a device that uses the information generated between the bioreceptor and the analyte and converts it into a quantifiable signal that is presented in terms of user-comprehensible graphs, numbers, or images. Most transducers generate either optical or electrical signals, which are typically proportional to the amount of interactions between analyte and bioreceptor. Various kinds of transducers used in biosensor devices are tabulated in Table 12.2.

Table 12.2: Various kinds of transducers used in biosensor devices.

Transducer	Measurement mode		Typical applications
Electrochemical	Amperometric	Enzyme electrodes	Immunological systems
		Conductometric	
	Potentiometric	Ion-selective electrodes	Ions in biological media, chemical vapors
		Gas-sensing electrodes	Gases, enzymes, organelles, cells, tissues
		Ion sensitive field-effect transistors	Ion concentrations in solution, cellular imaging, DNA detection
Electrical		Conductivity	Detecting movement of muscles
Optical		Luminescence	Antibodies
		Fluorescence	
		Resonance to surface plasmons	
Piezoelectric	Mass detection	Quartz crystal microbalance (QCM)	Antibodies
		Surface acoustic waves (SAW)	

12.2 Biosensor classifications based on transducer

12.2.1 *Electrochemical biosensors*

Electrochemical biosensors were studied extensively since the early 1960s when the first biosensor of glucose oxidase was established. These biosensors are involved with the dynamics of electrical parameters in relation to a specific chemical, physical or biological reaction. Even though biosensing devices use a wide range of recognition components such as antibodies, DNA/RNA, cells, and microorganisms, electrochemical detection techniques mainly use enzymes owing to their unique binding capacities and biocatalytic action. They employ complex redox reactions to quantify the amount of an analyte present and translate this biological signal into an electrical signal. This approach currently dominates the biosensing field as it offers several advantages such as stable output, low fabrication costs, low

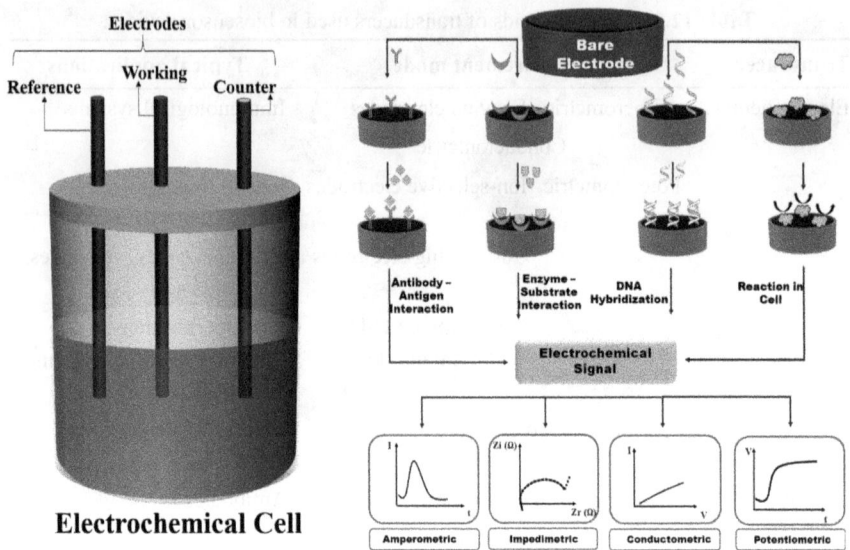

Figure 12.3: (Left) Graphic representation of the typical electrochemical biosensor cell; (Right) analyte detection using four types of transducer: amperometric, potentiometric, conductometric, and impedimetric (Bahadır *et al.*, 2015; Veloso *et al.*, 2012).

detection limit, specificity, simple design, ease of miniaturization, less external interferences, and ease of operation.

Electrochemical sensing involves three electrodes, and a schematic is shown in Figure 12.3. Since reactions are usually only found close to an electrode surface, electrodes themselves play an important role in the performance of electrochemical biosensors. Depending on the selected electrode, its detection ability may be greatly affected by the electrode content, its surface characteristics, and its proportions.

- **Reference electrode:** it is an electrode with a stable and established electrode potential. It is usually made up of Ag/AgCl, Hg/HgO, Ag/Ag$_2$SO$_4$, etc.
- **Working electrode:** recognized as *"indicator electrode"* where the electrochemical reactions of interest occur. In biosensors, it is the integration of a biomolecular recognition module and the physio-chemical transducer.
- **Counter electrode:** recognized as *"auxiliary electrode"* as it provides a means of applying input potential to the working electrode.

The working principle of electrical biosensors is based on the chemical reaction between immobilized biomolecules and target analyte. The reactions generate or ingest ions or electrons, which influence the solution's measurable electrical properties such as electric current or potential. Specifically, the electrochemical reaction would produce a quantifiable current (amperometric), an assessable potential difference (potentiometric), or a measurable change in the conductive properties (conductometric). A schematic of various kinds of biosensors is shown in Figure 12.3.

12.2.1.1 *Amperometric biosensors*

Amperometric (current at a fixed voltage) biosensors operate by applying a constant potential between the working electrode and reference electrode, and measuring the current induced by redox reactions. Specifically, measurement of current results from the analyte losing an electron (oxidation) or gaining an electron (reduction) while undergoing an electrochemical reaction. Amperometric biosensors can be used to identify electroactive solutes that are quickly reduced or oxidized. They have been used in glucose biosensing for over 35 years.

12.2.1.2 *Potentiometric biosensors*

Potentiometric (voltage at near-zero current) biosensors work under conditions of near-zero current flow. It detects the variation in potential difference between two electrodes, i.e., a the working electrode and reference electrode. The measured potential may then be used to ascertain the analytical quantity of interest, usually the concentration of any solution component. In other words, potentiometry provides elucidation about the ion movement (Ca^{2+}, Cl^-, K^+, and NH^{4+} ion-selective electrodes) in an electrochemical reaction.

12.2.1.3 *Conductometric biosensors*

Almost all electro-analytical systems are based on electrochemical reactions at the electrodes. However, conductometry is a process in which the electrodes have either no electrochemical reactions at all or minor secondary reactions that may be ignored. Most importantly, conductometric biosensors do not require the use of a reference electrode. These systems measure changes in the conductance of the medium due to the presence of the analyte. Conductometric biosensors cannot discriminate between different ions and have very limited use in biosensors.

12.2.2 *Optical biosensors*

Optical biosensors are effective analytical tools that provide major benefits over traditional analytical techniques. They allow many biological and chemical substances to be detected directly, in real-time, and label-free. These biosensors offer a wide range of advantages such as high specification, high sensitivity, ultra-small size, and cost-effectiveness.

Optical biosensors are primarily based on detection of the optical signals produced by biocatalytic or bio-affinitive reactions with the analyte. They measure the amount of light (ultraviolet, visible, and infrared) that has been transmitted, reflected, or emitted as a result of a biochemical reaction. Various optical phenomena such as absorption, refraction, fluorescence, luminescence, resonance to surface plasmons, etc., are utilized. A graphical representation of an optical biosensor is shown in Figure 12.4.

Optical biosensors are generally categorized as *label-free* and *label-based* modes. Through interaction of the analyte with the corresponding transducer, a *label-free* detection system emits the detected signal directly. On the other hand, a *label-based* system requires the use of a label that

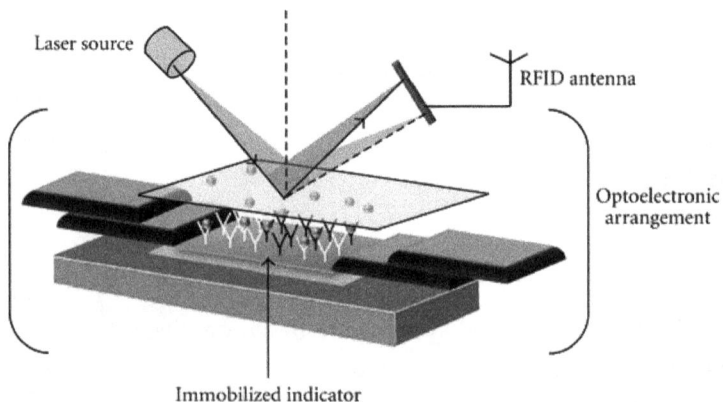

Figure 12.4:   Architecture of an optical biosensor (Dey *et al.*, 2011).

generates the optical signal via colorimetric, fluorescent, or luminescent means. Among these, colorimetric and surface plasmon-based biosensors are broadly investigated due to simplicity in detection of the visible color change and in exploitation of the evanescent field respectively.

12.2.2.1 *Surface plasmon resonance (SPR) biosensors*

Surface plasmon resonance (SPR) biosensors are developed to utilize the evanescent wave phenomena to determine binding quantities of biological macromolecules, including antibodies, proteins, DNAs, RNAs, and polysaccharides. In general, the SPR effect happens on a metal or any other conductive material at the interface of two media (typically dielectric constants of opposite signs) when polarized light strikes the surface under total internal reflection. The reflected photons generate an electrical field on the opposite side of the prism-metal interface (only when the prism is covered with a metal film). This field is called the evanescent field. Based on this phenomenon, SPR-based plasmonic tools have emerged as an effective and accurate clinical detection platform to detect the permittivity changes in biomolecular interactions, chemical detection, and immunoassays. The exciting ability of SPR sensing devices lies in the surface plasmons excited at a metal-dielectric interface with exceptionally high sensitivity to a minor variation in the refractive index of the dielectric. When a biomolecular interaction (e.g., specific binding of analytes) occurs, the refractive index is changed near the surface. The SPR sensor will then detect this change to the refractive index. A graphic representation showing analyses using antibodies as the biorecognition surface on the SPR platform is shown in Figure 12.5.

This label-free analyte system can be employed in real-time to learn the binding relationship between immobilized receptors and analytes by overseeing the fluctuations in surface optical properties, i.e., a shift in resonance angle because of variation in the interfacial refractive index. SPR in the visible and near-infrared wavelength range is of particular interest because optical containment at these wavelengths is effective. One of the most exciting applications of optical-based biosensors is fiber optics, which transform the emission signal to a measurable fluorescent signal to detect DNA.

Even though SPR-based biosensors are considered label-free, labeling is sometimes used as binding of analytes with a molecular weight

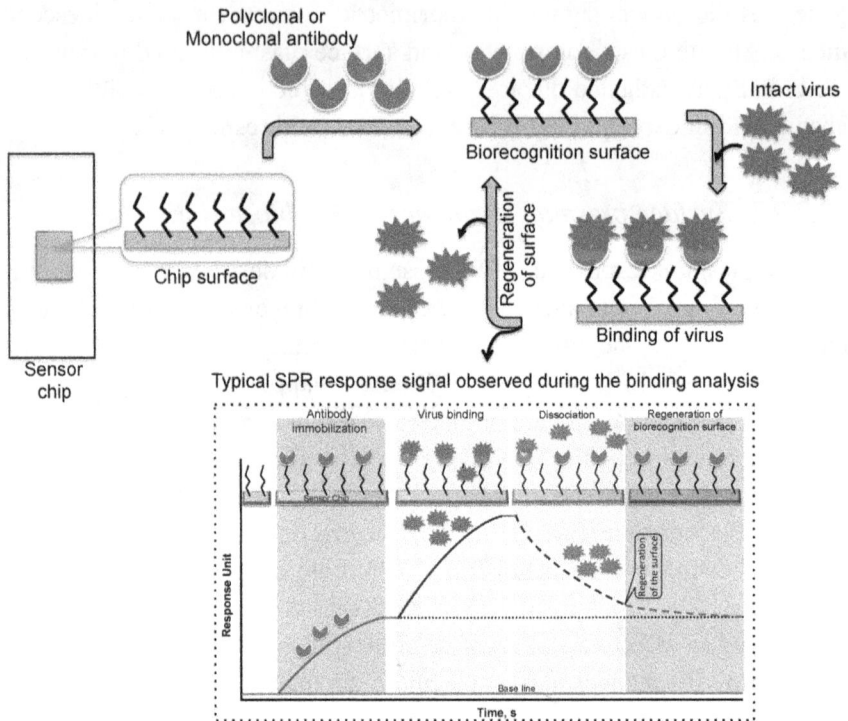

Figure 12.5: A graphic description showing analyses using antibodies as the biorecognition surface on the SPR platform (Homola *et al.*, 2002; Kumar, 2016).

(M_w) of less than 5000 Da on the SPR sensor chip sometimes produces no adequate change in the refractive index. This is because the change in resonance angle is proportionate to the analyte weight that attaches to the surface. It has been proved that the "*labeling*" of the analytes using secondary substitutes with high M_w achieved an improvement in sensor sensitivity for analytes with low M_w. For example, amplification of resonance angle shift was achieved by employing gold nanoparticles as a secondary labeling agent for antihuman immunoglobulin (anti-hIgG).

12.2.3 *Piezoelectric biosensors*

Piezoelectric sensors are mass-sensitive sensors that use piezoelectric crystals (Figure 12.6) for the detection of any change in mass arising because of biomolecular interactions. It is a well-understood fact that a

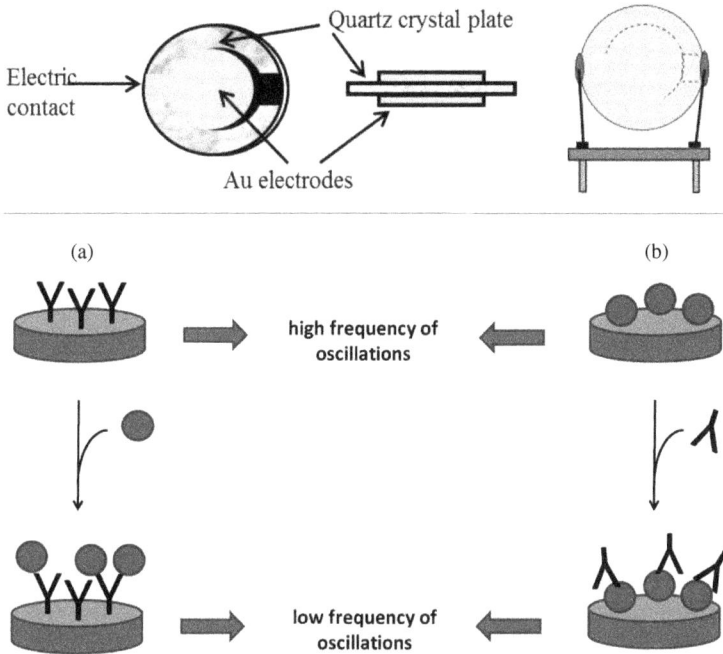

Figure 12.6: (Top) Schematic of a piezoelectric quartz crystal; (Bottom) piezoelectric immunosensors for the determination of (a) an antigen or (b) an antibody (Marrazza, 2014; Pohanka, 2018; Tombelli, 2012).

slight change of mass at the crystal surface will influence an oscillating piezoelectric crystal's resonant frequency. Piezoelectricity or piezoelectric effect is the physical phenomenon of a material's capacity to generate voltage or electrical signal in response to mechanical forces. The effect often operates in the opposite direction, meaning when voltage is provided to a piezoelectric material's surface, it induces mechanical stress or oscillation as the voltage alternates.

The quartz crystal microbalance (QCM) and the surface acoustic wave (SAW) designs are the most employed systems in piezoelectric biosensor devices and are classified as label-free technology biosensors. These are based on calculating changes in a piezoelectric crystal's resonance frequency due to the mass changes in the crystal structure. Piezoelectric devices produce vibrational waves, which are categorized as acoustic waves (vibration, sound, ultrasound, and infrasound waves). Depending on the depth propagation of these waves, they are further characterized as bulk acoustic waves, which are normally observed in QCM-based devices, and surface acoustic waves, which are just propagating on the substrate surface and are observed in SAW-based devices. Many commercial piezoelectric devices rely on the QCM phenomenon because of the drawbacks accompanied by SAW-based sensors. In SAW-based sensors, it is challenging to create a robust system because the frequency shift is influenced by many factors, such as the adsorbent's dielectric, conductive and elastic constants, and liquid conductivity.

12.2.3.1 *Quartz crystal microbalance*

A piezoelectric transducer makes use of QCM to detect the nanogram changes in mass in biologically sensitive materials. QCM examines variations in the vibration frequency triggered by a change in mass due to the target binding on the surface. A schematic of an electrochemical QCM apparatus is shown in Figure 12.7. The sensitive material is anchored onto the quartz crystal surface. When interaction between the substrate and the material occurs, this induces a change in the crystal's resonant frequency;

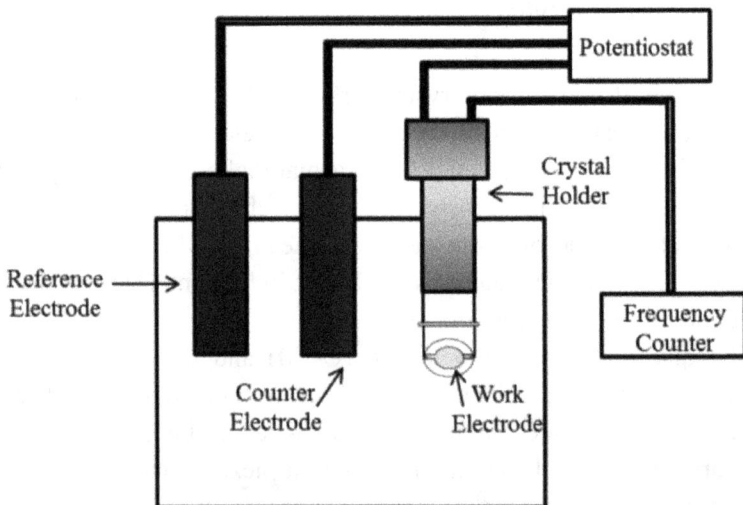

Figure 12.7:   Schematic of an electrochemical QCM apparatus (Marrazza, 2014; Zhang *et al.*, 2009).

thus, the changed crystal's mass or surface property is recorded in real-time. The detection principle is based on the relationship between an increase in mass and the change in frequency as expressed by the Sauerbrey equation:

$$\Delta f = \frac{2 f o 2}{A\sqrt{\rho\mu}} \Delta m$$

where Δf is frequency change in Hz; Δm is mass change; f_o is fundamental resonant frequency of the quartz in Hz; A is active crystal area of the QCM electrodes; ρ is mass density of the quartz; and μ is shear modulus of the quartz.

In practice, "*AT-cut quartz*" is predominantly used to prevent acoustic radiation losses due to the desirable low-temperature dependency of the resonant frequency. The equation shows that the variations in crystal oscillation frequency are not directly proportional to the fluctuations in mass. It implies that the analyte's introduction at the surface of the crystal altered by biologically active material results in the growth of its mass that affects the reduction in resonant frequency. This methodology has been applied to identify antibodies, large molecular weight proteins, small molecules to cells, and DNA. For DNA, a long string of nucleotides has a quantifiable amount of molecular mass, with some 100 basis pairs. The change in weight due to the hybridization of the nucleic acid probe with its complementary counterpart immobilized on the surface of a piezoelectric quartz crystal will result in an escalation in the crystal's resonance frequency.

12.2.3.2 *Surface Acoustic Wave*

In the case of SAW-based sensors, a surface acoustic wave is employed rather than a bulk acoustic wave. SAW devices use interdigitated transducers to produce acoustic waves on the surface of a piezoelectric crystal. Such systems allow the identification of biorelevant molecules in water or aqueous buffer solutions, which are extremely sensitive. However, the deployment of devices based on this understanding in biosensing applications has been limited.

12.3 Biosensor classifications based on bioreceptors

Bioreceptors are the most important tools for biosensor technology; they are the biological species designed to interact with the specific analyte of interest. The recognition of molecules is central to biosensing. Bioreceptors work on affinity and specificity. They enable binding affinity-based sensors to generate a measurable signal through the transducer, or produce/consume a component that the transducer of biocatalysis-based sensors can recognize. There are two classes of biosensors according to recognizable components: molecular and cellular biosensors.

12.3.1 *Molecule-based biosensors*

Molecule-based biosensors may use various kinds of antibodies, nucleic acids, enzymes, or ion channels. Because of immobilization of biological components, these are largely developed to react only to certain target molecules and thus possess very high sensitivity.

12.3.1.1 *Nucleic acid-based biosensors*

A biosensor based on nucleic acids incorporates nucleic acids as the bioreceptor and an electrode as the physicochemical transducer. Nucleic acids are known as natural biopolymers which encode hereditary material. Thesy include DNA, RNA, artificially synthesized peptide nucleic acid polymer, and aptamers (short DNA or RNA molecules). The nucleic acid-based biosensors were especially developed on a key fact that a single-stranded nucleic acid molecule can identify its corresponding strand in a sample and attach to it. The interaction comes from the formation of strong hydrogen bonds between the two strands. The immobilization and hybridization procedures are illustrated in Figure 12.8. Designing such nucleic acid detection is significant because of its employment in gene identification, molecular diagnosis, drug screening, and environmental defence. Almost all nucleic acid-based biosensors are developed by immobilizing nucleic acids to a solid support via various techniques such as adsorption, covalent bonding, ionic bonding, physicochemical method, and direct coupling to a transducer.

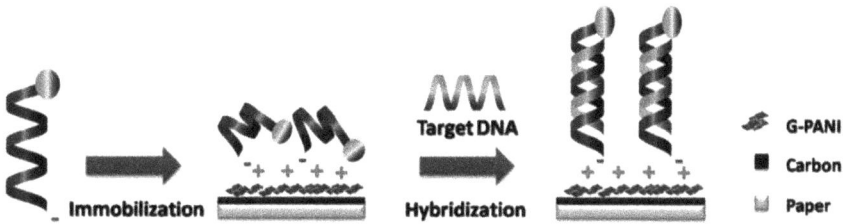

Figure 12.8: Immobilization and hybridization steps of paper-based electrochemical DNA biosensors (Teengam *et al.*, 2017).

DNA is probably the most significant of all biomolecules as it holds all genetic instructions in all living things. For the past couple of decades, genetic research has focused on the unique complementary structure of DNA between the adenine/thymine and cytosine/guanine nitrogenous base pairs. One of the crucial steps in DNA biosensor manufacturing is to use a distinct functional matrix to immobilize the single-stranded DNA probe effectively. For this reason, biopolymer-nanomaterial composites are used significantly. DNA-based SPR biosensors are used in monitoring the binding of low molecular weight ligands to DNA in real-time.

12.3.1.2 *Enzyme-based biosensors*

Enzymes are globular proteins that can catalyze biochemical reactions. In Table 12.3, some specific enzymes with their functions are summarized. The mode of action of enzyme-based biosensors involves oxidation or reduction which can be detected electrochemically, and is dependent on biological recognition of target substrate. This category of biosensors relies on inhibitor quantification, measuring the enzymatic activity in absence and presence of the inhibitor. As enzymes are not consumed in a reaction, these biosensors can be used for an extended period. The enzyme's catalytic activity does not restrict identification of the analyte, whereas the stability of the enzyme ultimately determines a sensor's lifetime.

Electrochemical biosensors based on enzymes are developed by the integration of an immobilized enzyme and a transducer. Most standard electrochemical enzyme biosensors are based on oxidoreductase enzymes

Table 12.3: Common enzymes with specific catalytic mechanisms (Zhao *et al.*, 2017).

Enzyme	Mechanism/Function
Oxidases (e.g., glucose oxidase)	Catalyze an oxidation-reduction reaction, usually O_2 is reduced to H_2O or H_2O_2
Peroxidases (e.g., horseradish peroxidase)	Catalyze the oxidization of substrate generally using H_2O_2 as the oxidizing agent
Phosphatases (e.g., alkaline phosphatase)	Eliminate phosphate groups from the substrate
Dehydrogenases (e.g., glucose dehydrogenase)	Oxidize a substrate by transferring H_2 to an electron acceptor
Acetylcholinesterase	Catalyzes the hydrolysis of acetylcholine and some other choline esters
β-galactosidase	Catalyzes the hydrolysis of β-galactosides into monosaccharides by breaking the glycosidic bond
Proteases/peptidases	Catalyze the hydrolysis of the peptide bonds that link amino acids together in a polypeptide chain
DNA ligases	Join DNA strands together by catalyzing the formation of a phosphodiester bond
DNA polymerases	Synthesize DNA molecules from nucleotides
Ribozymes (RNAzymes)	Catalyze specific biochemical reactions
Deoxyribozymes (DNAzymes)	Catalyze specific biochemical reactions

linked with amperometric detection. The immobilized enzyme recognizes a target molecule and catalyzes the reaction. Numerous electrochemical biosensors were introduced and used in the medical fields by integrating enzymatic reactions with electrochemical transducers. The most widely studied and commercialized enzyme-based electrochemical biosensor is the glucose self-monitoring system (measurement of glucose concentration in the blood) aimed at patients with metabolic disorders (e.g., diabetes). Apart from glucose, lactate and glutamate are two other important brain analytes that attracted considerable attention in enzyme-based biosensors. Voltammetric enzyme-based biosensors, especially cyclic voltammetry, are extensively applied to measure electrochemical responses of heme proteins (hemoglobin and myoglobin). Enzyme-based biosensors are more specific than cell-based biosensors (section 12.3.2). However, even after tremendous success, they still have many challenges. For example, it is hard and expensive to look for a new, highly effective, and active enzyme. Furthermore, sensitivity, reliability, and adaptability to various applications are often difficult.

12.3.1.3 *Antibody-based biosensors*

In response to the presence of foreign molecules (antigens), including pathogens, toxic agents, and others, antibodies are defensible immune proteins produced by the immune system. Antibody-based biosensors take advantage of the extraordinary affinity of antibodies to form a stable complex with their corresponding antigens, i.e., the antibodies directly attach to pathogens or toxins, or associate with immune system components of the host. Graphical representation of antibody-based biosensors using antibodies as bioreceptors is shown in Figure 12.9. These are also described as immunosensors. Immunosensors are affinity-based analytical devices that have an immense capacity to become a next-generation bio-analytical system. For immunosensing, various modified transducers are employed, including electrochemical, optical, and piezoelectric.

Immunosensing based on electrochemical transducers, especially amperometric transducers, provides an excellent biosensing tool for accurate biomarker assessment that incorporates the unique benefits of electro-analytical approaches such as quick and cost-effective determination of pathogens, cancerous molecules, bacteria, and viruses. The fundamental concept of the electrochemical immunosensor is to identify variations in the surface potential and oxidation state of an electroactive species. The signals are produced due to a shift in resistance, current, capacitance, etc.,

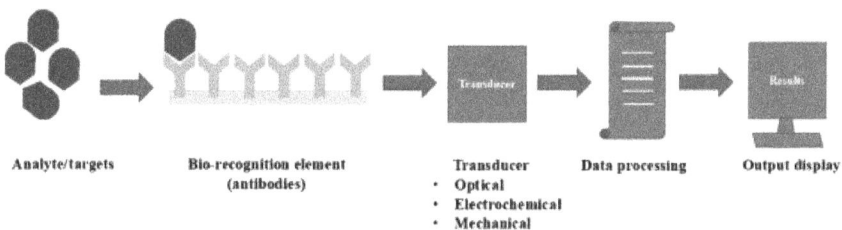

| Analyte/targets | Bio-recognition element (antibodies) | Transducer
• Optical
• Electrochemical
• Mechanical | Data processing | Output display |

Figure 12.9: Graphical representation of antibody-based biosensors using antibodies as bioreceptors (Jain *et al.*, 2019).

due to the production of an immunocomplex through antibody and antigen interaction.

12.3.1.4 *Aptamer-based biosensors*

Aptamers are short, chemically synthesized single-stranded DNA or RNA molecules that are created from the randomized nucleic acid store by three simple steps: binding, separation, and amplification. Aptamers can be used as biosensors because of key features such as small size, high specificity and sensitivity, strong affinity, and effective immobilization. The advantages of aptamers over antibodies in biosensor applications is shown in Table 12.4. Most aptamers are acquired through a combinatorial biology technique known as SELEX (systematic evolution of ligands by exponential enrichment). Aptamers can be considered as chemical

Table 12.4: Advantages of aptamers over antibodies in biosensor applications.

Property	Aptamers	Antibodies
Stability	Highly stable at high temperatures	Sensitive to temperature and quickly denatured for protein-based antibodies
	Can quickly recover and attach to targets after re-annealing	Experience irreversible denaturation
	Even under a wide range of buffer conditions, chemical stability is achieved	Require the use of stringent physiological conditions only
Target	Fast affinity to specific targets, for example enzymes and several protein classes	In some cases, labelling can lead to a loss in affinity
	Efficient immobilization	Difficult
Production	Can be synthesized *in vitro* in large quantities via chemical reactions cost-effectively	Very expensive and requires large-scale mammalian cell growth facility
Reactions	Low-immunogenic and low-toxic molecules	Considerably immunogenic but varies
	Kinetic parameters can be modified accordingly	Difficult to modify kinetic parameters

antibodies that connect tightly to a precise molecular target such as anti-gens. However, they have a much lower molecular weight than that of actual antibodies. Furthermore, they can bind to a broad variety of molec-ular targets such as proteins, viruses, bacteria, whole cells, and small molecules such as metal ions, organic dyes, drugs, amino acids, etc. Aptamer-based biosensors, therefore, depend mostly on the unique recog-nition mode of each aptamer-target pair. The bulk of these designs, how-ever, comes under two groups, namely single-site binding and dual-site binding (Figure 12.10).

Apart from being highly stable, aptamers can undergo a number of modifications on their molecular surfaces such as circularizing, linking, or clustering to customize their properties for different applications. The small molecular targets often gets hidden within the binding pockets of aptamer structures (Figure 12.10A), which leaves little or no space for interface with a secondary molecule. In contrast, larger molecules such as proteins can be structurally linked to aptamers via electrostatic interac-tions or hydrogen bonding. As a result, protein targets can be analyzed by both single-site (one aptamer) binding (Figure 12.10B) and dual-site (two aptamers) binding (Figure 12.10C). In some cases, a specific antibody can also be utilized as a second "aptamer" (Figure 12.10D). Aptamers may be labelled on both sides in aptamer-based biosensors (aptasensor) using an

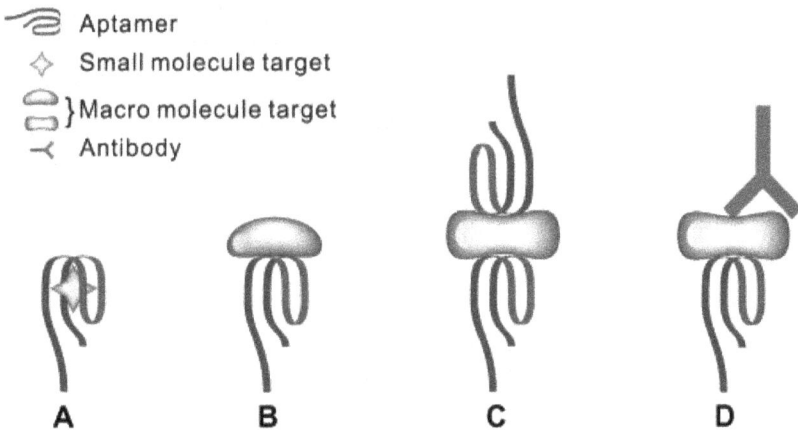

Figure 12.10: Aptamer-based assay formats (Song *et al.*, 2008).

electrochemical transducer. Due to protein binding, conformational changes in shape happen, leading to either a reduced or increased distance of the reporter agent (for example, methylene blue) from the electrode, thus resulting in an increase or decline in electron transfer. In optical-based aptasensors, SPR biosensor detection method is majorly used because of low sensitivity detection issues in colorimetric methods.

12.3.2 *Cell-based biosensors*

A cell-based biosensor uses cells as identification elements with an effective physicochemical transducer to identify cell physiological changes. Cellular biosensors provide alternatives to many challenges posed by molecular biosensors, such as molecular biosensors that do not detect molecules with identical functions. More specifically, when compared to molecular biosensors, cellular biosensors provide improved stability and biocatalytic activity.

Cells instinctively sense external stimuli as a way to adapt and thrive in their environment. By linking natural transcriptional responses to colorimetry or fluorescence, cellular biosensors can constantly sense and monitor analytes. Living cells express a broad range of molecules (receptors) in various amounts, which means that cells not only can provide a statistical response to specific stimuli in a given environment but can also help to empirically evaluate more than one analyte with reduced effort and cost. Cell-based biosensors employ microbial cells such as bacteria, yeast, fungi, algae, and living human cells as biospecific sensors to assess cellular physiological parameters, pharmaceutical effect, toxicity, etc. (Figure 12.11). Then they deliver a response through the association between stimuli and cell. In addition, living cells in a biosensor are often combined with external transducers to produce a quantified, readable signal. Choosing these transduction pathways depends on the functional approach and the type of cells used for biosensing (Figure 12.11).

Electrochemical and optical transducers are the most commonly employed for cell-based biosensors. Among these, impedance measurements of cells using miniature electrodes may provide valuable details in real-time about cell adhesion, proliferation and morphology, barrier

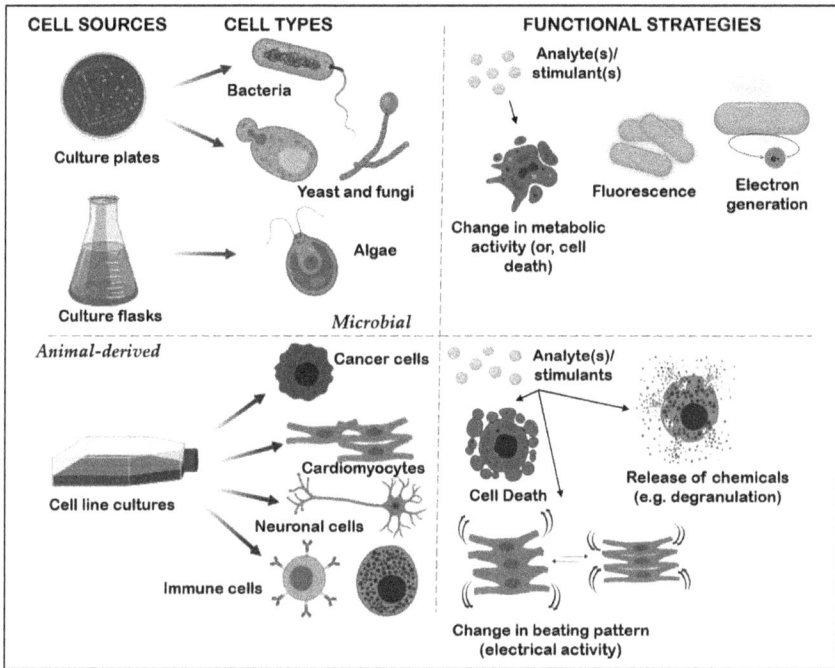

Figure 12.11: Graphical representation of different cell types (left) and functional strategies (right) utilized in cell-based biosensors (Gupta *et al.*, 2019).

function, and other activities addressed by the cytoskeleton. The electrical cell-substrate impedance sensor (ECIS) is a label-free, *in vitro* impedance-measuring system to examine the behavior of cells in tissue culture in real-time. As with all electrochemical sensors, an ECIS sensor is also composed of a working electrode, a counter electrode, and sometimes a reference electrode. The operating principle of the ECIS technique is relatively straightforward. In a typical setup, desired cells are full-grown in special culture spaces on top of opposing, circular gold electrodes. Then a slight alternating current (I) is applied across the electrodes. As cells grow over the electrodes, they act as insulators and block the flow of electricity, thereby resulting in a change of potential (V) across the electrodes. Based on Ohm's law ($Z = V/I$), the increase in electrical impedance (Z) in the circuit can be measured around the electrodes. This growing impedance can be used to understand the behavior of cells in the culture medium.

12.4 Multiple choice questions

1. Select the TRUE statement(s) regarding biosensor components.
   I. bioreceptor: material which analyses
   II. transducer: conversion of signal
   III. detector: reproducible response
      (a) only I
      (b) only II and III
      (c) only I and II
      (d) all of the above

2. Which of the following is NOT true about biosensors?
   (a) detects the analytes
   (b) provides output in the form of image
   (c) provides output in the form of signal
   (d) transducer converts the reaction into a readable output

3. A piezo-electrical crystal generates voltage when subjected to this force.
   (a) pressure
   (b) magnetic
   (c) electrical
   (d) mechanical

4. Which of the following about optical biosensors is/are TRUE?
   I. provide results in real-time
   II. have an option of label-free detection
   III. expensive
   IV. low specificity
      (a) only I
      (b) only II and IV
      (c) only I and II
      (d) only I, II and IV

5. Which of the following biosensors explore the "*evanescent wave phenomenon*"?
   (a) electrochemical biosensors
   (b) optical biosensors
   (c) piezoelectric biosensors
   (d) all of the above

6. In electrochemical biosensors, amperomertic biosensors measure
   (a) change in voltage
   (b) change in conductivity or resistance
   (c) change in current
   (d) all of the above

7. This acts as detector in optical sensors.
   (a) light emitting diode
   (b) photo diode
   (c) transistor
   (d) all of the above

8. The minimum detectable amount in biosensors is ascertained by
   (a) affinity of the biocomponent for the analyte
   (b) sensitivity of the transducer
   (c) sample volume
   (d) all of the above

References & Further Reading

Bahadır, E. B., & Sezgintürk, M. K. (2015). Electrochemical biosensors for hormone analyses. *Biosensors and Bioelectronics, 68*, 62–71. doi:10.1016/j.bios.2014.12.054.

Dey, D., & Goswami, T. (2011). Optical Biosensors: A Revolution Towards Quantum Nanoscale Electronics Device Fabrication. *Journal of Biomedicine and Biotechnology, 2011*, 348218. doi:10.1155/2011/348218.

Ensafi, A. A. (2019). Chapter 1 — An introduction to sensors and biosensors. In A. A. Ensafi (Ed.), *Electrochemical Biosensors* (pp. 1–10): Elsevier.

Gupta, N., Renugopalakrishnan, V., Liepmann, D., Paulmurugan, R., *et al.* (2019). Cell-based biosensors: Recent trends, challenges and future perspectives. *Biosensors and Bioelectronics, 141*, 111435. doi:10.1016/j.bios.2019.111435.

Homola, J., Yee, S. S., & Myszka, D. (2002). Chapter 7 — Surface Plasmon Resonance Biosensors. In F. S. Ligler & C. A. Rowe Taitt (Eds.), *Optical Biosensors* (pp. 207–251): Elsevier.

Jain, R., Miri, S., Pachapur, V. L., & Brar, S. K. (2019). Chapter 14 — Advances in antibody-based biosensors in environmental monitoring. In S. Kaur Brar, K. Hegde, & V. L. Pachapur (Eds.), *Tools, Techniques and Protocols for Monitoring Environmental Contaminants* (pp. 285–305): Elsevier.

Kumar, P. K. R. (2016). Monitoring Intact Viruses Using Aptamers. *Biosensors,* *6*(3), 40. doi:10.3390/bios6030040.

Marrazza, G. (2014). Piezoelectric Biosensors for Organophosphate and Carbamate Pesticides: A Review. *Biosensors, 4*(3), 301–317. doi:10.3390/ bios4030301.

Metkar, S. K., & Girigoswami, K. (2019). Diagnostic biosensors in medicine — A review. *Biocatalysis and Agricultural Biotechnology, 17*, 271–283. doi:10.1016/j.bcab.2018.11.029.

Parkhey, P., & Mohan, S. V. (2019). Chapter 6.1 — Biosensing Applications of Microbial Fuel Cell: Approach Toward Miniaturization. In S. V. Mohan, S. Varjani, & A. Pandey (Eds.), *Microbial Electrochemical Technology* (pp. 977–997): Elsevier.

Pohanka, M. (2018). Overview of Piezoelectric Biosensors, Immunosensors and DNA Sensors and Their Applications. *Materials, 11*(3), 448. doi:10.3390/ ma11030448.

Qian, L., Li, Q., Baryeh, K., Qiu, W., Li, K., Zhang, J., Yu, Q., Xu, D., Liu, W., Brand, R.E., Zhang, X., Chen, W., & Liu, G. (2019). Biosensors for early diagnosis of pancreatic cancer: a review. *Translational Research, 213*, 67–89. doi: 10.1016/j.trsl.2019.08.002.

Song, S., Wang, L., Li, J., Fan, C., *et al.* (2008). Aptamer-based biosensors. *TrAC Trends in Analytical Chemistry, 27*(2), 108–117. doi:10.1016/j. trac.2007.12.004.

Teengam, P., Siangproh, W., Tuantranont, A., Henry, C. S., *et al.* (2017). Electrochemical paper-based peptide nucleic acid biosensor for detecting human papillomavirus. *Analytica Chimica Acta, 952*, 32–40. doi:10.1016/j. aca.2016.11.071.

Tombelli, S. (2012). Chapter 2 — Piezoelectric biosensors for medical applications. In S. Higson (Ed.), *Biosensors for Medical Applications* (pp. 41–64): Woodhead Publishing.

Veloso, A. J., Cheng, X. R., & Kerman, K. (2012). Chapter 1 — Electrochemical biosensors for medical applications. In S. Higson (Ed.), *Biosensors for Medical Applications* (pp. 3–40): Woodhead Publishing.

Zhang, G., & Wu, C. (2009). Quartz Crystal Microbalance Studies on Conformational Change of Polymer Chains at Interface. *Macromolecular Rapid Communications, 30*(4–5), 328–335. doi:10.1002/marc.200800611.

Zhao, W.-W., Xu, J.-J., & Chen, H.-Y. (2017). Photoelectrochemical enzymatic biosensors. *Biosensors and Bioelectronics, 92*, 294–304. doi:10.1016/j. bios.2016.11.009.

Chapter 13
Additive manufacturing and bioprinting

13.1 Introduction

Additive manufacturing (AM), also known as "*3D printing*", "*rapid prototyping*", or "*solid free-form technology*", is receiving considerable attention in recent years. Although the phrases 3D printing and AM are frequently applied synonymously, 3D printing is primarily a subset of AM that uses the layer-by-layer approach to build up parts from scratch. Over the last two decades, 3D printing has contributed to progress in diverse sectors, including aerospace, biomedical, consumer goods, arts, and food. It is a family of processes that allows the fabrication of physical 3D devices by adding material layer-by-layer without using special tooling, molds, or fixtures. This technology is exemplified by the capability to construct single parts and complicated structures effectively and accurately with just a computer-aided design (CAD) file. Examples of dense and intricate designs generated by 3D printing techniques are shown in Figure 13.1. Even though the term "*3D Printing*" is commonly applied as an alternative word for the whole AM procedures, in reality the processes differ in their approach of layer deposition.

The 3D printing process is exactly in contrast to the well-known subtractive/traditional manufacturing techniques, where the process begins with more material than is needed, and the component is built by selectively eliminating any unnecessary material (either by hand carving or machining) until the final shape develops. AM technology thus offers considerable advantages such as shorter manufacturing times, less material wastage, and the potential to create complex parts. The important

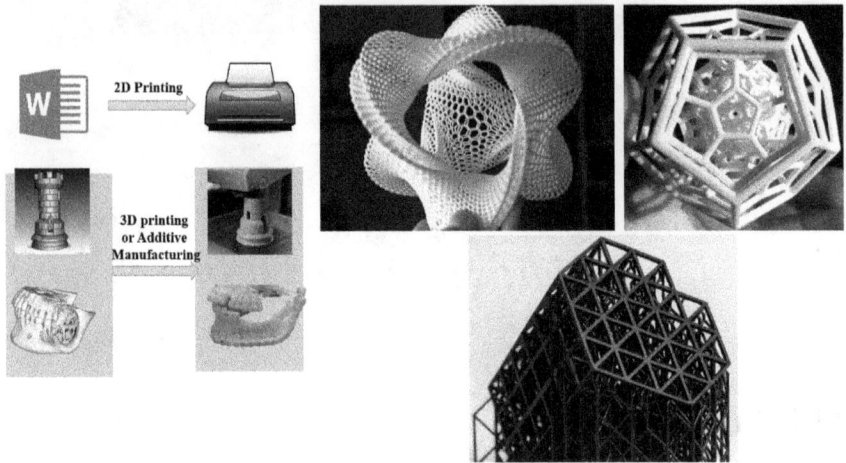

Figure 13.1: (Left) Typical differences between the common 2D printing and AM; (Right) examples of dense and intricate designs generated by 3D printing techniques (Image courtesy 3dhubs, Unimelb and Brewbooks (Flickr)). 3D printing is usually associated with printing by individuals at home or in the community and on a smaller scale. In contrast, AM usually refers to manufacturing technologies with large supply chains.

differences between traditional and additive manufacturing are presented in Table 13.1.

On the whole, the term "*additive manufacturing*" refers to technologies in which customized 3D complex systems are built one thin high-quality layer at a time. Each sequential layer of melted or incompletely melted material binds to the preceding layer. The digital sequence of the AM process chain is presented in Figure 13.2. The typical AM process chain consists of:

- **Step 1:** The first phase of the AM chain is the CAD model. It provides geometric data for the expected or desired component.
- **Step 2:** Next is CAD model translation into a standard .STL format. The data needed for the geometry of the components will be included in the file now. A simple surface geometry containing triangular elements known as *facets* characterizes the .STL file of the solid model. Each *facet* has three vertices, each of which is indicated by the x, y, z, and normal vector coordinates.

Table 13.1: Differences between traditional and additive manufacturing.

	Traditional manufacturing	**Additive manufacturing**
Typical process	Machining, casting, forging, extrusion, etc.	Layer-by-layer
Freedom of design	Less innovation of designs due to pre-established tooling; very difficult to create complex shapes	Allows innovation of design; creation of complex shapes is made easy
Material waste	More wastage of material due to tooling or machining	Incredibly resource-efficient; almost no wastage of the material
Material selection	Limited choice of materials	Offers wide material selection
Speed	Requires molds to be manufactured first; takes days and months to have the first part in hand	Desired part can be printed on-demand without any rampup or tooling; lead time as short as 2 or 3 days
Reproducibility	Highly reproducible	Relatively repeatable as long as the cycle is optimized
Secondary processing	Compulsory to attain the required surface finish	Not always required as some AM processes can fabricate models with exceptional surface finish

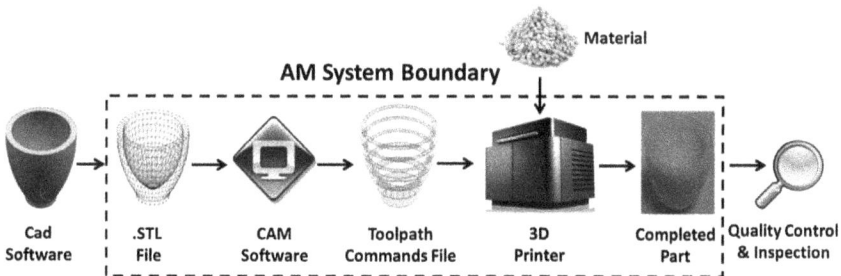

Figure 13.2: Additive manufacturing process chain (Sturm *et al.*, 2017).

- **Step 3:** The .STL file transforms the pre-designed framework into a number of layers and produces a toolpath. The toolpath file includes the controls that shift the axes and the deposition functions of the AM systems. It is theoretically similar to a computer programming language.

- **Step 4:** The final module in the AM part development sequence is the machine itself.

This technology allows the design and manufacture of 3D objects based on images acquired from medical imaging systems, such as computed tomography (CT) and magnetic resonance imaging (MRI). Various substances may be used for layering material such as metallic powder, polymers, ceramics, polymer-ceramic composites, bioinks, glass, and even chocolate-like edibles. The most significant advantage of industrial 3D printing is the freedom to design components, which do not rely on any tool or mold. AM technology provides significant strategic advantages for industries such as on-demand spare parts manufacturing, customized products, lightweight prototypes, practical integration, and formulation of entirely new ideas.

13.2 Overview of 3D printing technologies

The American Society for Testing and Materials (ISO/ASTM 52900:2015) has classified AM methods into seven core groups (Table 13.2). Even

Table 13.2:   Different AM technologies.

Method	Feedstock	Binding mechanism	Activation source
Vat photopolymerisation	Photosensitive resin (filler)	Photopolymerization	UV light
Powder bed fusion	Powders with spherical morphology with optimum size being 15–45 μm	Selectively melting or sintering particles together at specific points	High-energy thermal sources such as laser, electron beam, or infrared light
Material jetting	Liquid photoreactive material and casting wax	Photopolymerization	Radiation, thermal, or piezoelectric method; similar to stereolithography method
Material extrusion	Continuous filament of a thermoplastic material	Thermal bonding	Inbuilt heat

Table 13.2:   (*Continued*)

Method	Feedstock	Binding mechanism	Activation source
Binder jetting	Powder in granular form and binder	Binder acts as an adhesive between powder layers	Liquid binder
Directed energy deposition	Powder particles or wire	Metallurgical bond	Laser, electron beam, or plasma beam
Sheet lamination	Thin sheets of material	Adhesive bonding, thermal bonding, chemical reaction bonding, or ultrasonic connection	Ultrasonic welding (metals) or adhesives (paper)

though it is not specified, the classification is loosely based on the type of heat source used (laser, UV, electron beam, electric arc, etc.) or feedstock material (polymers, ceramics, metal powder, wire, thin metal sheet, etc.). The seven categories are (i) material extrusion, (ii) vat photopolymerization, (iii) material jetting, (iv) binder jetting, (v) sheet lamination, (vi) directed energy deposition (DED), and (vii) powder bed fusion (PBF). The first three techniques are commonly utilized for non-metallic materials. In contrast, binder jetting, DED, and PBF are used extensively for processing metallic parts.

13.2.1 *Vat photopolymerization*

Vat photopolymerization is a 3D printing technology used to fabricate solid parts from a liquid raw material via ultraviolet (UV) light. This technology is based upon photopolymerization or photoinitiated polymerization, which primarily uses radiation-curable resins or photopolymers as main components to initiate the chemical reaction. Upon irradiation, the uncured photopolymers are cross-linked together through a chain reaction, which is primarily instigated by free radicals or ions produced using a suitable light source. The ISO/ASTM definition states that "*vat photopolymerization is an AM process in which liquid photopolymer in a vat is selectively cured by light-activated polymerization*". Over the past few years, vat photopolymerization has evolved to include various techniques

Table 13.3:   Advantages and disadvantages of the vat photopolymerization process.

Advantages	Disadvantages
Very high resolution and accuracy	Only photopolymers can be used
High-speed fabrication and good surface finish	Poor mechanical strength
Unlike other techniques, no nozzle is required	For biomedical applications, sometimes UV light can induce toxicity to the cells; this process has issues in printing multicellular objects; damage to biological cells during photocuring is also reported
Intricate internal structures can be fabricated easily	

like stereolithography, digital light processing, continuous liquid interface production, and solid ground curing. The common element in all types of vat photopolymerization is that all procedures use special resins called photopolymers as the core printing material. Many photocurable resins have been studied and developed in vat photopolymerization processes, including epoxy, polyurethane, polyester, and acrylic resins. The advantages and disadvantages of the vat photopolymerization process are tabulated in Table 13.3.

- **Stereolithography (SLA):** It is one of the most common and extensively used techniques in the world of AM. 3D Systems Inc. built SLA equipment in 1988 based on the work of originator Charles Hull. The technique's fundamental concept is to solidify photocurable resin using a UV laser source and to use a layer-by-layer deposition technique to create the entire item. A schematic illustration of a photopolymerization-based SLA is presented in Figure 13.3a.
- **Digital Light Processing (DLP):** DLP was first introduced in 1993 by Texas Instruments. It is a technique that employs digital micromirror devices, a component made up of several micromirrors for masking the light that passes through and creating the desired pattern of a layer onto the bottom of the resin tank. DLP utilizes a more traditional light source, such as an arc lamp, together with a liquid crystal display panel.
- **Continuous Liquid Interface Production (CLIP):** In 2015, CLIP technology (Figure 13.3b) was developed as a novel alternative to the

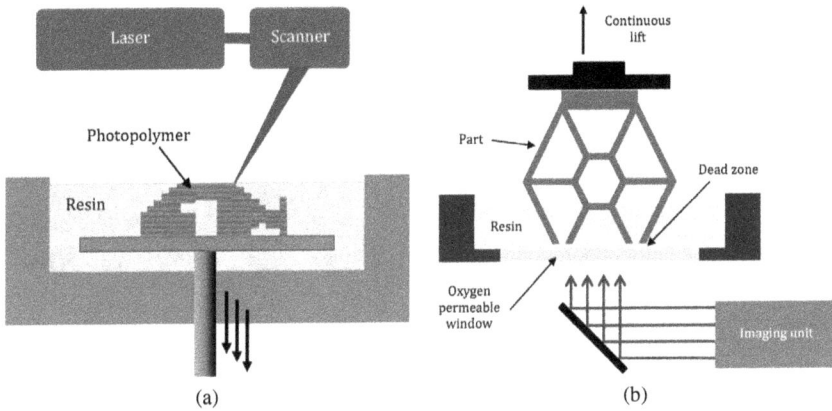

(a)   (b)

Figure 13.3: (a) Graphic illustration of a photopolymerization-based SLA process (top-down approach); (b) representation of a CLIP 'bottom-up' DLP device that uses a constant instead of stepwise manufacturing procedure to increase part production speed considerably (Stansbury *et al.*, 2016).

traditional layer-by-layer SLA process. It has been developed to overcome certain shortcomings in traditional 3D printing by achieving build speeds higher than normal layer-by-stage SLA processes. In CLIP technology, an oxygen-permeable projection window is used to create a slim polymerization-free zone (dead zone) in the resin at the bottom of the vat.

13.2.2 *Powder bed fusion*

Powder bed fusion (PBF) (Figure 13.4) is a subgroup of AM whereby a heat source (e.g., laser or electron beam) is employed to fuse or melt a bed of powder particles layer-by-layer to create a solid object. According to ISO/ASTM classification, PBF is termed *"an additive manufacturing process in which thermal energy selectively fuses regions of a powder bed"*. Based on the heat source applied, type of bonding between powder particles (sintering or melting), and vacuum environment or not, PBF technology is classified into selective laser melting, selective laser sintering, direct metal laser sintering, selective heat sintering, electron beam melting and direct metal laser melting. The advantages and disadvantages of powder bed fusion are presented in Table 13.4.

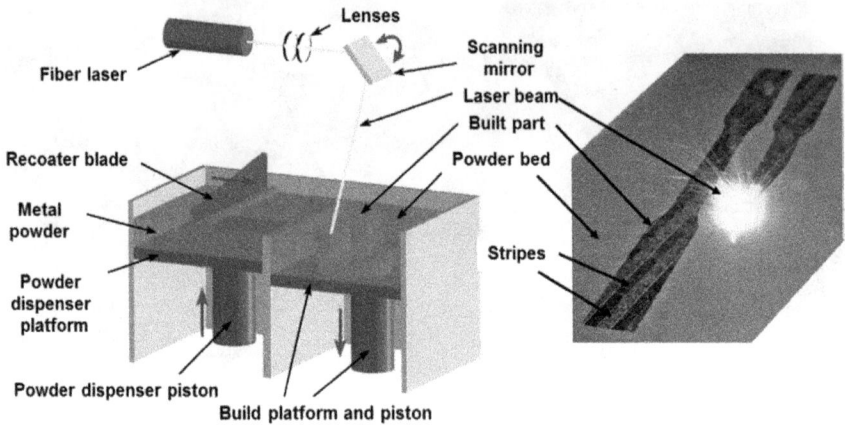

Figure 13.4:   Graphical illustration of laser PBF system (Direct Metal Laser Sintering by EOS GmbH) (Criales *et al.*, 2017).

Table 13.4:   Advantages and disadvantages of powder bed fusion.

Advantages	Disadvantages
No external support is required: powder itself acts as an integrated internal support structure	Relatively slow and long print time because of prerequisites for the process
More wastage of material due to tooling or machining	Multiple fusion steps can generate cracks into the material
Wide choice of materials: ceramics, glass, plastics, metals, and alloys	Voids arise from powder microstructure
Powder recycling	
Excellent mechanical properties	

- **Selective Laser Sintering (SLS):** In the SLS process, high power laser is employed as a heat source to selectively fuse or sinter powdered polymer, ceramic, or glass together to form a solid structure in a layer-wise deposition manner. The printed structures are usually of high quality and complex geometries.

- **Selective Laser Melting (SLM):** SLM is almost like SLS but goes a step further by utilizing the laser to achieve a full melt of the powder particles. Depending on the powder characteristics and desired structure, SLM laser power can be manipulated in the range of 100 W to 1 kW. At these high energies, the powder particles not only fuse together but are melted to form a homogeneous component. In a broader sense, when compared to SLS technology, parts fabricated by the SLM process have improved mechanical properties because of fewer or no voids. However, as melting of particles is involved, this technology is only practical when using single metal powder.

- **Electron Beam Melting (EBM):** EBM is comparable to SLM, substituting the laser with an electron gun. It uses an electron beam to fuse the metal powder together to build parts on a layer-by-layer basis. Due to the utilization of an electron beam, the building chamber uses a vacuum as an alternative to an inert environment.

13.2.3 *Material jetting*

In material jetting, droplets of the building material are preferentially discharged, which are then UV-curated. According to ISO/ASTM standards, material jetting is characterized as "*an additive manufacturing process in which droplets of build material are selectively dispensed*". Graphic illustration of the material jetting procedure is shown in Figure 13.5. Material

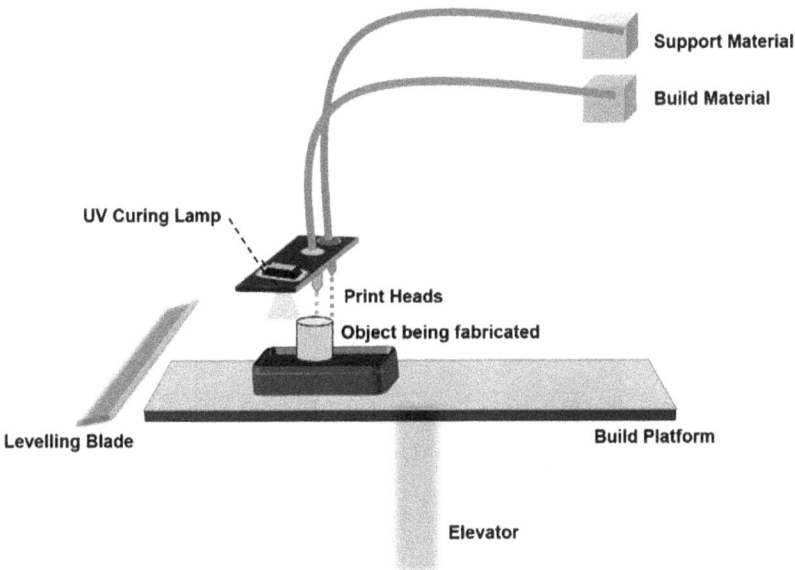

Figure 13.5: Graphic representation of the material jetting process (Sireesha *et al.*, 2018).

jetting is one of the few AM technologies that is capable of creating 3D structures with highest dimensional precision and great surface character-istics. In this procedure of layer-by-layer printing, wax-like melted mate-rials are jetted into the inkjet heads, and then cured and solidified to form 3D objects. The supporting material, which is typically made from differ-ent materials, may be removed during post-processing. Material jetting is unique in permitting various materials to be printed on the same product and in full color. Technologies such as photopolymer jetting or polyjet-ting, drop on demand, thermojet printing, inkjet printing, and multijet modeling/printing fall under the group of material jetting.

13.2.4 *Binder jetting*

Binder jetting (Figure 13.6a) was invented in 1993 at the Massachusetts Institute of Technology, and Z Corporation acquired permission for

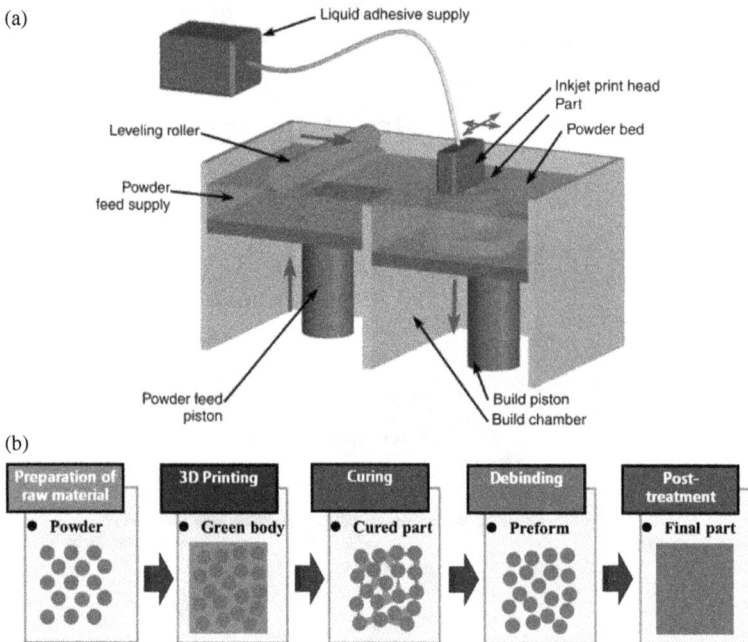

Figure 13.6: (a) Graphic representation of ink/binder jet 3D printing process and (b) steps of binder jet printing (Lv *et al.*, 2019; Moritz *et al.*, 2018).

commercialization. It works accordingly by discharging liquid binding agent / binding adhesive onto powder and then curing it to form the "*green*" part (Figure 13.6b). The final 3D object is accomplished by sintering the green part with an optional infiltration. According to ISO/ASTM standards, binder jetting is characterized as "*an additive manufacturing process in which a liquid bonding agent is selectively deposited to join powder materials*". Binder jetting works virtually with any powdered feedstock and can accommodate any functionally graded material. Since the binder jetting method only needs to print the binder material, the construction of the 3D object is relatively fast compared with other systems, such as material jetting.

13.2.5 *Material extrusion*

Material extrusion (Figure 13.7), also described as fused deposition modelling or fused filament fabrication, is one of the most common

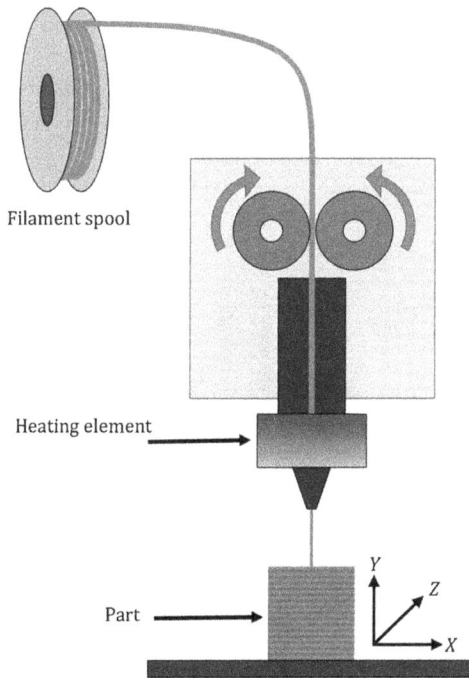

Figure 13.7:   Schematic of FDM (Stansbury *et al.*, 2016).

techniques in AM. In the process, pre-loaded material is extruded or drawn through a heated nozzle. As the bed moves vertically, the nozzle moves horizontally, permitting the molten raw material to be constructed layer-by-layer. Appropriate adhesion amongst layers is achieved by accurate control of temperature and, in some instances, using chemical bonding agents. According to ISO/ASTM standards, material extrusion is described as *"an additive manufacturing process in which material is selectively dispensed through a nozzle or orifice"*. This technique can be used to turn several types of materials such as thermoplastics and bioceramics into 3D objects.

13.2.6 *Direct energy deposition*

Direct energy deposition (DED) (Figure 13.8), also referred to as laser cladding, laser metal deposition, or laser-engineered net spacing (LENS), is a major AM technology employed to manufacture metal components. According to ISO/ASTM standards, DED is defined as *"an additive manufacturing process in which focused thermal energy is used to fuse materials by melting as they are deposited"*. During DED processing, a movable heat source with high intensity is employed to melt and fuse metal powders/wires together to print 3D objects.

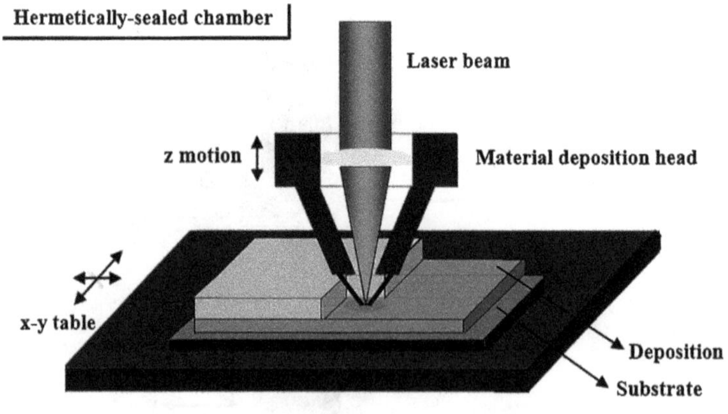

Figure 13.8: Schematic representation of LENS (Zhai *et al.*, 2016).

13.3 3D printing for biomedical applications

3D printing has become an extremely popular technique in the biomedical engineering field and has become a breakthrough technology for biomedical applications, particularly for tissue engineering and regenerative medicine. This is due to its ability to deliver patient-specific designs, freedom of materials (Table 13.5), ability to manufacture implants with high

Table 13.5: Typical materials for AM technologies.

Printing process	Method	Typical materials
Vat Photopolymerization	SLA	Acrylics and epoxies, PPF ceramics hydrogels, cells
	DLP	Polymers, composites, zirconia, elastomers
Powder Bed Fusion	SLS	Nylon, PEEK, PLGA, PCL, PLA, PVA, HA
	3D Printing (3DP)	Starch, cellulose, PLGA, PCL, PLA, Al_2O_3, shape-memory alloys
	SLM	Steel, cobalt-based alloys, Cp-Ti, Ti-6Al-4V, aluminum, ceramics
	EBM	Ti-6Al-4V, Co-Cr-Mo, Cp-Ti, β-Ti alloys, Inconel 718
	DMLS	Ti-6Al-4V, Co-Cr
Material Jetting	CIJ	PCL, ABS, polyamide, PLA and its composites
	DOD	
Binder Jetting	Binder Jetting	Steel, polymers, $BaTiO_3$, intermetallics, solid oxide fuel cells, magnetic materials, shape memory alloys, biodegradable alloys
Material Extrusion	DIW	PCL, HA, zirconia, aerogels, bioactive glasses
	FDM	ABS, polyamide, PLA and its composites
Sheet Lamination	LOM	Ceramics, aluminum, stainless steel, copper, titanium, plastics, fabrics, synthetic materials and composites
Directed Energy Deposition	LENS	Metals, permalloys, magnetic alloys, Ti-tungsten alloys
	EBAM	SS, cobalt alloys, nickel alloys, copper-nickel alloys, tantalum, titanium alloys

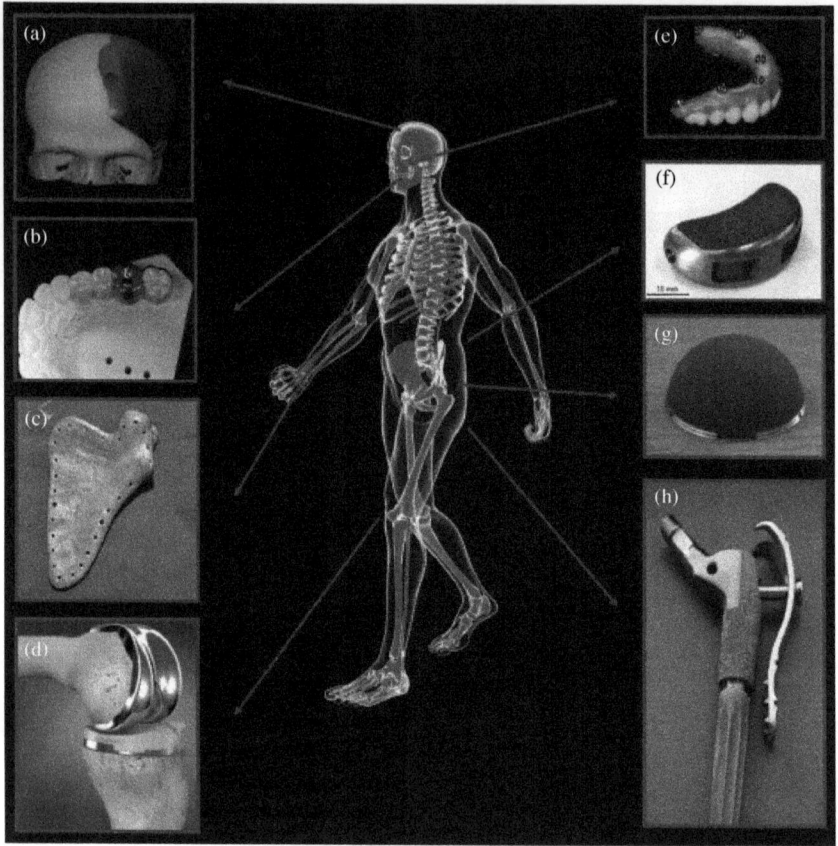

Figure 13.9:   Biomedical applications of 3D printing of biometals include (a) cranial prosthesis (Jardini *et al.*, 2016); (b) surgical guide (Almog *et al.*, 2001); (c) scapula prosthesis (Liu *et al.*, 2018); (d) knee prosthesis (Ibrahim *et al.*, 2017); (e) dental implants (Tischler *et al.*, 2018); (f) interbody fusion cage (Matsushita *et al.*, 2017); (g) acetabular cup (Saikko *et al.*, 2013); and (h) hip prosthesis (Hedlundh *et al.*, 2016). (Ni *et al.*, 2019).

structural complexity, design flexibility and quick customization, and personalization of medical products at a low cost. Based on these unique advantages, 3D printing has found applications in several biomedical categories (Figure 13.9) such as:

- restoration of anatomic defects (craniofacial implants) and designing of customized prosthetics
- dental implant design (molds, crowns, and caps)

- on-demand medical devices
- surgical models
- tissue regeneration scaffolds (skin and bone)
- organ printing (e.g., liver, lymphoid organs)
- drug discovery tissue models (pharmaceutical research)

The success of tissue engineering and regenerative medicine depends heavily on the design of the scaffold. The macro- and micro-architecture of the structures significantly influence the tissue regeneration process. Depending on whether cells are directly controlled before or during the construction process, two primary approaches are developed for producing scaffolds for tissue engineering: (i) chemically driven processes and (ii) computer-aided layered manufacturing-based processes. The details about chemically driven scaffold fabrication processes such as solvent casting, particulate leaching, solvent casting/particulate leaching, melt molding, gas foaming, freeze-drying, phase separation, self-assembly, and electrospinning were discussed in detail in Chapter 10. Scaffolds produced by these strategies produce distinct pore architecture with respect to shape, size, and orientation and serve as the most desired surfaces for cell adhesion, proliferation, and differentiation. It should be noted that in these methodologies scaffolds are first developed, while cells of interest are seeded in the next step. Some critical shortcomings are:

- absence of in-depth cellular infiltration
- low cell seeding efficiency at the initial stages
- huge inconsistent cellular proliferation within the scaffold matrix

Over the last decade, the scientific community has developed many methods to minimize these drawbacks. One such popular approach is to include cells directly within the design during the fabrication phase. This approach provides the benefit of integrating many synthesis procedures at one time, thereby assisting seeding capacity and uniform cell distribution issues. This method has taken off exponentially in recent times, with many manufacturing processes being built to create cellular constructions *in situ*.

13.4 3D bioprinting

3D bioprinting is one such exciting approach in AM technology that allows the user to fabricate cell patterns in a small confined space where the cell function and its viability are maintained in the printed scaffold. This approach has drawn considerable interest in tissue engineering, regenerative medicine, pharmacokinetics, and other biological fields by offering 3D designing or modelling of living cells, growth factors, and drugs. This contemporary deposition approach offers a highly efficient base for the manufacture of intricate bioengineered structures through a computer-aided layer-by-layer printing process using bioinks. A schematic of bioprinting and individual steps involved is shown in Figure 13.10.

Bioink is principally a printing biomaterial made up of specific biological products, i.e., cells, growth factors, or drugs that are embedded in a delivery medium such as cultures and hydrogels. It must be noted that bioink is not a rigid gel but is a viscous sol with flow properties. In general, the bioink or bioink mixture comprises three or four components depending on the application: an adequate condition with nutrients for the cells to survive and grow, a second element for improved viscosity, and stimuli such as growth factors or agents. Many bioinks are made

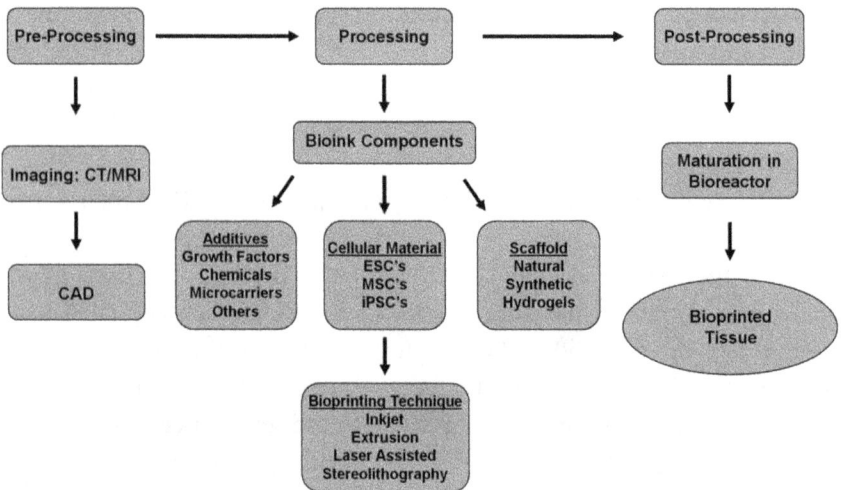

Figure 13.10:   Bioprinting overview schematic (Berry *et al.*, 2020; Bishop *et al.*, 2017).

from compatible materials such as polymers, ceramics, hydrogels, and composites. In particular, hydrogel inks have gained much more recognition compared with polymer and ceramic, and substantial progress has already been made in developing new formulations of inks.

Different AM techniques with bioprinting capabilities are developed to combine cells, growth factors, and biomaterials to construct complex tissue structures to mimic native tissues in a highly reproducible manner. Besides, 3D bioprinting technologies have surfaced as an innovative method for the manufacture of many tissues and organs, including skin, cardiac tissue, bone, liver, tubular tissue, and cartilage. CAD-based layered 3D bioprinting techniques (Figure 13.11) include (i) droplet-based bioprinting, (ii) extrusion-based bioprinting, and (iii) laser-based bioprinting (stereolithography and its modifications), which allow the fabrication of such complex tissues with unique spatial control over the deposition of cells and biomolecules. Inkjet and extrusion printing are nozzle-based procedures, while light-assisted bioprinting does not require any nozzle. The differences among the three bioprinting techniques are tabulated in Table 13.5.

13.4.1 *Droplet-based bioprinting*

Droplet-based bioprinting, a non-contact printing system, is a unique and most compelling method in all 3D-based bioprinting techniques. This method is known for its simplicity and agility that precisely deposits pico-liter to nanoliter droplets of bioink onto a substrate for the construction of operational tissues and organs. This technology is loosely built on the traditional inkjet process (home/office inkjet printers), where individual

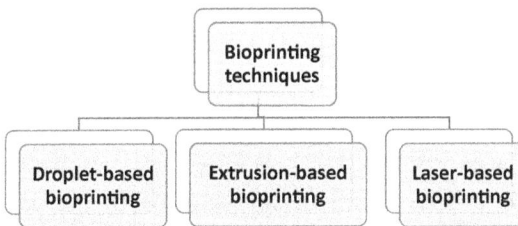

Figure 13.11: Different bioprinting techniques.

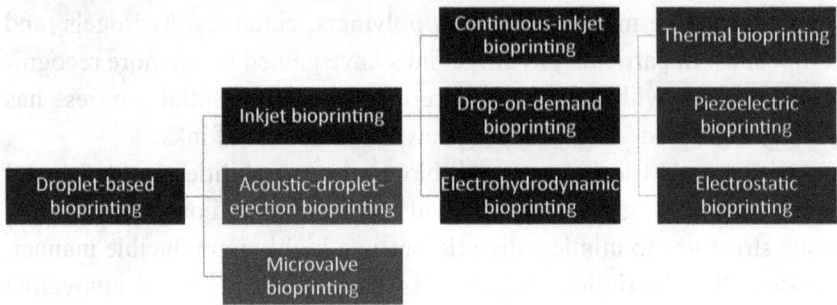

Figure 13.12: Droplet-based bioprinting types.

droplets are used to model or design a substrate. Droplet-based bioprinting heavily depends on physical parameters such as gravity, atmospheric pressure, and fluid mechanics to substantially influence bioink to generate droplets, and then eject them onto a receiving substrate. The bioink is contained in a cartridge attached to the print head. There are three fundamental approaches (Figure 13.12) to droplet-based bioprinting: (i) inkjet bioprinting, (ii) acoustic-droplet-ejection, and (iii) microvalve bioprinting. Details of droplet-based bioprinting and their subsets are shown in Figure 13.12. For effective deposition, all these techniques largely depend on the physical properties of the bioinks such as density, viscosity, and surface tension.

13.4.1.1 *Inkjet bioprinting*

Inkjet bioprinting (Figure 13.13) can be further divided into three important categories, i.e., continuous inkjet (CIJ), drop-on-demand (DOD), and electrohydrodynamic bioprinting (EHD).

- In CIJ bioprinting, continuous droplets are developed by forcing the ink onto the surface via a small nozzle in the presence of electrostatic force.
- DOD generates droplets only when needed by generating a pressure pulse within a microfluidic chamber. Due to the pulsed nature of printing and more user control, this approach is preferred over CIJ. Based on the droplet generation mechanism, DOD technology is

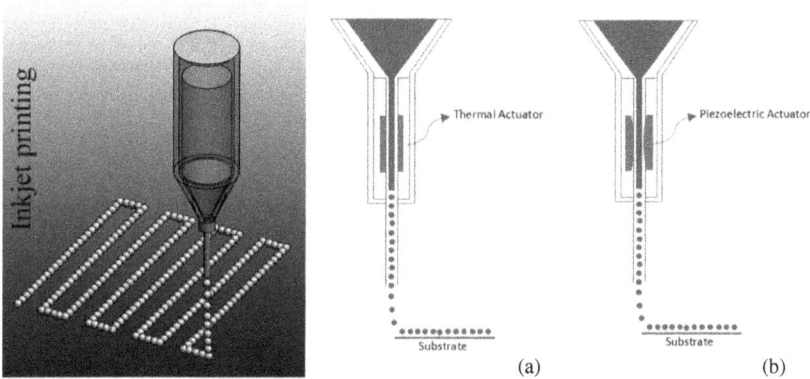

Figure 13.13: Schematic diagram of the DOD inkjet printing technique using (A) thermal and (B) piezoelectric actuators (Derakhshanfar *et al.*, 2018; Kholgh Eshkalak *et al.*, 2020).

further classified into (i) thermal inkjet (produce droplets by means of a thermal actuator) (Figure 13.13a), (ii) piezoelectric inkjet (produce droplets by means of a piezoelectric actuator) (Figure 13.13b), and (iii) electrostatic bioprinting (produce droplets by utilizing an electrostatic force). However, the high pressures involved in DOD techniques can be harmful to biological cells.

- EHD jet bioprinters use Coulomb force to drag the bioink out of the orifice, thereby avoiding the need for high pressure. EHD jet bioprinters limit the shear stress-induced cell damage.

13.4.1.2 *Acoustic-droplet-ejection bioprinting*

Acoustic-droplet-ejection (ADE) bioprinting applies mild or soft sound energy produced by an acoustic actuator to discharge a series of microdroplets (e.g., nanoliter or picoliter). Propulsion of liquid or suspended solid of a bioink solution happens from an "*open infinite pool*" instead of a nozzle. Droplet size is regulated by the wavelength of the sound emitted. Focusing sound follows principles similar to those for focusing light. Unlike other inkjet-based techniques in ADE bioprinting, bioink and the constituent cells are not exposed to extreme heat, high pressure, applied voltage, or considerable shear stress during droplet ejection. A schematic representation of ADE bioprinting is shown in Figure 13.14a.

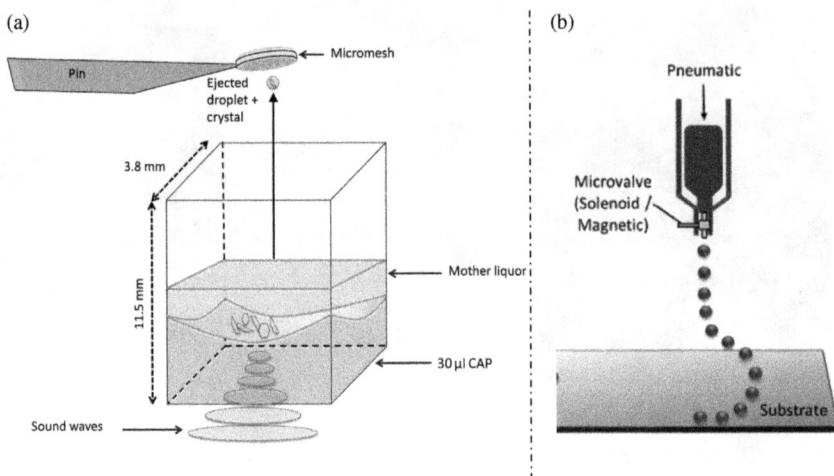

Figure 13.14: Schematics of (a) ADE bioprinting and (b) MAB bioprinting (Cuttitta *et al.*, 2015; Vijayavenkataraman *et al.*, 2018). ADE bioprinting image is reproduced with permission of the International Union of Crystallography.

13.4.1.3 *Microvalve-assisted bioprinting*

Microvalve-assisted bioprinting (MAB) (Figure 13.14b) makes use of an electromechanical valve to produce droplets. This technology holds enormous potential in the fabrication of tissues/organs. However, through the MAB technique, it is only possible to print hydrogels within a limited range of viscosities (1–200 mPa s).

13.4.2 *Extrusion-based bioprinting*

The extrusion-based bioprinting process has progressed significantly through the printing of various biologic products in the past decade, such as cells, tissues, tissue structures, organ modules, and microfluidic devices. For extrusion, this fluid-dispensing system is driven either by mechanical (piston or screw) or pneumatic pressure mechanisms. Extrusion-based printheads presenting extrusion via pneumatic, piston, and screw dispensing are shown in Figure 13.15. In a pneumatic mechanism, pressurized air (valve-free or valve-based) offers the necessary push. In contrast, in the piston and screw-driven mechanisms, vertical and rotational mechanical forces set off the extrusion of the liquid bioink,

Pneumatic   **Mechanical**

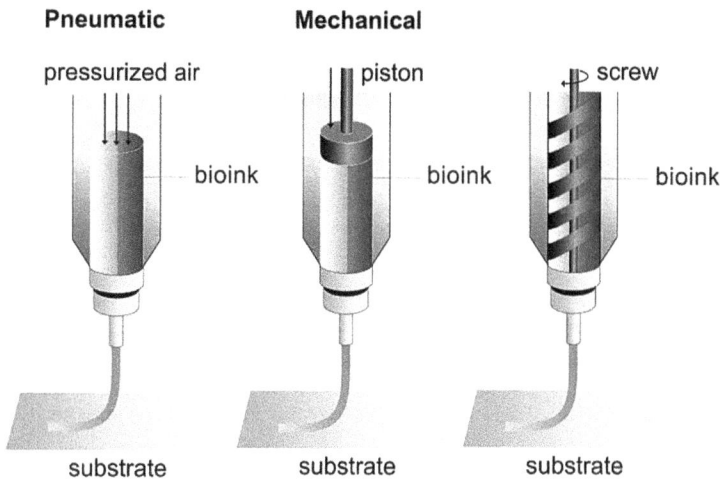

Figure 13.15: Schematics of extrusion-based printheads indicating extrusion via pneumatic pressure, piston, and screw dispensing (Włodarczyk-Biegun *et al.*, 2017).

respectively. All of these approaches result in continuous pressure on the device that allows thin filaments to be extruded, although each technique has its own individual strengths and limitations.

Pneumatic printers contain a pneumatic dispenser, which uses compressed gas to push bioink from a syringe nozzle. Such systems have straightforward components that permit highly viscous materials to be spread over a wide range of pressures. Hydrogels with thinning properties work best in pneumatically-driven extrusion-based bioprinting because after extrusion, the gel-like substance maintains the form of a filament.

The piston-driven design typically offers more control of bioink flow from the nozzle and physical deposition due to direct mechanical movement. However, this technique is constrained in the extent of pressure it can generate, making it inappropriate for some high viscosity bioinks. Screw-driven design provides more spatial control and has shown to be excellent for delivering higher viscosity bioinks. However, the screw-driven design will create higher pressure drops along with the nozzle, which could theoretically damage the stacked cells. In all three processes, cells embedded inside the ink experience mechanical stress within nozzles due to the extremely high variable pressure. If the increased shear stress is not controlled, it may ultimately lead to cell death in bioinks.

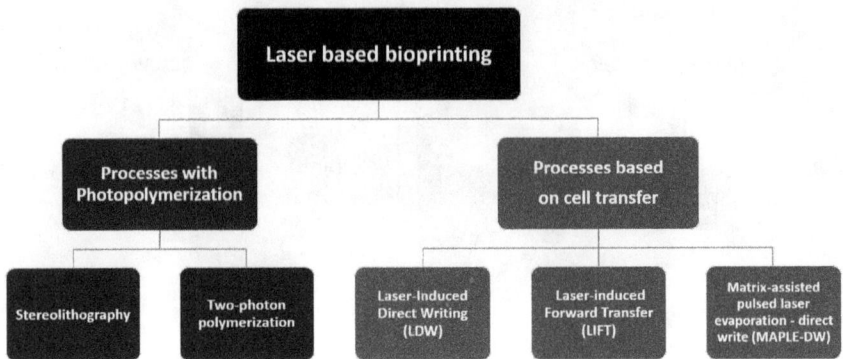

Figure 13.16:   Classification of laser-based bioprinting techniques.

13.4.3 *Laser-based bioprinting*

Laser-based bioprinting (LAB) is a group of procedures (Figure 13.16) that uses a pulsed laser source to deposit biological components and multiple cells onto a substrate. This method is often referred to as biological laser printing. Since it is a nozzle-free method, there are many benefits compared to inkjet and extrusion-based printing. The advantages include high-resolution printing of small droplets, printing of extremely viscous liquids, high cell survival rate, and high cell densities (approximately 100,000 cells per second). LAB uses UV or near-UV wavelengths as energy sources to print a variety of hydrogel solutions, microbeads, cells, proteins, and nucleic acids. The method typically involves three components: a pulsed laser source, a substrate covering liquid biological materials, and a receiving substrate.

The LAB system entails a complex laser-substance interaction mechanism, which involves energy conversion and phase transitions. Prior to laser exposure, the upper slide, called "*donor slide*", is coated with an energy absorption layer, which is transparent to the laser radiation wavelength. A thin layer of the desired bioink (usually a sol with embedded cells or proteins), usually in the range of 0.1–100 μm, is either coated or adhered to a biological polymer onto the rear side. The receiving substrate is placed just beneath the bioink-coated side. The transfer of this bioink onto the receiving substrate is induced by focusing one or more laser pulses on to the absorption layer. The schematics are shown in Figure 13.17.

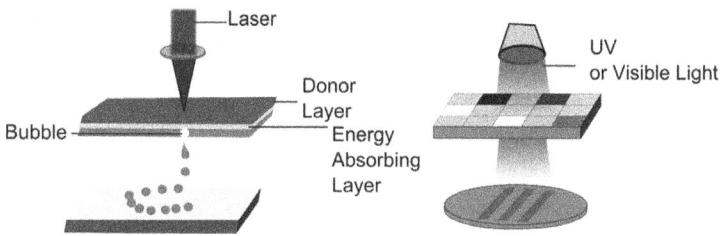

Figure 13.17:   Examples of laser-assisted bioprinting and stereolithography bioprinters (Foyt *et al.*, 2018).

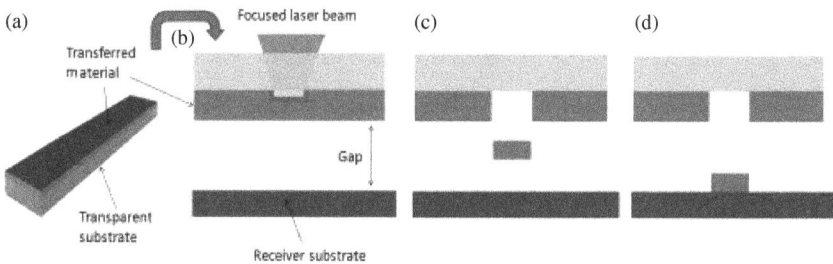

Figure 13.18:   The principle of LIFT printing. (a) A sketch of the donor, which contains a transparent substrate coated with a thin metal layer to be printed; (b) a focused laser pulse is absorbed in the metal layer leading to local heating; (c) the thermal energy provides the conditions for the transfer of part of the layer material; and (d) transferred pixel landing on the receiver (Zenou *et al.*, 2018).

This basic working theory covers widely used LAB processes such as laser-induced forward transfer (LIFT), absorbing film-assisted LIFT, biological laser processing, and matrix-assisted pulsed laser evaporation-direct writing (MAPLE-DW). Among all, LIFT is the most common nozzle-free LAB technique that involves a pixellated transfer of material by locally heating a transparent substrate using a laser pulse. The high-powered focused pulsed laser beam generates a high-pressure bubble that pushes the bioink in the direction of the receiving substrate placed nearby. The principle of LIFT printing is shown in Figure 13.18. Unlike LIFT technology, in the MAPLE-DW process, a low-powered pulsed laser and a laser absorbent interfacial layer are used to facilitate viable cell transfer between the target plate and bioink.

Table 13.6: Differences between various bioprinting techniques.

	Droplet-based	**Extrusion-based**	**Laser-based**
Resolution	Low (50 μm)	Medium (5 μm to mm)	High (100–600 μm)
Bioink	Liquids and hydrogels	Hydrogels	Cells in the medium
Cell viability	Medium (85%)	Very low (40–80%)	Very high (> 95%)
Gelation method	Chemical and photocross-linking	Chemical, physical, and photocross-linking	Chemical and photocross-linking
Advantage	Affordable	Multiple compositions	High accuracy
Disadvantage	Viscosity issues	Shear stress on the nozzle tip	The laser can sometimes result in cell death

13.5 3D printing for orthopaedic implants

AM has been used for more than a decade in medical procedures, mostly in surgical subspecialties such as cranio-maxillofacial reconstruction, cardiothoracic surgery, joint (hip and knee) arthroplasty, and orthopaedic surgery. The greatest advantage offered in medical applications by 3D printers is the ability to manufacture customized medical devices and instruments. In biomedical engineering, the capability to design highly complex patient-specific 3D biomedical devices is crucial. The layout includes the designing and repairing 3D anatomic defects, restoration or rebuilding of complex organs, and synthesis of scaffolds for stem cell differentiation.

Metal AM processes such as powder bed fusion, directed energy deposition, and binder jetting are widely used to manufacture models for hard tissue surgeries with each offering different capabilities.

13.5.1 *Customized implants*

The application of AM technology in orthopedic treatment has resulted in highly accurate and comprehensive production of patient-specific prosthetics (Figure 13.19a) and implants via 3D scanning, modelling, and digital processing of patient information (Figure 13.19b). Most existing implants are uniformly shaped and have consistent dimensions (widths and thicknesses). In some cases, there is a significant bone loss (due to

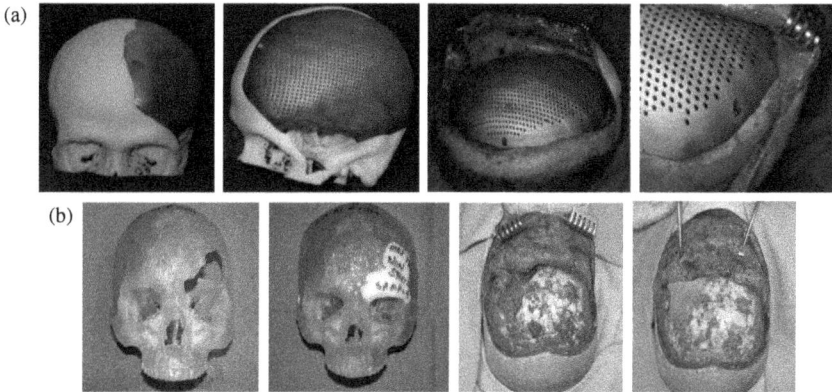

Figure 13.19: (a) Bio-models for cranial reconstruction surgery and prostheses to deliver an aesthetically pleasing forehead contour; (b) (from left to right) 3D model demonstrating supraorbital rim deformity; CAD/CAM implants used for supraorbital rim deformity; intraoperative view of supraorbital rim deformity; after implant placement (Jardini *et al.*, 2016; Lee *et al.*, 2020).

bone tumor resection, bone fracture), so the use of market-available ortho-pedic implants is not recommended. In such situations, custom implants are essential, i.e., the adaptivity to each individual is crucial. Using SLM, EBM, or FDM metal technologies, complicated mesh structures with enhanced design and functionality are made possible. Metallic biomateri-als such as stainless steel (316L), Co-Cr alloys, and titanium and its alloys (Ti–6Al–4V) are well-suited for customized load-bearing implants owing to their favorable biomechanical properties.

13.5.2 *Joint replacements (hip and knee)*

Total hip replacement (THR) or total hip arthroplasty (THA) is a standard and extremely effective surgical method that enhances joint functionality. The demand for these kinds of operations is relatively huge as they help patients move with minimal pain and have a more active lifestyle. One of the major complications of arthroplasty surgery is the loosening of the prosthesis from the bone. Different metal AM technologies can resolve this issue by manufacturing porous scaffolds appropriate for THR and THA. This permits natural bone ingrowth, guaranteeing higher stability of

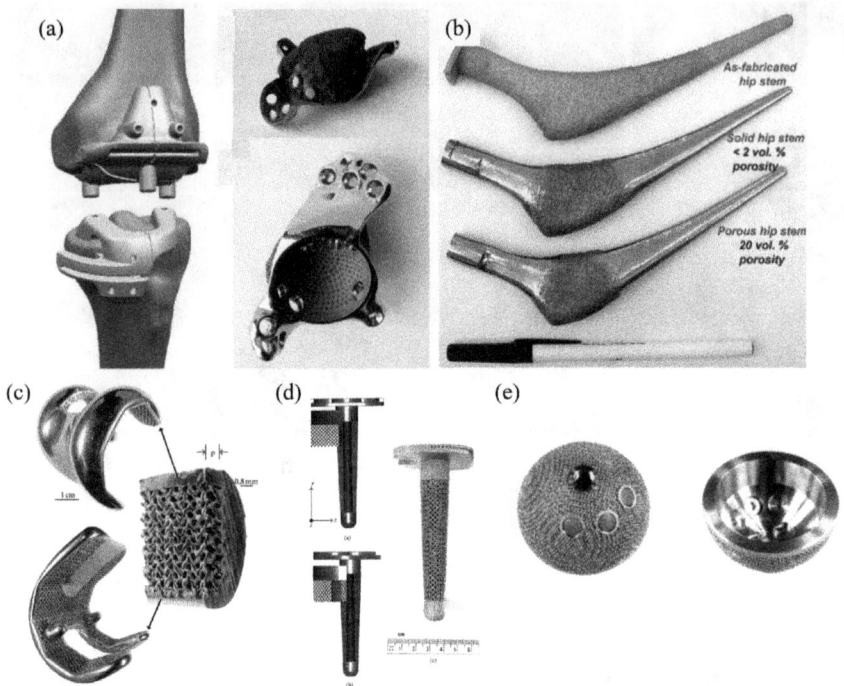

Figure 13.20: (a) Patient-specific saw guides for total knee arthroplasty (Smith & Nephew, USA) and custom-made Ti acetabulum implant with screw planning (Materialise, Belgium); (b) functional hip stems with designed porosity fabricated using LENS™; (c) Co-29Cr-6Mo alloy femoral knee implant prototype fabricated by EBM and HIPed; (d) tibial (knee) Ti-6Al-4V stem; (e) 3D printed cups (Dall'Ava *et al.*, 2019; Krishna *et al.*, 2007; Mok *et al.*, 2016; Murr *et al.*, 2012).

the implant. Knee implants frequently employ a cast Co-29Cr-6Mo alloy for femoral application. Patient-specific saw guides for THR and THA are shown in Figure 13.20.

13.5.3 *Anatomic models*

3D printed bio-models are frequently used for pre-operative preparation, practicing in medical procedures, surgical training, new product testing, new biomedical technology production and design, and design for pre-operative implants. Various kinds of surgical models are shown in

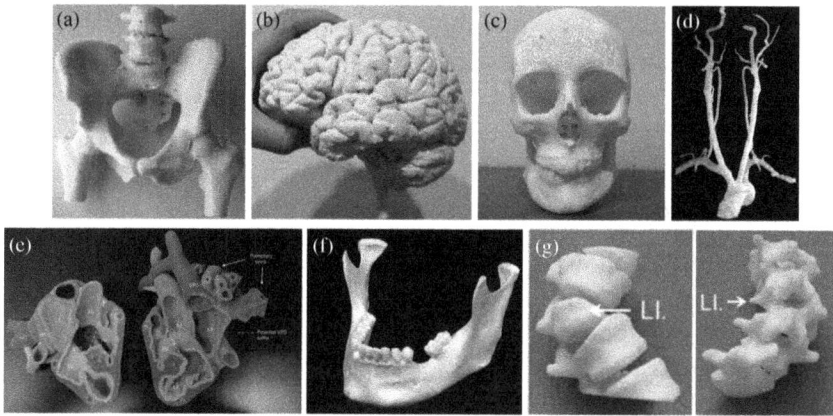

Figure 13.21: (a) 3D printed human pelvis showing a traumatic defect in sacrum; (b) 3D printed brain; (c) 3D printed skull; (d) 3D printed arcus aorta, carotid and vertebrals from MRA; (e) 3D model of heart; (f) mandibular 3D model; (g) 3D printed thoraco-lumbar section (Anwar *et al.*, 2018; Dilmen, 2015; Eltes *et al.*, 2020; Msallem *et al.*, 2020; Nevit, 2016).

Figure 13.21. Surgical operations are sometimes challenging even to skilled surgeons as they involve unpredictable circumstances, prompt actions, and unforeseeable outcomes. 3D printed models come to assist in these situations by allowing surgeons to practise on an exact replica before the actual surgical procedure. Many studies have shown an increased probability of success for the first time of surgery if 3D models were used. When performing cardiovascular surgery (especially for congenital heart disease), neurosurgery (intra-cranial neuropathological disease), and maxillofacial surgery, this 3D printed organ-based, physically replicated part is being used to visualize patient anatomy and disorders and understand inter-tissue relationships.

13.6 Multiple choice questions

1. What type of materials are used in photolithography?
   (a) any polymer with high molecular weight
   (b) photoreactive polymers
   (c) any polymer with low molecular weight
   (d) all ceramics and metals

2. Select the TRUE statement about 3D bioprinting.
    (a) fabrication of biological constructs similar to their native counter-parts
    (b) developing biological constructs for use as an anatomical model
    (c) developing biological constructs for use in display
    (d) no biological components are used

3. Which of the following is TRUE about bioinks?
    (a) they are created by combining cultured cells and various non-biocompatible materials
    (b) they are created by combining polymers and various nanoparticles
    (c) they are core materials used to produce live tissue using 3D print-ing
    (d) any material that can be in a semi-liquid form is known as bioink

4. Increasing the concentration of bioinks in inkjet and extrusion-based bioprinting
    I. affects cell viability
    II. has no effect on cell viability as there is no ejection of solution from nozzle
    III. makes the inks highly viscous which clogs the nozzle and has effect on mechanical properties
    (a) only I
    (b) only I and II
    (c) all of the above
    (d) only I and III

5. In laser-assisted bioprinting technology, viscosity of solution
    (a) should be as low as possible
    (b) should be as high as possible
    (c) is not a critical parameter because there is no ejection of solution from the nozzle
    (d) none of the above

6. Select the TRUE statement(s) regarding extrusion-based bioprinting.
    I. resolution is very limited
    II. high temperature could damage the cells
    III. no temperature is involved
    IV. very high cell densities can be printed

    (a) only I and IV
    (b) only I, III and IV
    (c) only II and IV
    (d) only I, II and IV

7. In extrusion-based printing, low cell survivability is due to
    (a) high temperatures
    (b) shear stress during printing
    (c) low viscosity of the liquid
    (d) all of the above

8. Select the TRUE statement(s) regarding laser-assisted bioprinting.
    (a) it is a nozzle-free technology
    (b) works only with limited viscosity solutions
    (c) independent of viscosity of the solution
    (d) all of the above

9. Which of the following is/are NOT true about stereolithography bioprinting?
    (a) fabricates biological components at a very low resolution
    (b) requires very little material, implies less wastage of material
    (c) long processing time
    (d) all of the above

References & Further Reading

Almog, D. M., Torrado, E., & Meitner, S. W. J. (2001). Fabrication of imaging and surgical guides for dental implants. *Journal of Prosthetic Dentistry, 85*(5), 504–508. doi:10.1067/mpr.2001.115388.

Anwar, S., Singh, G. K., Miller, J., Sharma, M., *et al.* (2018). 3D Printing is a Transformative Technology in Congenital Heart Disease. *JACC: Basic to Translational Science, 3*(2), 294–312. doi:10.1016/j.jacbts.2017.10.003.

Berry, D. B., Yu, C., & Chen, S. (2020). Chapter 75 — Biofabricated three-dimensional tissue models. In R. Lanza, R. Langer, J. P. Vacanti, & A. Atala (Eds.), *Principles of Tissue Engineering (Fifth Edition)* (pp. 1417–1441): Academic Press.

Bishop, E. S., Mostafa, S., Pakvasa, M., Luu, H. H., *et al.* (2017). 3D bioprinting technologies in tissue engineering and regenerative medicine: Current and future trends. *Genes & Diseases,* *4*(4), 185–195. doi:10.1016/j. gendis.2017.10.002.

Criales, L. E., Arısoy, Y. M., Lane, B., Moylan, S., *et al.* (2017). Laser powder bed fusion of nickel alloy 625: Experimental investigations of effects of process parameters on melt pool size and shape with spatter analysis. *International Journal of Machine Tools and Manufacture, 121,* 22–36. doi:10.1016/j.ijmachtools.2017.03.004.

Cuttitta, C. M., Ericson, D. L., Scalia, A., Roessler, C. G., *et al.* (2015). Acoustic transfer of protein crystals from agarose pedestals to micromeshes for high-throughput screening. *Acta Crystallographica Section D, D71,* 94–103. doi:10.1107/S1399004714013728.

Dall'Ava, L., Hothi, H., Di Laura, A., Henckel, J., *et al.* (2019). 3D Printed Acetabular Cups for Total Hip Arthroplasty: A Review Article. *Metals, 9*(7), 729. doi:10.3390/met9070729.

Derakhshanfar, S., Mbeleck, R., Xu, K., Zhang, X., *et al.* (2018). 3D bioprinting for biomedical devices and tissue engineering: A review of recent trends and advances. *Bioactive Materials, 3*(2), 144–156. doi:10.1016/j.bioactmat. 2017.11.008.

Dilmen, N. (2015). 3D printed human pelvis showing traumatic defect in sacrum. 10 cm height. *Creative Commons Attribution-Share Alike 3.0 Unported license.*

Eltes, P. E., Kiss, L., Bartos, M., Gyorgy, Z. M., *et al.* (2020). Geometrical accuracy evaluation of an affordable 3D printing technology for spine physical models. *Journal of Clinical Neuroscience, 72,* 438–446. doi:10.1016/j.jocn. 2019.12.027.

Foyt, D. A., Norman, M. D. A., Yu, T. T. L., & Gentleman, E. (2018). Exploiting Advanced Hydrogel Technologies to Address Key Challenges in Regenerative Medicine. *Advanced Healthcare Materials, 7*(8), 1700939. doi:10.1002/ adhm.201700939.

Hedlundh, U., & Karlsson, L. J. (2016). Combining a hip arthroplasty stem with trochanteric reattachment bolt and a polyaxial locking plate in the treatment of a periprosthetic fracture below a well-integrated implant. *Arthroplasty Today, 2*(4), 141–145. doi:10.1016/j.artd.2016.02.002.

Ibrahim, M. Z., Sarhan, A. A., Yusuf, F., & Hamdi, M. J. (2017). Biomedical materials and techniques to improve the tribological, mechanical and bio-medical properties of orthopedic implants — A review article. *Journal of Alloys and Compounds, 714,* 636–667. doi:10.1016/j.jallcom.2017.04.231.

Jardini, A., Larosa, M., Macedo, M., Bernardes, L., Lambert, C., Zavaglia, C., Maciel Filho, R., Calderoni, D., Ghizoni, E., & Kharmandayan, P. J. (2016). Improvement in cranioplasty: advanced prosthesis biomanufacturing. *Procedia CIRP, 49*, 203–208. doi:10.1016/j.procir.2015.11.017.

Kholgh Eshkalak, S., Rezvani Ghomi, E., Dai, Y., Choudhury, D., *et al.* (2020). The role of three-dimensional printing in healthcare and medicine. *Materials & Design, 194*, 108940. doi:10.1016/j.matdes.2020.108940.

Krishna, B. V., Bose, S., & Bandyopadhyay, A. (2007). Low stiffness porous Ti structures for load-bearing implants. *Acta Biomaterialia, 3*(6), 997–1006. doi:10.1016/j.actbio.2007.03.008.

Lee, J., Gordon, C., & Yaremchuk, M. J. (2020). Chapter 3.12 — Custom Craniofacial Implants. In A. H. Dorafshar, E. D. Rodriguez, & P. N. Manson (Eds.), *Facial Trauma Surgery* (pp. 463–470): Elsevier.

Liu, D., Fu, J., Fan, H., Li, D., Dong, E., Xiao, X., Wang, L., & Guo, Z. J. (2018). Application of 3D-printed PEEK scapula prosthesis in the treatment of scapular benign fibrous histiocytoma: a case report. *Journal of Bone Oncology, 12*, 78–82. doi:10.1016/j.jbo.2018.07.012.

Lv, X., Ye, F., Cheng, L., Fan, S., *et al.* (2019). Binder jetting of ceramics: Powders, binders, printing parameters, equipment, and post-treatment. *Ceramics International, 45*(10), 12609–12624. doi:10.1016/j.ceramint.2019.04.012.

Matsushita, T., Fujibayashi, S., & Kokubo, T. (2017). Chapter 4 — Titanium foam for bone tissue engineering. In C. Wen (Ed.), *Metallic Foam Bone* (pp. 111–130): Elsevier.

Mok, S.-W., Nizak, R., Fu, S.-C., Ho, K.-W. K., *et al.* (2016). From the printer: Potential of three-dimensional printing for orthopaedic applications. *Journal of Orthopaedic Translation, 6*, 42–49. doi:10.1016/j.jot.2016.04.003.

Moritz, T., & Maleksaeedi, S. (2018). Chapter 4 — Additive manufacturing of ceramic components. In J. Zhang & Y.-G. Jung (Eds.), *Additive Manufacturing* (pp. 105–161): Butterworth-Heinemann.

Msallem, B., Sharma, N., Cao, S., Halbeisen, F. S., *et al.* (2020). Evaluation of the Dimensional Accuracy of 3D-Printed Anatomical Mandibular Models Using FFF, SLA, SLS, MJ, and BJ Printing Technology. *Journal of Clinical Medicine, 9*(3), 817. doi:10.3390/jcm9030817.

Murr, L. E., Gaytan, S. M., Martinez, E., Medina, F., *et al.* (2012). Next Generation Orthopaedic Implants by Additive Manufacturing Using Electron Beam Melting. *International Journal of Biomaterials, 2012*, 245727. doi:10.1155/2012/245727.

Nevit. (2016). 3D printed Brain. *Creative Commons Attribution-Share Alike 3.0 Unported license.*

Ni, J., Ling, H., Zhang, S., Wang, Z., *et al.* (2019). Three-dimensional printing of metals for biomedical applications. *Materials Today Bio, 3,* 100024. doi:10.1016/j.mtbio.2019.100024.

Saikko, V., Ahlroos, T., Revitzer, H., Ryti, O., & Kuosmanen, P. J. (2013). The effect of acetabular cup position on wear of a large-diameter metal-on-metal prosthesis studied with a hip joint simulator. *Tribology International, 60,* 70–76. doi:10.1016/j.triboint.2012.10.011.

Sireesha, M., Lee, J., Kranthi Kiran, A. S., Babu, V. J., *et al.* (2018). A review on additive manufacturing and its way into the oil and gas industry. *RSC Advances, 8*(40), 22460–22468. doi:10.1039/C8RA03194K.

Stansbury, J. W., & Idacavage, M. J. (2016). 3D printing with polymers: Challenges among expanding options and opportunities. *Dental Materials, 32*(1), 54–64. doi:10.1016/j.dental.2015.09.018.

Sturm, L. D., Williams, C. B., Camelio, J. A., White, J., *et al.* (2017). Cyber-physical vulnerabilities in additive manufacturing systems: A case study attack on the .STL file with human subjects. *Journal of Manufacturing Systems, 44,* 154–164. doi:10.1016/j.jmsy.2017.05.007.

Tischler, M., Patch, C., & Bidra, A. S. J. (2018). Rehabilitation of edentulous jaws with zirconia complete-arch fixed implant-supported prostheses: an up to 4-year retrospective clinical study. *Journal of Prosthetic Dentistry, 120*(2), 204–209. doi:10.1016/j.prosdent.2017.12.010.

Vijayavenkataraman, S., Yan, W.-C., Lu, W. F., Wang, C.-H., *et al.* (2018). 3D bioprinting of tissues and organs for regenerative medicine. *Advanced Drug Delivery Reviews, 132,* 296–332. doi:10.1016/j.addr.2018.07.004.

Włodarczyk-Biegun, M. K., & del Campo, A. (2017). 3D bioprinting of structural proteins. *Biomaterials, 134,* 180–201. doi:10.1016/j.biomaterials.2017.04.019.

Zenou, M., & Grainger, L. (2018). 3 — Additive manufacturing of metallic materials. In J. Zhang & Y.-G. Jung (Eds.), *Additive Manufacturing* (pp. 53–103): Butterworth-Heinemann.

Zhai, Y., Lados, D. A., Brown, E. J., & Vigilante, G. N. (2016). Fatigue crack growth behavior and microstructural mechanisms in Ti-6Al-4V manufactured by laser engineered net shaping. *International Journal of Fatigue, 93,* 51–63. doi:10.1016/j.ijfatigue.2016.08.009.

Answers to Questions

Chapter 1

1. The term "cell" is not applicable for
   (a) algae
   (b) bacteria
   (c) virus
   (d) fungi

2. Which of the following about angiogenesis is TRUE?
   (a) it is the process of formation of new blood vessels
   (b) endothelial cell is responsible for proliferation and migration
   (c) it involves matrix degradation and cell signaling
   (d) all of the above

3. The spherical defined organelle that comprises the genetic material is the
   (a) cell wall
   (b) ribosome
   (c) nucleus
   (d) mitochondria

4. What is the mechanism by which material absorption in cells takes place through the plasma membrane?
   (a) egestion
   (b) diffusion
   (c) mitosis
   (d) endocytosis

5. What portion of the human eye is implanted into a living person from a deceased donor?
   (a) **cornea**
   (b) retina
   (c) iris
   (d) sclera

6. Which of the following sequences about the human body is correct in increasing order?
   (a) **chemicals, cells, tissues, organ, organ system, organism**
   (b) organism, cells, chemicals, organ system, tissues, organ
   (c) organism, cells, organ, tissue, chemicals, organ system
   (d) tissues, cells, organism, chemicals, organ system, organ

7. Which of the following is NOT true?
   (a) the human body is composed of trillions of cells
   (b) cells contain the body's hereditary material
   (c) cells survive, grow, reproduce, and die on their own
   (d) **a group of cells with similar structure and function is called an organ**

8. What nutrient(s) become(s) part of the bone matrix?
   (a) only calcium
   (b) **calcium and phosphorus**
   (c) only phosphorus
   (d) calcium, phosphorus, vitamins A, B and D

9. An example of a ball and socket joint is found in between
   (a) femur and tibia
   (b) **femur and pelvis**
   (c) ankle bones
   (d) tibia and fibula

10. Which of the following is NOT true?
    (a) the ligaments of the hip joint act to increase stability
    (b) hip is the largest ball-and-socket joint in the human body

(c) in the hip joint, the ball femoral head, and the socket is the acetabulum

(d) the only weight-bearing bone in the lower leg is the femur (it is the tibia)

11. The receptors which detect movement of the body are located in the ___, and the first part of the eye that refracts light rays is the ___
    (a) vestibule; retina
    (b) semi-circular canals; cornea
    (c) middle ear; lens
    (d) organ of corti; optical nerve

12. Which part of the brain begins voluntary movement, and which neurons carry impulses from receptors to the central nervous system?
    (a) cerebellum; sensory
    (b) occipital lobes; mixed
    (c) temporal lobes; motor
    (d) frontal lobes; sensory

13. What are blood clots made up of, and which mineral is accountable for blood clotting?
    (a) fibrin; calcium
    (b) collagen; sodium
    (c) thrombin; phosphorus
    (d) albumin; magnesium

14. The mineral crystal found within the matrix of bone is called
    (a) calcium carbonate
    (b) hydroxyapatite
    (c) calcium phosphate hydrate
    (d) tricalcium ortho phosphate

15. The widening of blood vessels is known as
    (a) vasoconstriction
    (b) atherosclerosis
    (c) vasodilation
    (d) thrombosis

Chapter 2

1. Disease existing at or before birth is
   (a) congenital
   (b) communicable
   (c) non-communicable
   (d) none of the above

2. The immune system comprises
   (a) humoral and fibrous systems
   (b) humoral and cell-mediated systems
   (c) antigens
   (d) lymphocytes

3. Researchers believe that Paget disease may be caused by
   (a) virus
   (b) parasite
   (c) an abnormal gene
   (d) A and C

4. Gum disease is associated with
   (a) pregnancy
   (b) heart disease and stroke
   (c) diabetes
   (d) all of the above

5. Human Immunodeficiency Virus causes AIDS by attacking a type of white blood cell called
   (a) CD4
   (b) CD3
   (c) CD8
   (d) none of the above

6. Which of the following is a viral disease?
   (a) type 1 diabetes
   (b) type 2 diabetes
   (c) blood cancer
   (d) influenza

7. The hardest material in the human body is the
   (a) bone
   (b) enamel
   (c) dentin
   (d) skull

8. When the individual is unable to recognise everyday objects and name them correctly, this is known as
   (a) prosopagnosia
   (b) anomia
   (c) agnosia
   (d) aphosonomia

9. If the lens in the eye becomes opaque, the disease is called
   (a) myopia
   (b) astigmatism
   (c) glaucoma
   (d) cataract

10. Hypertension is the term used for
    (a) increase in heart rate
    (b) decrease in heart rate
    (c) decrease in blood pressure
    (d) increase in blood pressure

Chapter 3

1. Which of the following is TRUE?
   (a) collagen fibers in the ECM have higher Young's modulus than elastin
   (b) collagen is protein fiber found in the minimum amount throughout our body
   (c) fibrin is responsible for strength and cushioning in human body
   (d) collagen is arranged as simple bundles and has a limited length

366 An Introduction to Biomaterials Science and Engineering

2. Which of the following is NOT true?
   (a) ECM is a molecule network composed of various proteins, glycosaminoglycan, and glycoconjugate
   (b) ECM is a structural scaffold that aids in enhancing cellular properties
   (c) ECM is as it is, does not undergo any remodeling
   (d) ECM controls communication between cells

3. Which of the following tissues cannot be formed from embryonic stem cells?
   (a) connective tissue
   (b) epithelial tissue
   (c) endodermal tissue
   (d) none of the above

4. What is the least invasive source of stem cells from the human body?
   (a) adipose tissue
   (b) bone marrow
   (c) umbilical cord blood
   (d) liver

5. A stem cell has the ability to
   I. produce daughter cells that are an exact replica of itself
   II. develop only into certain cell types
   III. produce daughter cells that are dedicated to differentiation
   IV. develop into many cell types
      (a) only I and II
      (b) only I and III
      (c) only I, III and IV
      (d) none of the above

6. Which of the following proteins are abundant in the ECM, and which of the cells do not reside in the ECM?
   (a) actin; mesenchymal stem cells
   (b) elastin; fibroblasts
   (c) collagen; hepatocytes
   (d) laminin; adipose cells

7. Which of the following is/are TRUE about integrins?
   I. integrins are the principal receptors
   II. integrins regulate the interaction between a cell and its microenvironment to control cell fate
   (a) only I
   (b) all of the above
   (c) none of the above
   (d) only II

8. In a developing embryo, stem cells differentiate into
   (a) ectoderm
   (b) endoderm
   (c) mesoderm
   (d) all of the above
   (e) none of the above

9. What is the role of adult stem cells in the human body?
   (a) always offer the source of cells for diagnosing diseases
   (b) play a role as repair system for the body
   (c) regulate the functioning of an organ
   (d) all of the above

10. Which of the following is correct for ESCs?
    (a) they are multipotent
    (b) they are already differentiated inner mass cells of a human embryo
    (c) they have the potential for self-renewal
    (d) they have the ability to become any type of cell in the body

11. Which of the following is NOT true regarding growth factors?
    (a) growth factors are naturally occurring substances and can also be produced by genetic engineering
    (b) growth factors typically act as signaling molecules between cells
    (c) cytokines and hormones are growth factors
    (d) growth factors do not have binding capacity

12. Which adult cells can be transformed into iPS cells?
    (a) bone cells
    (b) nerve cells

    (c) no cells can convert themselves into iPS cells
    (d) any adult cell which has a capability of dividing

13. Which of the following techniques is facing bioethical issues?
    (a) embryonic stem cell therapy
    (b) cell therapy
    (c) DNA microarray
    (d) all of the above

14. Which term describes grafts from other humans?
    (a) allografts
    (b) allogeneic
    (c) xenogeneic
    (d) none of the above

Chapter 4

1. Biomaterials
    (a) are always synthetic materials; natural materials are not employed
    (b) are always natural materials; synthetic materials are not employed
    (c) can be natural or synthetic materials
    (d) are always polymeric materials

2. Select the statement which correctly relates to biocompatibility.
    (a) a biocompatible material should provide healing characters
    (b) a biocompatible material should have therapeutic characteristics
    (c) a material is considered as a biocompatible material as long as it causes no harm to the host body
    (d) a biocompatible material should have the exact dimensions as the damaged tissue or part

3. Select the option(s) which do(es) NOT come under the class of biocompatible materials.
    (a) eyeglasses; wheelchair
    (b) contact lenses; dental implants

(c) orthopedic implant; stents

(d) external hip prosthesis; massage footwear

4. Which of the following has the best osteointegration properties?

(a) SS316

(b) porous titanium

(c) Co-Cr alloys

(d) all of the above

5. Which of the following is/are biomaterial(s)?

I. materials used for tooth filling

II. materials used for cardiovascular repairs

III. glucose meters and stethoscopes

IV. materials used for hip implants

    (a) only I

    (b) only I, II and IV

    (c) only I, III and IV

    (d) only III

6. Select the option(s) which is/are TRUE about biodegradation.

(a) it depends on the molecular architecture

(b) it is a precise breakdown of the material over time

(c) metals biodegrade faster than polymeric materials

(d) all of the above

7. Which class of biomaterials has chemical structures similar to bone?

(a) polymeric biomaterials

(b) ceramic biomaterials

(c) metallic biomaterials

(d) all of the above

8. Which class of biomaterials encourages bonding with surrounding tissues and stimulates new bone growth?

(a) bioinert ceramics

(b) bioactive ceramics

(c) Co-Cr alloys

(d) all of the above

9. Which of the following is TRUE?
    (a) ceramics possess excellent wear and friction properties
    (b) SS316, Co-Cr and Ti alloys form a protective oxide layer on their surfaces
    (c) bioceramics are more reactive then certain metallic implants
    (d) all of the above

Chapter 5

1. Increasing molecular weight of a polymer usually
    (a) increases the strength of the polymer
    (b) decreases the strength of the polymer
    (c) has no effect on the strength of the polymer
    (d) none of the above

2. Which of these polymers cannot be recycled, and which is the strongest polymer group?
    (a) thermoplasts; thermosets
    (b) thermosets; thermosets
    (c) elastomers; thermoplasts
    (d) all polymers; elastomers

3. Which of the following is/are NOT true about polymers?
    I. high mechanical strength
    II. high-temperature stability on par with ceramics
    III. high elongation with viscoelastic behaviour
    (a) only I and II
    (b) only II
    (c) only I and III
    (d) all of the above

4. Which compound is made up of many monomers joined in long chains, and which pattern is not a copolymer?
    (a) ethanol; BBAABBAABBAABB
    (b) methanol; ABCABCABCABC
    (c) cellulose; CCCCCCCCCCC
    (d) fibrin; AACAACAACAA

5. Which of the following is/are TRUE?
   I. a thermosetting polymer will not melt
   II. a thermoplastic will melt and be malleable into any desired shape
   (a) only I
   (b) only II
   (c) all of the above
   (d) none of the above

6. Which is the best method to store degradable hydrogels?
   (a) storing in a refrigerator at 4°C or under alcohol
   (b) storing in a beaker at 20°C
   (c) physicochemical properties of hydrogels are not dependent on storage
   (d) all of the above

7. Composite materials are classified based on
   (a) type of matrix
   (b) size and shape of reinforcement
   (c) melting points
   (d) mechanical and biological properties

8. The calculation of number average (M_n) and weight average (M_w) depends, respectively, on
   (a) total weight of all polymer chains; molecular weight of each molecule
   (b) molecular weight of each molecule; total weight of all polymer chains
   (c) individual weight of each polymer chain; total weight of all polymer chains
   (d) none of the above

9. Which of the following is NOT a polymeric biomaterial?
   (a) chitosan
   (b) hydroxyapatite
   (c) polylactic-co-glycolic acid
   (d) polymethyl methacrylate

10. Which of the following is TRUE?
    (a) degradation rate of PCL is very fast
    (b) PCL is an amorphous polymer
    (c) crystallinity of a polymer affects the degradation rate
    (d) all of the above

Chapter 6

1. Ceramic head is favoured over metal head against the UHMWPE acetabular cup because of
    (a) longer lifetimes and lower wear rates
    (b) high melting temperatures
    (c) brittleness
    (d) none of the above

2. Which type of atomic bonding characterizes the ceramics?
    (a) covalent bonding
    (b) ionic bonding and metallic bonding
    (c) covalent and ionic bonding
    (d) metallic bonding

3. Which of the following is TRUE regarding characteristic properties of ceramic materials?
    (a) high-temperature stability; high mechanical strength; low elongation; low hardness
    (b) high-temperature stability; high mechanical strength; low elongation; high hardness
    (c) low-temperature stability; high mechanical strength; high elongation; low hardness
    (d) low-temperature stability; low mechanical strength; high elongation; high hardness

4. Which of the following is NOT true of crystalline solids?
    (a) they have long-range and short-range order
    (b) they contain a repeating pattern of atoms or ions or molecules
    (c) they contain a random arrangement of constituents
    (d) they have well-defined melting points

5. Which type of material, with example, upon placement in human body starts to dissolve slowly and is replaced by advancing tissue?
   (a) bioinert; alumina
   (b) bioactive; hydroxyapatite
   (c) bioresorable; tricalcium phosphate
   (d) bioinert; tricalcium phosphate

6. Which type of material, with example, has minimum interaction with surrounding tissue?
   (a) bioinert; alumina
   (b) all biomaterials
   (c) bioresorable; tricalcium phosphate
   (d) bioinert; tricalcium phosphate

7. Which of the following classes of bioinert materials is used as coating component on metallic biomaterials to enhance biological properties?
   (a) bioceramics
   (b) biopolymers
   (c) titanium
   (d) particulate suspension

8. During sintering, densification is not due to
   (a) atomic diffusion
   (b) surface diffusion
   (c) bulk diffusion
   (d) grain growth

9. Which of the following is TRUE about biodegradation of bioceramic bone fillers?
   (a) biodegradation of the component should match the healing rate of the bone
   (b) the component can degrade faster irrespective of healing
   (c) no relation between biodegradation and bone healing
   (d) faster biodegradation of component will help bone to heal faster

10. Which of the following is/are NOT true about bioglass?
    I. carbonate-substituted hydroxyapatite enhances bioactivity and biocompatibility
    II. thin oxide layer of TiO_2 is formed on the substrate
    III. the rate of ion release from the bioglass surface is determined by the Ca:P ratio
    IV. bioglass composition and microstructure do not have any role in determining bioactivity
        (a) only I and III
        (b) only III
        (c) only II and IV
        (d) only I, II and IV

11. Which of the following is/are TRUE regarding HCA of bioglass?
    I. HCA enhances bioactivity and biocompatibility
    II. HCA crystals provide a base for adsorption of components of ECM
    III. HCA crystals improve melting temperature of bioglass
    IV. HCA crystals facilitate chemical bonding with neighbouring bone
        (a) only I and II
        (b) all of the above
        (c) only I, III and IV
        (d) only I, II, and IV

12. Which of the following is/are NOT true about hydroxyapatite?
    I. used in bone tissue engineering owing to its chemical similarity to the mineral of bone
    II. cannot be used in bone repair due to low melting point
    III. also used as coating material on metallic implants to improve bio-active properties
    IV. does not have any effect on improving osseointegration
        (a) only III and IV
        (b) only I, II and IV
        (c) only I and II
        (d) only II and IV

13. An example of amorphous material is
    (a) **glass**
    (b) zinc
    (c) carbon
    (d) iron

14. Select the TRUE statement(s) about hydroxyapatite phase.
    (a) **it has low solubility under physiological conditions (pH 7.4)**
    (b) it has high solubility under physiological conditions (pH 7.4)
    (c) **it has higher dissolution in acidic conditions (pH 6.5)**
    (d) it has lower dissolution in acidic conditions (pH 6.5)

15. Select the TRUE statement(s) about effect of crystallinity of hydroxyapatite.
    (a) **has an influence on solubility**
    (b) does not have an influence on solubility
    (c) **affects protein adsorption**
    (d) does not have an effect on protein adsorption

Chapter 7

1. Select the statement(s) which is/are TRUE about metallic implants.
    I. metallic implants do not encounter any issue with wear
    II. metallic implants comprise two or more metals
    III. a thin stable oxide layer is formed on top of biometals which further resists corrosion
    IV. metallic implants are used as bone fillers
    (a) only I
    (b) only II and IV
    (c) **only II and III**
    (d) all of the above

2. Stress shielding usually occurs in
    (a) polymeric biomaterials
    (b) bioceramics
    (c) **metallic implant materials**
    (d) any biomaterial

3. High elastic modulus in materials arises from
   (a) **high strength of metallic bonds**
   (b) hydrogen bonds
   (c) covalent bonds
   (d) none of the above

4. Which of the following is/are NOT true about stress shielding?
   I. it usually occurs due to modulus mismatch between bone and implanted material
   II. it is associated with polymeric scaffold materials
   III. the lower modulus provides for the possibility of less stress shielding effects
   IV. it leads to implant stabilization
      (a) only I
      (b) **only II and IV**
      (c) only II, III and IV
      (d) only IV

5. Which of the following is/are TRUE?
   I. Ti-6Al-4V alloy has less stress shielding effect than α alloy
   II. β alloys for orthopaedics are developed to increase melting temperature
   III. β alloys have lower stress shielding effect than α and $\alpha + \beta$ alloys
      (a) only I
      (b) **only III**
      (c) only II and III
      (d) all of the above

6. Which is a *unique* characteristic about Ti implants which is NOT present in other metallic implant materials?
   (a) **osseointegration**
   (b) formation of a native oxide layer
   (c) used for permanent implants as internal and external fixation devices
   (d) biocompatibility

7. Implants for hard tissue engineering are most often made of
   (a) titanium
   (b) hydroxyapatite
   (c) calcium carbonate
   (d) alumina and zirconia

8. Select the TRUE statement(s) about magnesium alloys for bone tissue engineering.
   (a) have lower Young's modulus compared to other Ti SS316 alloys
   (b) have unique osseointegration properties
   (c) reduce the stress shielding-related problems of orthopaedic/ cardiovascular implants
   (d) all of the above

9. Select the TRUE issue(s) about magnesium alloys when utilized for bone tissue engineering.
   (a) fast corrosion rate in physiological environment
   (b) evolution of H_2 gas in physiological environment
   (c) low Young's modulus
   (d) all of the above

10. Which of the following is TRUE regarding the formation of $Mg(OH)_2$ on Mg alloys?
    (a) enhances the osteointegration bone bonding like TiO_2 layer
    (b) accelerates corrosion because of reaction with Cl^- in physiological conditions
    (c) improves bone-tissue integration
    (d) all of the above

11. Which type of stainless steel is commonly used in orthopaedic implants?
    (a) austenitic stainless steel
    (b) ferritic stainless steel
    (c) martensitic stainless steel
    (d) duplex stainless steel

12. In stainless steel, this element is added for improving corrosion resistance; and the presence of hydrogen in steel causes this effect.
    (a) tungsten; increases corrosion resistance
    (b) magnesium; improves cell adhesion
    (c) carbon; decreases cell adhesion
    (d) chromium; embrittlement

13. Capability of an orthodontic wire to spring back to its original shape is assessed by
    (a) Young's modulus
    (b) stiffness
    (c) resilience
    (d) elasticity and plasticity

Chapter 8

1. Sterilization is a process
   (a) by which the microbial burden on objects is reduced or completely removed
   (b) by which the microbial burden on objects is increased
   (c) used to improve surface properties of the object
   (d) used to change the surface topography of the object

2. The absence of all forms of microbial life, including spores, is known as
   (a) cleaning
   (b) sanitization
   (c) disinfection
   (d) sterilization

3. The temperature-pressure combination for typical autoclaving is
   (a) 99°C and 9 psi
   (b) 121°C and 15 psi
   (c) 114°C and 10 psi
   (d) 141°C and 13 psi

4. Which of the following is an accepted sterilant?
   (a) chlorhexidine
   (b) chloroform
   (c) ethylene oxide
   (d) benzene

5. Which of the following is NOT a sterilization method?
   (a) aqueous glutaraldehyde for 10 hours
   (b) dry heating at 180°C for 1–2 hours
   (c) water boiling of medical device at 100°C for 20–25 minutes
   (d) using electrons for sterilization

6. Which of the following is TRUE regarding heat conduction in dry air?
   (a) slower than in steam
   (b) quicker than in steam
   (c) similar to steam
   (d) none of these

7. Which order of reaction describe the destruction of microorganisms by moist heat?
   (a) first-order
   (b) zero-order
   (c) fourth-order
   (d) fifth-order

8. Cell-sensitive media comprising bacterial spores and heat-sensitive materials are usually sterilized by
   (a) autoclaving
   (b) dry heat
   (c) UV radiation
   (d) chemical treatments

9. Which of the following about EtO sterilization is NOT true?
   (a) kills all bacterial spores
   (b) kills all microorganisms
   (c) performed at temperatures identical to autoclaving
   (d) long cycles

10. The long exposure of batch sterilization may cause the following consequence:
    (a) purification of media may happen
    (b) revival of media may happen
    (c) product degradation
    (d) quality of the device may improve

Chapter 9

1. Select the TRUE statement(s) regarding surface modifications of biomaterials.
   (a) to improve the performance of bioimplants
   (b) to enhance the relation of material towards biocompatibility and bondability
   (c) to increase material core properties such as melting point
   (d) to improve tribological properties of the material

2. Arrange the wound healing phases in increasing order of occurrence.
   (a) proliferative; inflammatory; hemostasis; remodeling
   (b) inflammatory; proliferative; remodeling; hemostasis
   (c) hemostasis; inflammatory; proliferative; remodeling
   (d) inflammatory; remodeling; proliferative; hemostasis

3. The first incident that occurs during blood-material interaction is
   (a) cellular attachment
   (b) platelet interaction
   (c) adsorption of plasma proteins
   (d) absorption of plasma proteins

4. Treatment of the implant surface by acid etching and grit blasting
   (a) increases surface roughness and increases cell adhesion
   (b) decreases surface roughness and increases cell adhesion
   (c) increases surface roughness and decreases cell adhesion
   (d) decreases surface roughness and decreases cell adhesion

5. Which of these factors influences healing of a wound?
   (a) vascular insufficiency
   (b) diabetes mellitus
   (c) site of wound
   (d) all of the above

6. Rough surface of the implant material usually
   (a) does not have any effect on cellular properties
   (b) is avoided because it has negative effect on cellular properties
   (c) is desirable as it enhances cellular adhesion and proliferation properties
   (d) all of the above

7. Which of the following is/are NOT true regarding acid treatment on substrate?
   I. produces a clean and uniform surface
   II. eliminates the oxide layer and contamination
   III. improves osteoconductive properties
   IV. provides unfavourable growth conditions for cells
      (a) only I
      (b) only II and III
      (c) only I and IV
      (d) only IV

8. The main reason to perform alkali treatment on substrates is to
   (a) enhance the bioactivity and increase cell adhesion and proliferation
   (b) increase melting temperature of the sample
   (c) decrease osteoblast cell adhesion and proliferation
   (d) increase or decrease Young's modulus

9. What is the end stage of the healing process after biomaterial implantation?
   (a) fibrous encapsulation
   (b) coagulation and hemostasis
   (c) proliferative phase
   (d) epithelialization

10. Plasma-sprayed coatings on metallic implants such as Co-Cr and Ti, and bioceramics such as Al_2O_3
    (a) increase surface roughness and bone bonding; no effect on hardness
    (b) increase surface roughness and bone bonding; increase hardness
    (c) no effect on surface roughness; decrease hardness
    (d) no effect on bone bonding; increase hardness

11. Which of the following is/are TRUE about microporosity and particle size?
    I. higher microporosity induces better protein adsorption
    II. smaller particle size induces better protein adsorption
    III. lower microporosity induces better protein adsorption
    IV. larger particle size induces better protein adsorption
       (a) only I and IV
       (b) only II and III
       (c) only III and IV
       (d) only I and II

12. Coating the surface of hip implants
    (a) significantly reduces failure rates
    (b) increases wear rates
    (c) decreases implant-bone bonding
    (d) none of the above

Chapter 10

1. Imagine you have prepared electrospun nanofibers, and you are optimizing parameters. How do you image and measure the porosity quickly?
    (a) by doing basic image analysis using microscope
    (b) by doing image analysis using transmission electron microscopy
    (c) by using X-ray diffraction analysis
    (d) none of the above

2. Which of the following is considered *least* when designing a scaffold for bone tissue engineering?
   (a) biodegradation properties
   (b) mechanical properties
   (c) pore size and pore morphology
   (d) none of the above

3. An ideal scaffold should have the following properties:
   (a) biodegradable properties irrespective of application
   (b) mechanical stability, non-toxicity and suitable biodegradation
   (c) toxicity and non-biodegradability
   (d) immunogenic and low strength

4. A scaffold material should
   (a) remain longer than needed in the body and provide mechanical support even after tissue is regenerated
   (b) potentially stress-shield the tissue
   (c) have mechanical properties more than required
   (d) gradually degrade with time as new tissue formation increases

5. Issues with conventional fabricated scaffolds for tissue engineering include
   I. pore size control
   II. toxicity induced by biodegraded products
   III. weak mechanical properties
      (a) only I
      (b) only II and III
      (c) all of the above
      (d) only I and II

6. In solvent casting and particulate leaching, internal architecture is determined by
   (a) polymer matrix
   (b) solvent
   (c) embedded salts in the dissolved polymer matrix
   (d) none of the above

7. Pore diameter in solvent casting and particulate leaching is controlled by
    (a) **size of the salt particles**
    (b) molecular weight of polymer matrix
    (c) size of the mold
    (d) none of the above

8. Select the main issue(s) with conventional fabrication techniques:
    (a) no or less control in pore geometry
    (b) no or less control in precise pore size
    (c) difficulty in construction of the internal architecture
    (d) **all of the above**

9. Which of the following is NOT true about the electrospinning technique?
    (a) it yields a three-dimensional scaffold that mimics the ECM matrix
    (b) **evaporation of solvent does not happen during the electro-spinning process**
    (c) rotating mandrel yields aligned nanofibers
    (d) the process involves the use of a high-voltage power supply

Chapter 11

1. Drug delivery is significant as conventional methods result in
    (a) **low bioavailability**
    (b) no side effects
    (c) high efficacy
    (d) all of the above

2. Typical properties of carrier-mediated drug transport include
    I. non-saturability
    II. active transport
    III. chemical specificity
    (a) only I
    (b) only I and II
    (c) **only II and III**
    (d) all of the above

3. Which of the following is/are TRUE for using nanocarriers in drug delivery?
   I. have improved solubilization and can be delivered non-invasively
   II. deliver to site-specific targets
   III. induce damage to the surrounding tissue considerably
   (a) only I
   (b) only I and III
   (c) only I and II
   (d) only III

4. Which of the following is/are NOT true about drugs?
   I. drugs can only be hydrophobic but not hydrophilic
   II. hydrophobic drugs are easily wetted
   III. hydrophobic drugs have low solubility in water
   IV. hydrophilic drugs can easily pass through membrane bilayers
   (a) only I, II and III
   (b) only I and II
   (c) only II, III and IV
   (d) only III

5. Which of the following is NOT true about drug release?
   (a) drug release pattern can be altered by changing geometry and the device
   (b) sustained drug release is possible in monolithic matrix systems
   (c) drug release from reservoir systems normally follow zero-order kinetics
   (d) in membrane-controlled reservoir systems drug is either in liquid or powdered form

6. Which of the following about burst release of drug is/are TRUE?
   I. has short half-life *in vivo*
   II. patient does not require frequent dosing
   III. unpredictable and difficult to control
   IV. high release rates can be reached in the initial stages after activation
   (a) only I
   (b) only I, III and IV
   (c) only I, II and IV
   (d) only I, II and III

7. Which of the following is not a route of drug administration?
    (a) intravenous
    (b) subcutaneous
    (c) intramuscular
    (d) dissolution

8. Which of the following is TRUE for implantable drug delivery devices?
    I. requires invasive surgery
    II. possibility of dose dumping
    III. low bioavailability
    IV. high concentration of drug is delivered at the implantation site
        (a) only I, II and IV
        (b) all of the above
        (c) only III and IV
        (d) only II and IV

9. From which type of diffusion-controlled device will release rate decrease with time?
    (a) monolithic diffusion device
    (b) membrane-controlled reservoir systems
    (c) all of the above
    (d) none of the above

10. Which of the following is most extensively utilized by the drug industry in forming drug salts for water solubilization?
    (a) sodium
    (b) magnesium
    (c) calcium
    (d) phosphorus

11. Encapsulation of a drug usually involves
    (a) suspensions
    (b) association colloids and emulsions
    (c) micelles
    (d) liposomes

12. Polymeric micelles are extensively used for
    (a) delivery of poorly water-soluble drugs
    (b) delivery of highly water-soluble drugs
    (c) any kind of drug, irrespective of solubility
    (d) all of the above

13. In polymeric micelles, drugs are loaded
    (a) on the external surface
    (b) into the hydrophilic cores
    (c) into the hydrophobic cores
    (d) into the hydrophilic tails

Chapter 12

1. Select the TRUE statement(s) regarding biosensor components.
    I. bioreceptor: material which analyses
    II. transducer: conversion of signal
    III. detector: reproducible response
        (a) only I
        (b) only II and III
        (c) only I and II
        (d) all of the above

2. Which of the following is NOT true about biosensors?
    (a) detects the analytes
    (b) provides output in the form of image
    (c) provides output in the form of signal
    (d) transducer converts the reaction into a readable output

3. A piezo-electrical crystal generates voltage when subjected to this force.
    (a) pressure
    (b) magnetic
    (c) electrical
    (d) mechanical

4. Which of the following about optical biosensors is/are TRUE?
   I. provide results in real-time
   II. have an option of label-free detection
   III. expensive
   IV. low specificity
      (a) only I
      (b) only II and IV
      (c) only I and II
      (d) only I, II and IV

5. Which of the following biosensors explore the *"evanescent wave phenomenon"*?
   (a) electrochemical biosensors
   (b) optical biosensors
   (c) piezoelectric biosensors
   (d) all of the above

6. In electrochemical biosensors, amperomertic biosensors measure
   (a) change in voltage
   (b) change in conductivity or resistance
   (c) change in current
   (d) all of the above

7. This acts as detector in optical sensors.
   (a) light emitting diode
   (b) photo diode
   (c) transistor
   (d) all of the above

8. The minimum detectable amount in biosensors is ascertained by
   (a) affinity of the biocomponent for the analyte
   (b) sensitivity of the transducer
   (c) sample volume
   (d) all of the above

Chapter 13

1. What type of materials are used in photolithography?
    (a) any polymer with high molecular weight
    (b) photoreactive polymers
    (c) any polymer with low molecular weight
    (d) all ceramics and metals

2. Select the TRUE statement about 3D bioprinting.
    (a) fabrication of biological constructs similar to their native counterparts
    (b) developing biological constructs for use as an anatomical model
    (c) developing biological constructs for use in display
    (d) no biological components are used

3. Which of the following is TRUE about bioinks?
    (a) they are created by combining cultured cells and various non-biocompatible materials
    (b) they are created by combining polymers and various nanoparticles
    (c) they are core materials used to produce live tissue using 3D printing
    (d) any material that can be in a semi-liquid form is known as bioink

4. Increasing the concentration of bioinks in inkjet and extrusion-based bioprinting
    I. affects cell viability
    II. has no effect on cell viability as there is no ejection of solution from nozzle
    III. makes the inks highly viscous which clogs the nozzle and has effect on mechanical properties
    (a) only I
    (b) only I and II
    (c) all of the above
    (d) only I and III

5. In laser-assisted bioprinting technology, viscosity of solution
   (a) should be as low as possible
   (b) should be as high as possible
   (c) is not a critical parameter because there is no ejection of solution from the nozzle
   (d) none of the above

6. Select the TRUE statement(s) regarding extrusion-based bioprinting.
   I. resolution is very limited
   II. high temperature could damage the cells
   III. no temperature is involved
   IV. very high cell densities can be printed
      (a) only I and IV
      (b) only I, III and IV
      (c) only II and IV
      (d) only I, II and IV

7. In extrusion-based printing, low cell survivability is due to
   (a) high temperatures
   (b) shear stress during printing
   (c) low viscosity of the liquid
   (d) all of the above

8. Select the TRUE statement(s) regarding laser-assisted bioprinting.
   (a) it is a nozzle-free technology
   (b) works only with limited viscosity solutions
   (c) independent of viscosity of the solution
   (d) all of the above

9. Which of the following is/are NOT true about stereolithography bioprinting?
   (a) fabricates biological components at a very low resolution
   (b) requires very little material, implies less wastage of material
   (c) long processing time
   (d) all of the above

Index

www.ingramcontent.com/pod-product-compliance
Lightning Source LLC
Chambersburg PA
CBHW050535190326
41458CB00007B/1790